WHITNEY GOETSCH

Waves

A Memoir of Perseverance in Battling Chronic Lyme Disease

First edition

Editing by Robyn Mulder

This book was professionally typeset on Reedsy.
Find out more at reedsy.com

To Timothy
Thank you for loving me enough to stand by my side . . .
you have shown me what it feels like to truly be loved.

"There are some things in life that we just can't control . . . it's not up to us. But . . . we can control how we choose to respond."

-Dad

Contents

Foreword

You Will Know My Name

You will wake up in the morning
And never feel the same.
I am the beast inside of you
And you will know my name.

I will steal your hopes and dreams
And confine you to your bed.
Every doctor you see
Will say it's in your head.

I will rip apart your body
Every cell deep within.
I will inflame your brain so badly
You won't know where to begin.

The fog will rap around you
Making every day a blur.
I will steal your personality
And everything you were.

You will feel my power
As you tremor deep inside.
And when you try to kill me
I will change my form and hide.

I will make you wish for death
While you pray for God to save you.
I will put your faith in question
And while you suffer I'll pursue.

I will make your ears ring loudly
Not even your screams can silence me.
I will whisper in your ear
You will never be free.

Your nerves will feel on fire
While you wake in the dark night drenched.
Always feeling like you're drunk
But your thirst will never be quenched.

Every single step you take
Will feel like an impossible feat.
Your body will react to every food
Making it nearly impossible to eat.

No one will understand
The way you feel inside.
Many will leave you
Instead of standing by your side.

I will steal away your vision
And make it hard to see a future.
Everything around you
Will become a blur.

The ripping pain inside of you
Will remind you that I am there.
You will suffer every day

Making life hard to bear.

I will harm you so badly
You will be unable to breathe.
You will suffocate daily
And beg of me to leave.

And if I was inside of you
While you were forming life.
I will go after your child
And this will cause a bitter strife.

"What is your name!?!"
You will scream in desperation.
Bartonella, Babesia, and I am *LYME.*
You pray that you have found me at just the right time.

Whitney Helen Goetsch

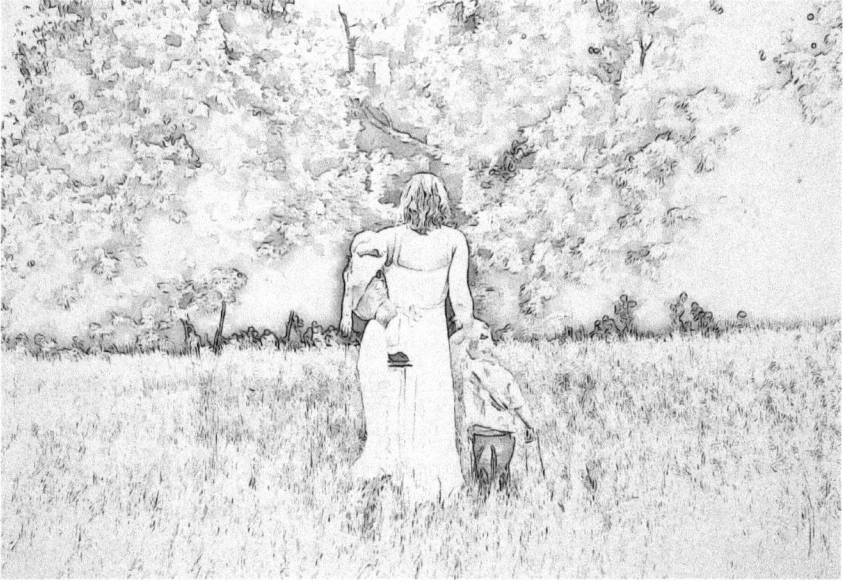

. . . you pray that you have found me at just the right time.

Preface

THE DREAM

One night I had a dream. I was swimming in the unforgiving waters of an ocean. The *waves* were slowly crashing into me. Ahead of me I could see a large mass of land. It seemed impossibly far away. With every stroke I took, the *waves* pushed me back, moving me further away from the land. The water terrified me. I felt a sense of impending doom because I knew what was beneath the surface.

As I drew closer to shore, the tip of a fin cut through the dark water. I stopped as fear overtook me. I could not escape it. The *waves* began to calm, but as I moved forward more fins erupted through the surface. It was then that I knew I had to make a *choice*. I could swim through the sharks or give up and never make it. I would surely drown . . . or worse.

I lunged myself forward through the creatures as *waves* crashed around me. Some sharks tried to evade me while others came at me with defiance. When they realized that I would not back down they surrendered and cleared a path for me. *Except one.* This shark challenged me after I thought the others had backed down. They hadn't. Instead, they turned in unison with their leader and stood before me, blocking my path. Heart pounding, I was frozen in the *waves,* knowing that if I kept pushing I may have a chance of getting past them. But if I stayed I would surely die.

I felt them all around me, as if they were a part of me. *I chose to go forward.*

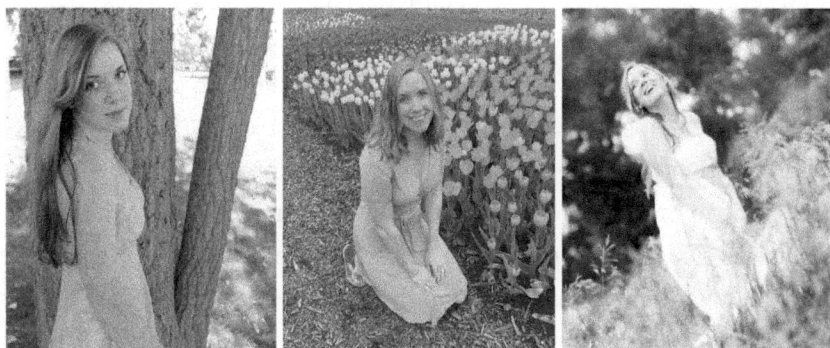

I loved many parts of my life . . .

THE CALM BEFORE THE *WAVES*

I awoke to the cry of my younger son, Eliot, who had recently turned one year old. He still refused to sleep through the night and I never felt fully rested. I couldn't shake the feelings from my dream. I felt very alarmed, as if it were a reality that I was trapped inside of. I got out of bed, grabbed my son from his crib, and brought him into my room to nurse. Yes, I still nursed my one-year-old son. I had to cut my firstborn off at around three because of the onset of hyperemesis gravidarum. This severe pregnancy illness was absolutely terrible, but I always told myself to be grateful because I had struggled for several years with infertility issues and a miscarriage.

So as I would be throwing up everything I ate or drank—including water—or dry heaving because there was nothing left, I would repeatedly tell myself: Be *grateful . . . don't complain . . . you will get through this.* Or my favorite: *This too shall pass.*

* * *

The first few years with my little ones were a bit of a blur mixed with a lot of happy memories. Neither of my children were good sleepers. I felt like a cow most of the time . . . constantly breastfeeding, and if I drove them anywhere it would result in them either crying or getting carsick. *But how I loved being a mother.* And how very *grateful* I was.

What I enjoyed most was the bliss of viewing the world through a child's eyes. That's not to say I wasn't ever exhausted or stressed. But a lot of what I did with them was so *magical.* Playing in the snow, taking them to the zoo, going to the lake, going on walks down our gravel road with our dog, Annabelle. She would run alongside us and we wouldn't see her for a while until she would jump and fly through the golden wheat fields. She was always by our side as our loyal companion. I loved adventuring with my children and experienced a euphoric joy of living in the country, or "the village," as my older son called it.

I was extremely particular as a mother and very protective of my children. I observed everything. I remember the first time I decided to change all of my cleaning supplies. I had just finished mopping my kitchen floor with Lysol when Russell came crawling onto the wet linoleum. He shoved his little fists right into his mouth and I thought *Well, that can't be good for him.*

I made most of their baby food from scratch, breastfed exclusively for the first six months, looked meticulously at every ingredient in products, cloth diapered, made sure we spent most of our time outside, and I could never let them cry it out.

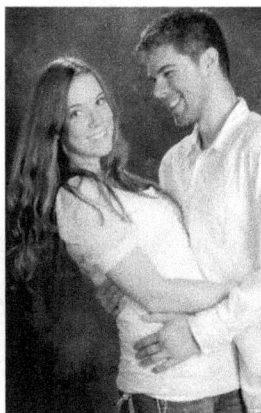

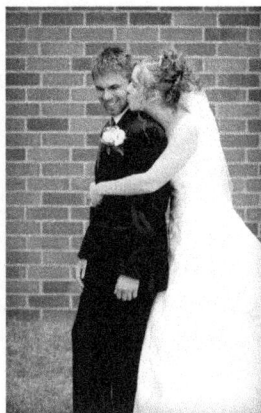

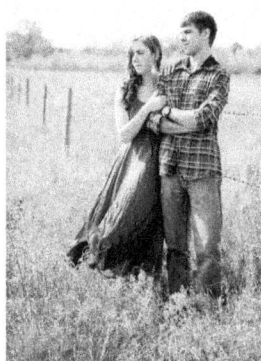

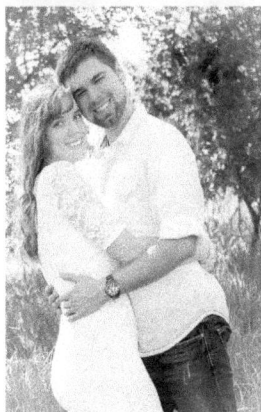

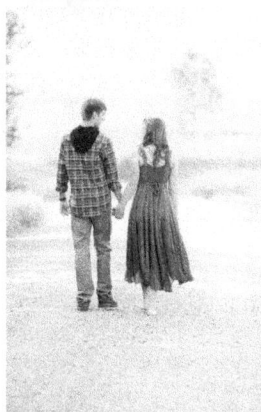

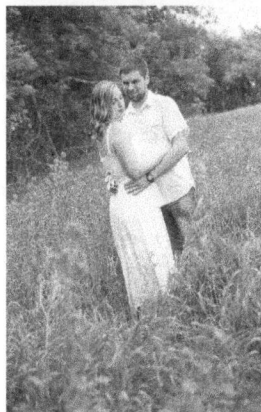

All I ever wanted was to be a mother . . .

When I fell in love with my husband, Timothy, all I ever wanted was to be a mother. So when I did struggle with infertility it was absolutely heartbreaking. At one point I could not even see a pregnant woman out in public without crying when I got home. *Why me?* I would ask myself. I remember one time specifically, after about two years of negative tests, I threw myself to the floor in tears and sobbed for a long time. *Please God . . . bless me with a child! Please . . .*

I had asked many times in the two years of my infertility journey, but this time, as I sobbed on the living room floor, *I screamed it.* I told God all of the reasons I wanted this. I told him how good I would be as a mother. The big difference this time was that I *screamed* it out loud. Shortly after this *"prayer,"* I took a pregnancy test and, sure enough, there were two faint lines. *Thank you!* Later I learned that not all prayers work that way.

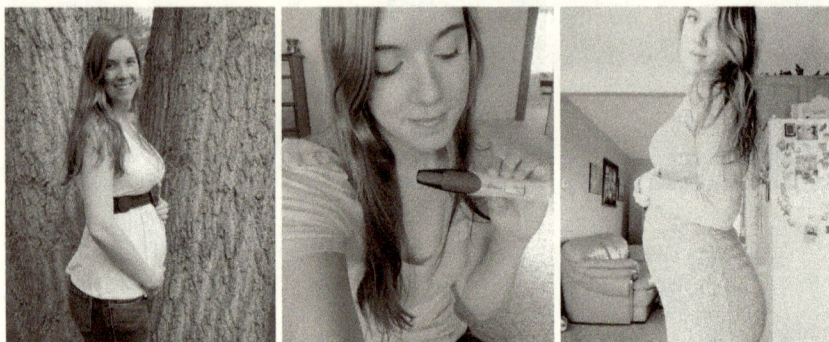

I took a pregnancy test and, sure enough, there were two faint lines. Thank you!

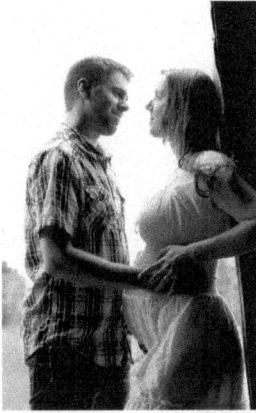

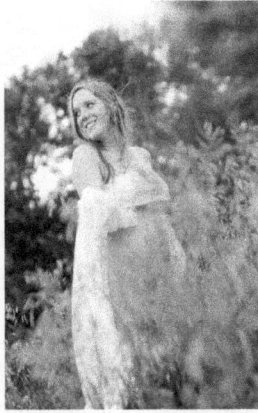

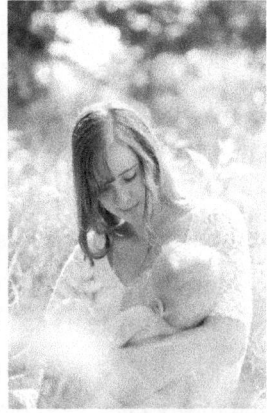

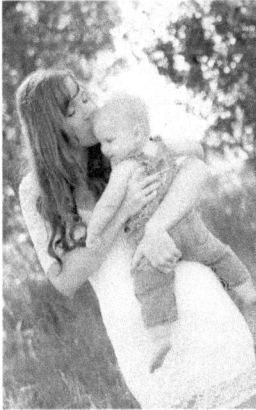

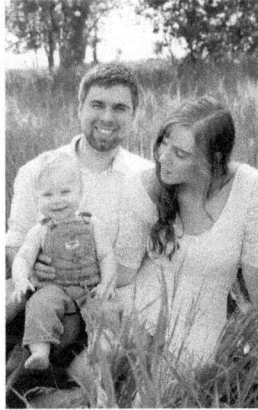

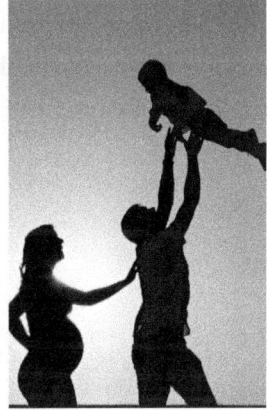

Please God, bless me with a child! Please . . .

When I was blessed with children, I took my job as a mother, homemaker, and caretaker very seriously. The chores were done, the house was immaculate, and my family had healthy, homemade meals. Supper was always hot on the table as soon as my husband walked in the door from work. *My dream had come true.*

I know many of you may laugh at my dream and at my idea of happiness . . . but if you had grown up spending most of your time alone because of family circumstances . . . and had sat at an empty table with a Hot Pocket for your supper . . . *you would understand.*

I usually filled the void of loneliness by escaping to my cat shed in the backyard. Friends would make fun of me about all of the cats, but they got to go home after school every day to a mom and dad and *I did not.* I sat with my dog as my companion. My cats made me feel warm and safe. I read Harry Potter books or immersed myself in Zelda games . . . I imagined that I was in their world instead of my own.

Sometimes, though, as my dad would pull out of the driveway to leave for another week away at work . . . the loneliness was too much, and I would hide my tears as I ran to the backyard and buried my sorrows in my dog. My prayer was simple. *Please God, send someone to love me . . . who stays by my side . . . so that I never have to be alone again . . .*

But that was a different season in my life. I was truly happy in my current season. And yes, having hot meals ready and on the table to enjoy with my family was my dream. I was not alone anymore. God had answered my prayers.

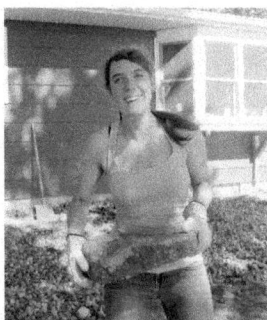

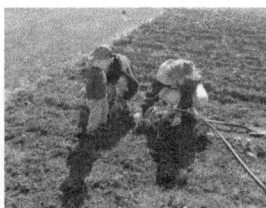

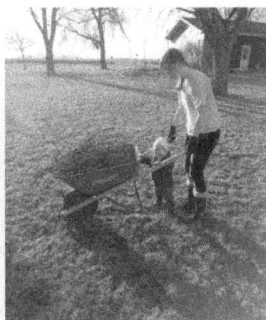

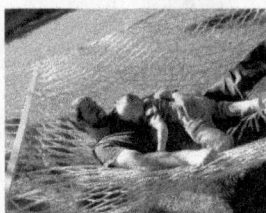

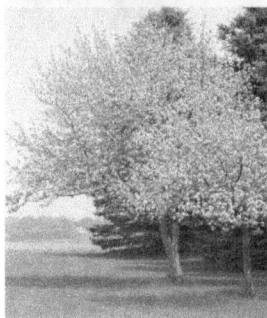

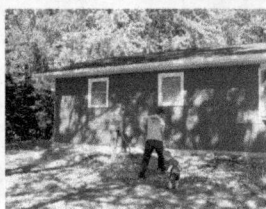

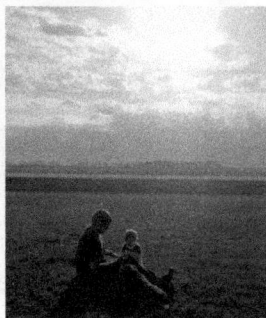

Send someone to love me . . . who stays by my side . . . so that I never have to be alone again . . .

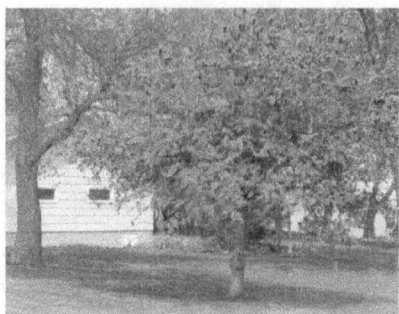

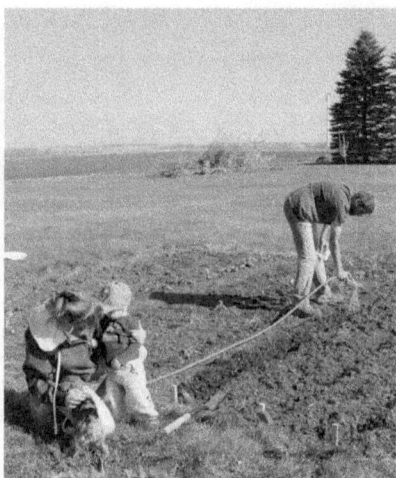

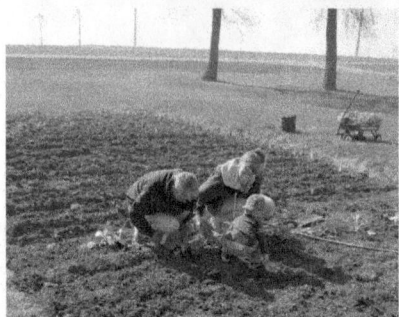

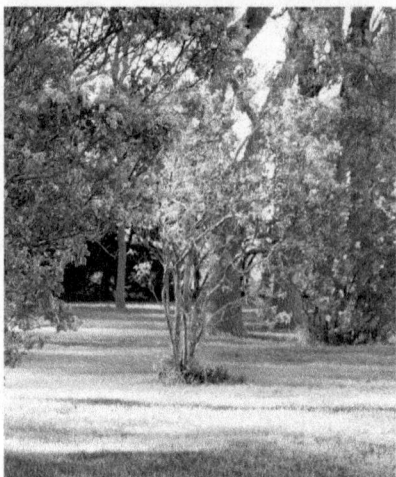

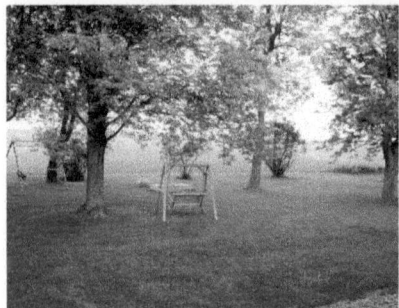

Oh how grateful I was to have my dream home with my family . . .

That entire decade was the happiest season of my life. My prayers were answered when I fell in love with *Timothy.* Our love story didn't happen easily. You would think it would have because we attended the smallest school ever together . . . but I was a social introvert and he . . . was not. It took a foreign exchange student from Japan to travel all the way to small-town South Dakota before Tim and I even noticed each other.

After Itoko went back to Japan she would email me, insisting I go on a date with *"Timothy."* Little did I know, she was emailing him the same thing about me. I didn't know this until years later, after I had our children.

I kept saying *no* to his persistent requests to take me out on a date. We *didn't have anything in common.* He was the hot drummer, and I was the nerd who spent all of her time in the library reading Harry Potter books and drawing pictures . . . and I'm sure he heard all about my *cats*.

It was because of Itoko that we ended up together. She didn't want to see *Timothy* alone because she cared about him deeply. She cared about me as well and knew how lonely I was. I think she *knew* that when she went back to Japan it left an empty space in both of our hearts.

My *prayers were answered* in a very unpredictable way. I was finally with someone who cared and loved me deeply. I was not alone any longer . . .

I will forever be *grateful* for Itoko.

* * *

During the entire pregnancy with Eliot, I suffered so much with hyperemesis gravidarum that Tim and I both agreed that two were enough. But as soon as Eliot came out my husband looked at me and told me he wanted another one. I wanted to slap him but instead I smirked. It's funny because all of the *suffering* vanishes when you see your baby. And a part of me wondered if maybe I should have another one someday . . . but not until Eliot turned five, that way Russell would be eight and old enough to help out. That was my rule. *I would never get that.*

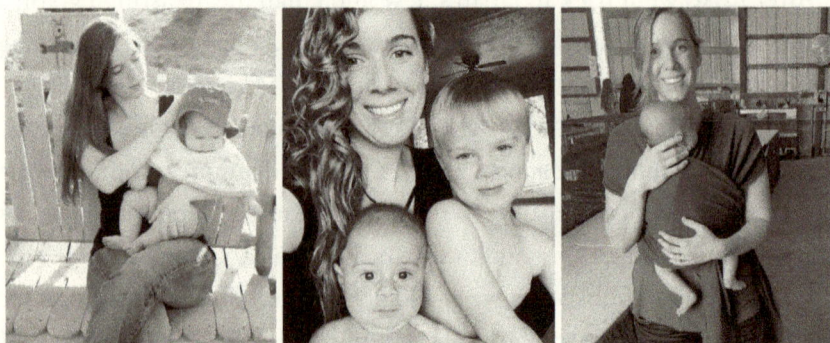

My prayers were answered . . .

I loved many parts of my life and during this new season my freedom expanded. Both of my sons had outgrown breastfeeding and were finally sleeping so well. Because they were sleeping I was finally getting enough sleep.

We lived in our dream home in the country, we grew our own vegetables, and I was getting more time to myself and could leave the house with ease.

Tim and I started to have more time for each other as well. We even dressed up as Danny and Sandy from the movie *Grease* for a Halloween party. We had never dressed up or attended a Halloween party before, but he had the perfect chin dimple and we couldn't resist. We stayed out late, snacked on delicious food, danced a few times, and had so many laughs with our friends. I remembered what it was like to be with my best friend again.

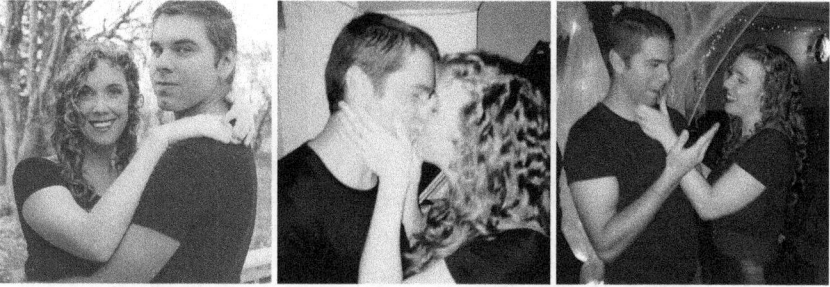

We could finally have fun again.

That summer we finished up some home repairs and I had more time for myself. Every morning, shortly after waking, I would exercise for an hour downstairs and laugh as my one-year-old would copy my sit-ups. Often I would go on long walks down the gravel road, pushing the stroller containing my two children. I was strong and healthy and not in a constant state of exhaustion anymore.

We also had more time for fun activities with our kids and spent the whole day at a water park in the hot sun with our four-year-old. We had so much fun together that day. I remember being out in the sun for hours, swimming in the pools and floating down the lazy river. I could do everything I wanted.

* * *

Sometimes living in the country would get lonely and I always felt guilty about that because it was my dream and my husband made it a reality. I knew, though, that it would only get easier as my children got older.

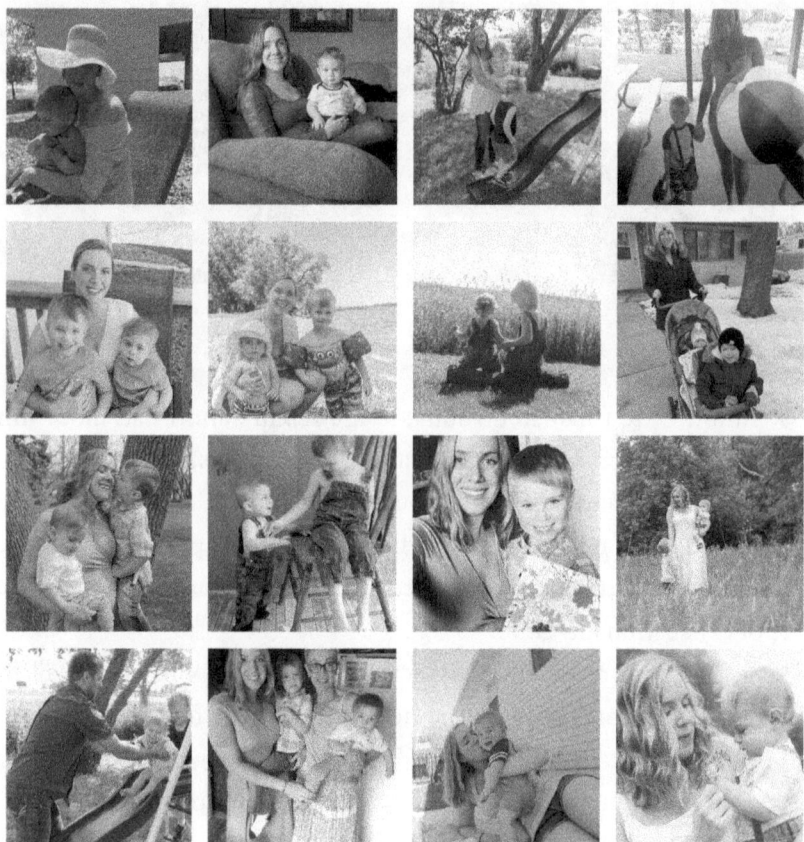

Oh . . . how I loved being a mother.

And it did get easier. My husband and I continued to have more intimate times together. *Like the old days.* I loved every moment that I was able to spend with my *best friend.*

We traveled all the way to D.C. together for a friend's wedding. This was our first time riding in an airplane. We stayed at a few fancy hotels, toured briefly, and dressed up for the fancy evening parties. On the wedding night, we spent our time dancing and laughing with friends. It was *magical* and I remember just wanting to stay forever in his arms as we danced the night away. I worried about my babies off and on, but I knew they were in good hands with my mother and sister-in-law. I still remember our trip as one of the best times I have had with my husband apart from our wedding. I loved being with him.

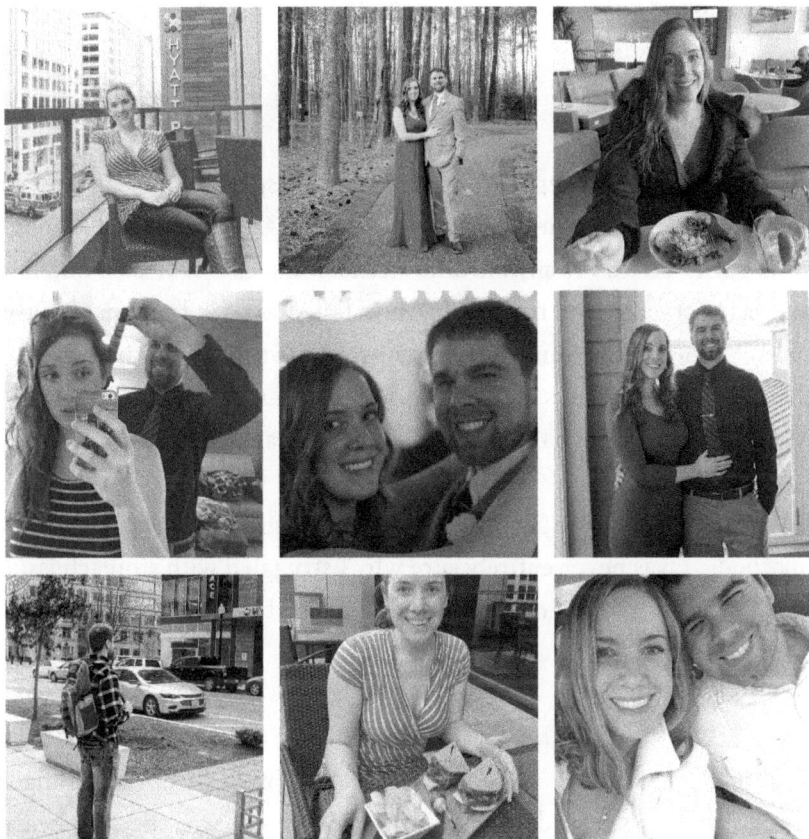

He is my best friend . . .

We spent a lot of time traveling as our kids became easier to haul around. My husband and I loaded up the car that summer and traveled to his mom's (Terri's) house for a brief visit before a trip to Rapid City. It was so hot when we got there, but my mom (Sandra) and I loved walking in the heat and needed to stretch our legs after the long drive. I remember the sweat just pouring off of me, but we walked a long distance before heading back to the house. During our stay we went to many parks, ate a lot of pie, and enjoyed watching the kids play together in the backyard. When we got to Rapid City, our trip was unfortunately cut short because we caught some kind of bug in between visits and drove home with fevers.

* * *

Oddly, that summer I kept getting viruses and I spent a lot of time feeling like I was getting sick but then getting better. It was strange, and I thought it was partly related to my chronic stomach issues so I tried a bunch of fad diets to try and heal my gut. I always failed to stick to them because I was still breastfeeding and starving most of the time. I also had so many cravings for sugar and salt, it was ridiculous. I still remember the juice fast I attempted. I got halfway through the day and then ate a handful of M&M's.

In my adult years I ate fairly healthy, but as a child I ate lots of sweets and junk foods. I was never entirely sure why I struggled with stomach issues, but it would come and go and it was difficult to bear when I had pain.

* * *

Later that summer we were also a part of Tim's sister's wedding in Minnesota. I was a bridesmaid and our older son was the ring bearer. My kids and I got sick right before the wedding with some virus and had mild fevers. During the photos, my husband pulled a red tick off of the back of my leg and *crushed it on the pavement* and we continued taking pictures. I still remember seeing how the blood smeared against the concrete. I didn't think much of it. Growing up I had ticks on and off and we always did the same, crushed them and moved on with our day.

I remember running into a bunch of ticks while fishing with my dad as a child. I would struggle through the tall grasses to keep up with his long strides. I followed quickly after him and went straight through a tick nest. They were all over me and Dad meticulously picked them off. He always told me that you had to make sure to get the head out of your skin. Despite his efforts, later I found a couple of ticks behind my ears. I picked them off myself and pinched them between my fingers. I examined them closely. Their little legs squirmed as they tried to escape. They were the ugliest things I had ever seen. I ended their squirming by crushing them with a sharp rock and watched my blood soak into the gravel road.

Then there was the time when my dad finally felt comfortable enough to let my sister and I stay at a two-week-long camp. Our camp counselors told us to tape any ticks we found to our nightstands. It almost became a game for us as kids. We wanted to see who would have the longest line of ticks. So when one kid would find a tick they would pull it off excitedly as they added another trophy to their line. I was bummed that I only had one taped on my nightstand by the end. I picked this one off myself and wasn't sure if I got the head out . . . that was the only time I didn't smear a tick into the concrete like my Dad always told us to do, and the next morning somehow my one tick had escaped.

I can recall a time when our cousin's dog got loose and we found her a week later covered in ticks of all different sizes. Some you could hardly see, while others were large and engorged. I remember my dad picking them off of her one by one using a tweezers and a small comb. It took hours. My sister and I dropped the fat ones onto the ground and popped them with our shoes.

My dad hollered, "Would ya just leave those things alone and throw them in the water bucket!"

I disobeyed him by popping more ticks against the concrete. Unfortunately, the dog became sick and it was not long after that that I briefly learned about Lyme disease.

I remember learning about Lyme disease in school, too, and I thought it was odd that my camp counselors basically let us play with them as kids. I always felt resilient, though, as you do when you are young, and never thought Lyme disease could happen to me. I never worried about my exposure to ticks. It was a normal thing to get them and I was told most don't carry the disease in South Dakota.

* * *

After I smeared the tick against the concrete at the wedding, I forgot all about it. That night we stayed up late dancing. I enjoyed our time but spent the remainder of the night in drenching sweats that I associated with the virus we had. I remember wishing I felt better and felt bad that the boys were up so late when they didn't feel the best either.

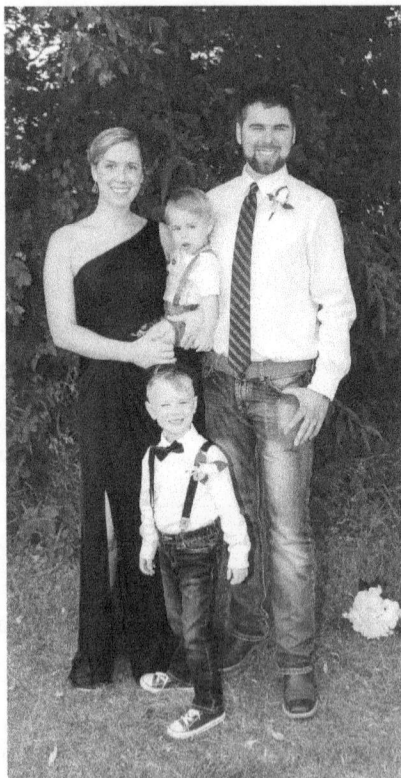

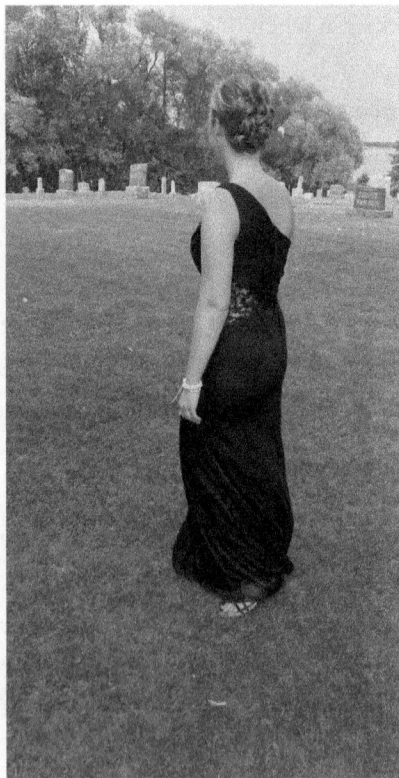

We pulled the tick off of the back of my leg and crushed it on the pavement . . .

FIRST SIGNS

My life really changed that summer. My mom and I would often have karaoke nights and I would treat her to a meal as a thank you for babysitting. I started to experience really scary symptoms after drinking a beer with my cheeseburger. My heart would jump around and begin to race and I would feel flushed. My abdomen would bloat and I would feel like I *couldn't breathe*.

I thought I was having a heart attack once and had my mom check my heart rate. "It is really high. Maybe try walking around a bit."

So I did. I got up and went to the bathroom and it resolved on its own. *That's weird . . .* I thought. I hardly ever drank alcohol and wondered if maybe that's why it happened.

The same thing happened to me twice that summer and fall and my stomach issues became debilitating. One time, while shopping downtown with my mom, I had to lie on the floor in the dressing room in excruciating pain. We had just finished a lunch of burgers, veggies, and Alfredo and I could not figure out which food was causing my extreme pain.

* * *

In November, we went to Terri's house for Thanksgiving. We went to *Christmas at the Capitol* and saw the Christmas tree light show. It was so beautiful. After the light show, my boys threw bread into the river for the geese. Their faces lit up as they watched the geese and continued to marvel at the beauty of the giant Christmas trees. I experienced similar emotions that weekend but noticed that I felt *off*. I didn't understand what I was feeling and couldn't quite place my symptoms, but I remember feeling uncomfortable on and off and just wanted to go home.

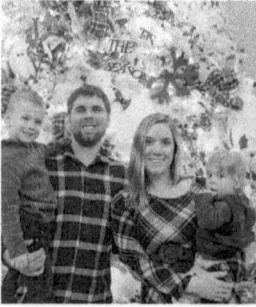

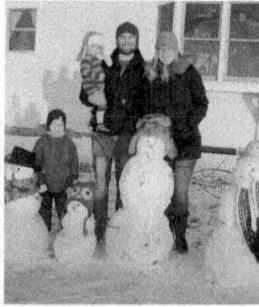

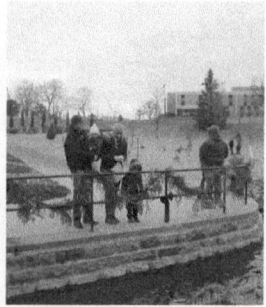

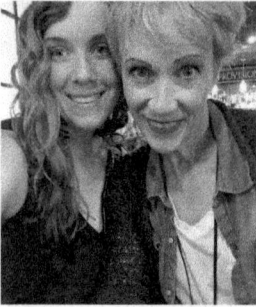

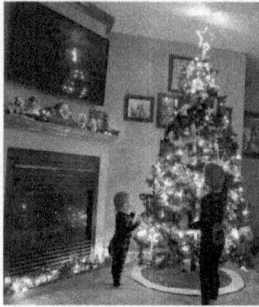

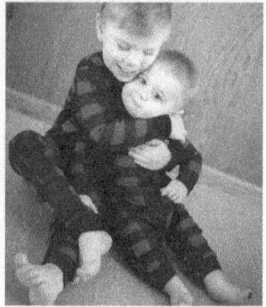

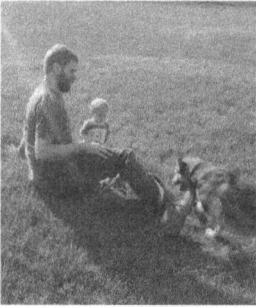

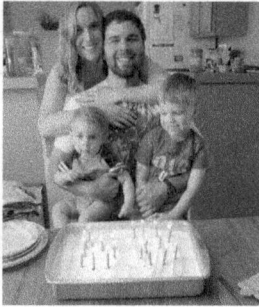

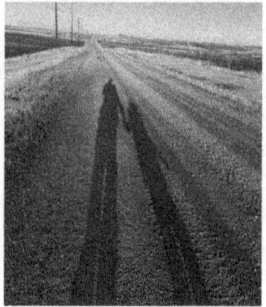

My life changed rapidly after that.

When we arrived home after our trip, I took my boys to the Children's Museum. We purchased a yearly membership and would go once a week together. We spent the whole day playing and I even picked up a few groceries on the way home. When we pulled into the driveway, I noticed how perfect the snow was for snowmen. The sun was starting to lower but I couldn't miss out on an opportunity like this. The snow gleamed as the sun set and I made four snowmen to represent each member of our family.

I remember how strong I felt and how joyful I was at seeing my children's eyes light up while we made them. I had the ability to do so much. I didn't realize it then, but I would soon lose that ability very rapidly.

Sometimes when I look back at the pictures that were taken right before my health decline, I wish I could warn myself about what was to come. But we were not taught that these things could happen and I had no idea of the magnitude of suffering I would endure.

* * *

My health decline began shortly after I thought I had overcome it. The heart rate episodes had seemed to resolve as I hadn't had one since early November. The last one happened after drinking alcohol again and I decided I just wouldn't drink anymore. But I still battled the chronic stomach issues which we had been trying to resolve with my doctor on and off for years. The pain was becoming worse and more frustrating.

My periods were still so bad and my doctor thought it would be best to put me on a high estrogen birth control pill to treat my symptoms. I went on the pill that morning and by night I felt very off. I couldn't quite understand what I was feeling but my feet were *buzzing*. It was as if a cell phone were under them. I often had issues with my feet burning or feeling really cold and looking purple when standing . . . but this was very *different*. I felt a very odd sensation of doom too. I didn't feel right, and when I lay down I wondered about the birth control. I went to sleep anyway, thinking *in the morning I will feel better.*

The next morning I still didn't feel right. Christmas was just a couple of days away and my son and I were recovering from a bout of food poisoning. I put my son in an Epson salt bath and as the water was running, I noticed my hands started to feel buzzy and numb off and on. I thought about the birth control pill again and wondered if that was the cause. I knew that, rarely, birth control pills could cause blood clots or strokes. This seemed unlikely to me since I had just started them a few days prior. My feet felt worse and the sensations were going up into my legs. I jumped in the bath with my son and tried to see if the hot water would help the sensation go away. *It did not . . .*

Acknowledgments

Many people kept me going and they do not even realize it. I experienced a big shift in my fight when I found a primary care provider who *actually* believed me. She often felt intimidated by the fact that I was working with functional medicine doctors, but the small things she did and still does during my many acute care visits pushed me to keep fighting during the darkest of times. She was a light in a dark tunnel for myself. She never made me feel *small* or *crazy*. She *restored* some of my *faith* in medical doctors. After about four years of suffering, she and another one of my advocating doctors—whom I met through my acupuncturist—opened their own clinic. I finally felt *safe* if I ever had to go to a doctor for an acute issue. They opened up an IV infusion room and told me people with POTS (postural orthostatic tachycardia syndrome) are welcome to get fluids whenever their body needs it. I finally had a place to go if I needed additional fluids for acute illness. *I can finally feel safe, UN-judged.* There *are* good doctors out there. You know who you are and I am forever *grateful* for you. To the many doctors and chiropractors who were kind to me, *I thank you.* To my functional medicine doctors who were determined to help me find the root cause, and found many, *I thank you.* For your *dedication*, I will *forever* be *grateful*. For the health coaches who guide me in giving myself *grace* and *self-compassion, I thank you.* To my brain health specialist who helped me so many times during vestibular flares, *I thank you.* To everyone who is helping me right now at the Lyme centers. I have never met a kinder group of people who are so dedicated to helping chronic Lyme patients heal. You have given me *new hope. I thank you.*

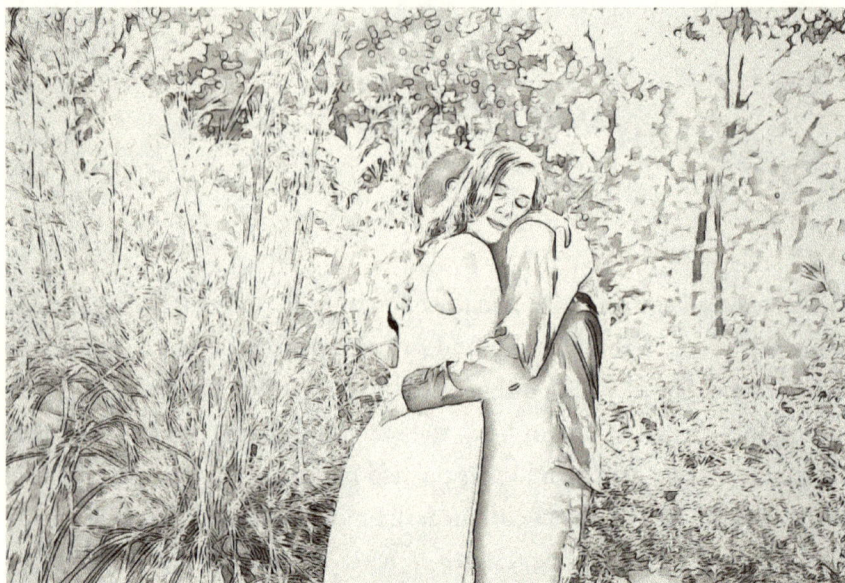

Thank you to those who made me feel safe . . . My husband, who attended every doctor visit. My children, who kept me fighting. My mother, who was there for me and my children more days than I can count. My father, who first demonstrated perseverance. My family and friends, who stood by my side. My sisters and sister-in-law, who tried their best to understand. Tim's mother, who helped me care for my children when I could not. The people who hardly knew me but cared enough to listen and pray for me. To the Lyme Warriors who reached out to me. My Lyme group moderator . . . thank you for caring enough to comment on my video. To my church members, who pray for me. To my healers. And I especially thank my acupuncturist, who was and still is a very big advocate for me. I have been to top doctors all over, including Mayo Clinic, and he is still at the top of the list. Above all, I thank God for carrying me on my darkest of days.

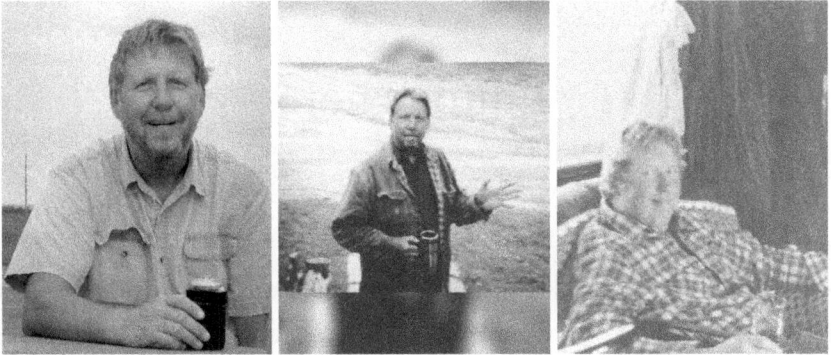

My father, who first demonstrated *perseverance.*

Editor's note

When Whitney gave me her manuscript to edit, I was surprised to find that it was over 100,000 words in length. I worried about telling her that we should try to get that down to about 75,000 words so the reader wouldn't feel overwhelmed. I mentioned that possibility to her, but I decided to read the whole thing before I pushed her to delete anything.

As a reader, I *was* overwhelmed, but it wasn't with the word count. I was touched by everything she's had to go through in the past five years. Which 25,000 words could we cut from her story? What if some of those words included a thought that would comfort or encourage a fellow sufferer? I decided most of those 25,000 words could be left in.

I made suggestions to explain some concepts earlier in the book, but for the most part I decided to just check for errors in spelling, punctuation, and grammar and correct those things. I'm not a medical professional, but I did my best to make sure the multitude of symptoms, syndromes, diseases, and treatments were all spelled correctly (don't blame Whitney if I missed anything).

I made or suggested changes to the wording in some places, but I left much of it just as Whitney wrote it. After all, most of the book is based on her journal entries. I even left in almost all of the ellipses . . . because so much of her story involved uncertainty and long periods of waiting for answers.

You may notice the timeline skipping around once in a while, but I even decided to leave that alone. Whitney's journey has not been a straight line from first symptom to final diagnosis (you'll notice that Lyme disease isn't even confirmed until halfway through the book!). Instead, she has had to tell her story even while suffering from the effects of Lyme and other health concerns. You may feel confused by the disturbing symptoms, the moments of hope, the changes in doctors and treatments, and the frustrating search for answers. Now just imagine being the one living through all of that.

I'm proud of my friend for her perseverance as she has had to deal with so much—and she's written a book in the midst of it all. I'm praying it can help many who are suffering and searching for answers.

~Robyn Mulder

Author's note

This book is based on five years of journal entries by the author. The medical providers' names are kept private and some names are fictionalized. I wrote this book to describe my own experience with chronic illness and Lyme disease, not with any malicious intent to humiliate doctors or the medical system.

I describe many tests, treatments, medications, and other methods of care received over the span of my illness. I am not a medical doctor, but I wrote from my perspective of what I learned from many specialists throughout my journey to reach a diagnosis. I describe many hard topics, including suicidal thoughts, anxiety, and depression. I am not offering medical advice, and I strongly caution my readers to not rely on my book for their own unique medical problems. The reader should find care and advice from qualified medical professionals.

I

Part One

My entire body was tremoring and I couldn't understand what was happening to me. I hoped that when it left my body things would improve. It did not.

1

I Want to Be Normal

December 27, 2018

You will not win.
I am in a battle . . . a battle against myself.
Trying to gain control over the person I once was.
A battle of the mind.
A battle of the heart.
Anxiety. Depression. You will not win.
My children and husband need me.
I am strong. I can do this.
I will win.

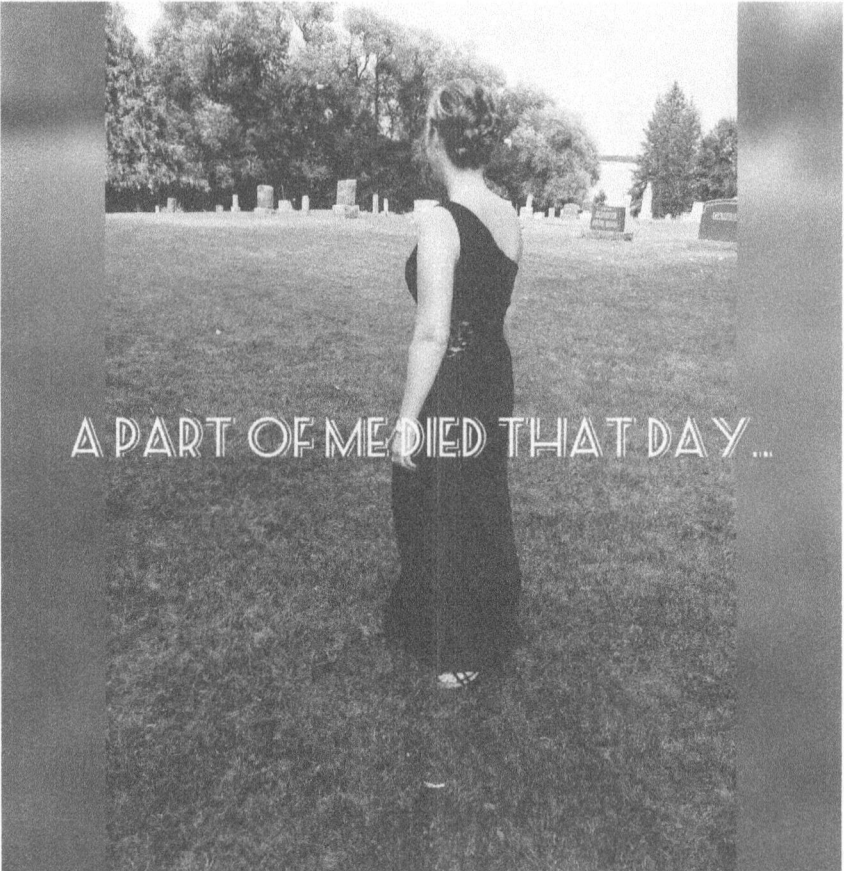

A part of me died that day . . .

Birth control entered my body on Tuesday, December 18. It wreaked havoc just a few days later. This was the most traumatizing day of my life. The pill was supposed to help my hormonal issues but, instead seemed to have taken over my body and mind . . . sending tremors and shakes throughout every inch of my body. Fear engulfed me. After the tingling sensations came on, everything went numb. I could not feel my feet and hands. My muscles constricted, causing my fingers to look deformed and it felt like my heart was being crushed.

4

* * *

It all started on a cold winter morning, just a few days before Christmas. I had just finished all of my gift wrapping the night before and the boys and I enjoyed several magical nights lying under the Christmas tree, looking up at the lights. The house smelled like fresh-baked cookies and gingerbread, and I couldn't wait until Christmas morning so that I could watch my boys open all of their gifts.

Sudden feelings of impending doom began a few nights after the birth control had entered my body. The following morning I put Eliot in the bathtub and as I sat on the edge I noticed my feet starting to tingle on the left side. Then the numbness set in and a feeling of *fear*. *Maybe the warm water will help.* I jumped into the bathtub with him. I stuck my feet under the tap and watched as the water rippled and formed into *waves* around my feet. Eliot was happily splashing in the water as the odd sensations started to overcome my body.

The sensations started to move to my hands and I began to lose feeling in them. I began to feel more panicked as the numb sensation crawled up my left arm and then into my face and chest. I got out of the water and tried to call my mom, but there was no answer. I called my husband. No answer. The sensations were getting worse and I started to feel faint and thought to myself *if something happens my son might drown.* I grabbed him out of the water and wrapped us up in blankets. He wasn't ready to get out and started to cry.

My symptoms were getting worse and I was thinking about dialing 911, but before I dialed the number my husband called. I sat on the bathroom floor with my naked baby in my arms. I calmed him down enough for my husband to hear me. I tried to stay calm, but he knew right away that something wasn't right by the sound of my voice. The most I could get out was my concerns about the birth control I had just started. I knew it must be a side effect but didn't know exactly what was happening. I was starting to worry about a stroke.

I got us dressed as best as I could, but the sensations in my arm and chest

5

were getting worse. I kept getting sharp pains in my chest, and waiting for my husband to get home felt like an eternity. I somehow managed to get us partly dressed and I didn't say much when my husband walked in the door. I just got into the car as he buckled the boys in with a worried look on his face. I could tell I was beginning to lose control of my mind. I could not think clearly and my speech was muddled. We started our 15-minute drive to town and my symptoms began to increase. I was terrified and as we approached the interstate things got worse and then everything started to constrict. It was as if my muscles were in a vice and it was slowly cranking inward. My entire left arm and both of my hands and feet all the way up to my chest were numb. *What's happening?!* I couldn't breathe well and felt faint.

I was trying to tell my husband, as calmly as I could, what was happening, while he was on the phone with 911. He sped up on the interstate and I could hear my older son in the background repeating everything I said to my husband back to me with worry in his small voice.

I kept saying, "It's okay, Mommy is going to be okay."

Won't I? As I was completely losing control over my body I still wanted to comfort my son. *Is this a stroke . . . a heart attack?* I remember being so afraid and telling Tim, *"I want my mom."* Funny how even when we are adults we want our mom when we are in pain or afraid . . .

We were about halfway there when my chest felt like it was being crushed. My arms came into a forward cripple and were stuck as if dried in concrete. I was losing my vision on and off and my husband stopped when he saw a patrol car parked along the interstate.

The officer took one look at me and all he said was, "Do you have any aspirin?!"

My husband shook his head no and the patrol officer told us to keep going and he would follow. I kept telling Tim to go faster . . . we had to get there. My husband was shaking in the driver's seat. I had tunnel vision and everything was jumping around. I could not breathe.

"My eyes flicked up to the reflection of my children in the mirror, and I remember scenes of my life flashing in front of me just like they show you in the movies. As I watched them flash before me, I felt determined to survive. *I wanted to live.*

We just got into town when we saw the ambulance and pulled over. They ripped me out of the vehicle. My son saw everything.

I still managed to get out, "Mommy is going to be okay . . ."

I did not really know if I would be okay, but I was trying to be strong for him and reassure him even when I felt like I was on the brink of death.

I was almost sure at this time that I was having a heart attack or stroke from the birth control. The rest of what happened after that was a blur. The paramedics worked quickly and asked me lots of questions. The most I could get out was that I had just started birth control and had recently gotten over food poisoning. I remember monitors being attached to me and a lot of noise and lights.

We later wheeled into the ER. The ER doctor had me hooked up to fluids and asked a bunch of questions about my stress levels and if I had been dealing with any major anxiety. I told him *no.* I was trying to think of anything going on in my life emotionally that could have caused this. My life was going so well. *I was happy.* I weakly replied that maybe I had a little stress about the upcoming holidays, but nothing major. He wrote it down and this was the first time that *panic disorder* was written in my chart. With no tests done other than the EKG and "normal" blood work, I was surprised they blamed it on anxiety so quickly.

The ER doctor said it was a panic attack and the blood work only showed abnormal bilirubin levels. We requested a CT scan to at least make sure I wasn't having a stroke, which they eventually did agree to do, but not without saying that this seemed like anxiety first. The results of that showed nothing remarkable, no signs of a stroke. The blood tests to rule out a blood clot were normal. *Thank God.* I was given fluids and a benzo (*benzodiazepines, also known as "benzos", are a class of depressant drugs that are used to decrease nervous system activity resulting in hypnosis, relieving anxiety and muscle spasms, relieving panic attacks, and reducing seizures.)* medication in my IV, which made me feel tired but didn't take away the air hunger or weird buzzing sensations all throughout my body.

Part of me was very relieved that I didn't have any life-threatening issues showing up. But the other part was scared and confused because I still didn't feel *normal*.

Since then, it has been an up-and-down battle.

I left the ER still not feeling right but with a workup scheduled with my primary doctor to discuss an anxiety disorder. This left me flabbergasted as I had no history of anxiety or depression. My mother did, which many doctors took interest in later, and they often used that fact to get out of doing any other labs. My mother was abused in her lifetime, though, and her situation was entirely different from mine. The only time I struggled with any type of anxiety was socially in my early teen years. I was very shy and unsure of myself. Everyone was maturing around me. I didn't know what I was doing without my mom around, and I was really self-conscious about my body. But a lot of girls go through that when all they have for female role models are the women they see on magazine covers. It didn't explain my present situation. I was skeptical about this being anxiety related.

January 1, 2019

I never thought I would have a New Year's resolution to return to the old me. These last two weeks have been incredibly hard. It has been an up-and-down battle.

When I went home, I continued to have the episodes until I could get in to see my primary care provider. He agreed that the birth control may have triggered this, but it would have completely left my system by now. He said I am left with a panic disorder which needs to be treated with medication. He prescribed a benzo for the attacks and an SSRI (*selective serotonin reuptake inhibitor, and it's a type of antidepressant medication that treats depression and other mental health conditions* for the disorder.) I mentioned to him that I was having a menstrual cycle that started after the birth control. The bleeding was so terrible I was passing clots the size of tennis balls. He didn't have much to say concerning this and he never checked my iron levels.

I felt the hormones in my body were causing this because I had just had a period a week before starting birth control. I'm bleeding all of the time. I feel so weak. My body must be fighting to remove the hormones. He still wrote up an order for a later MRI, but he sent me home with the prescriptions, but I didn't take the SSRI.

Later we did a CT of my chest and aorta because of my father's history of aortic dissection. My primary care doctor told me that my aorta was fine, and the only thing they saw were nodules in the lungs and a slightly enlarged liver. He didn't seem overly concerned, but I knew the liver is partly responsible for hormone production and wondered if being on the birth control is what caused the enlargement. I was also concerned about the nodules in my lungs . . . *why were they there?* I had such air hunger every day and often felt like I was fighting a lung infection.

I attended Christmas in a state of dizziness, severe air hunger, and adrenaline surges. I didn't know what else to do but take the benzo, which made me sleepy but didn't improve a lot of symptoms. My entire body was tremoring and I couldn't understand what was happening to me. I hoped it was the birth control and that when it left my body things would improve. It *didn't*.

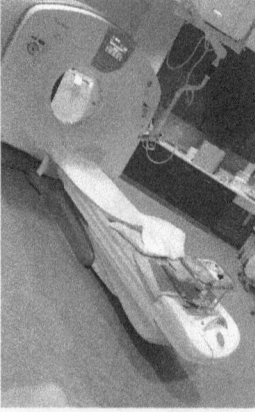

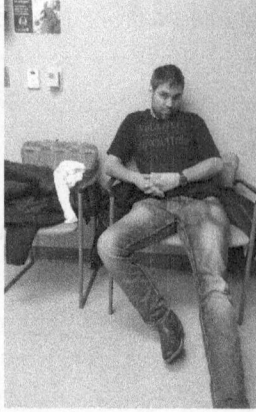

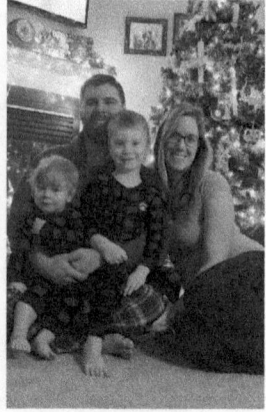

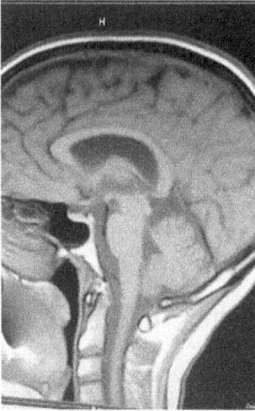

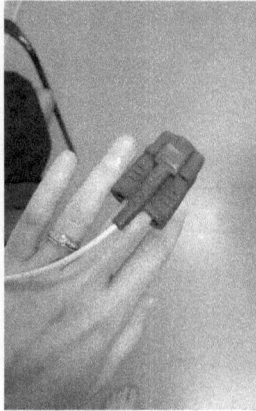

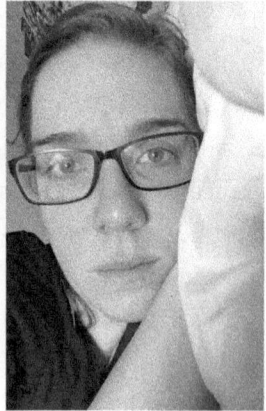

I hoped it was the birth control and when it left my body things would improve. It didn't.

The week after Christmas, an MRI with contrast—as well as a spinal tap—was done to rule out some infections. I didn't like the spinal tap. I did it sitting upright on the table and they sent me home right afterward. The last time I had a needle in my spine was when I had done an epidural during during Eliot's birth, and the doctor hit a nerve. I lost feeling on the right side of my body for 24 hours. It was very scary and I worried it would paralyze me. Thankfully it didn't.

I don't know why, but after the MRI my body started to burn and my legs felt heavy. I've had worse symptoms since . . . tremors and terrible pressure headaches behind my eyes. When I got home, I felt worse and I started to have increased symptoms and my legs began to feel increasingly heavy. The internal tremors were even worse and this was the onset of debilitating pressure headaches.

The pressure was unbearable. I would look at my husband and tell him something was not right . . . it felt as if the pressure behind my eyes were going to make my eyes burst. *Is this a brain aneurysm?* I would often have him hold my head in a tight vice-like grip and asked him to squeeze my head . . . that was the only way I would have any relief. The lights became so unbearable, I could hardly look outside anymore without them piercing through me, causing intense migraines and pressure attacks. The severity of these attacks were terrifying. *Could these be signs of a brain aneurysm?* The tests came back showing nothing remarkable. But my health continued to decline and I couldn't even look out of the window anymore without extreme pain. Everything began to overstimulate me, putting my body into uncontrollable episodes. *What was happening to me?*

It's hard for me to believe that a simple thing like birth control could wreak such havoc on the body. One minute I am questioning whether or not I have a serious anxiety disorder and the next minute I think, *No, there is something more to this!* This happened to me after a birth control pill was put into my body. I was not like this before. I had common anxieties, never crippling ones over nothing.

* * *

I have always had to be strong in life, which makes me wonder if maybe all of the tough stuff I dealt with over the last years made me this way and the birth control is just coincidental . . . but those thoughts push into my mind when I have sudden feelings that I cannot control. Then later, I know there is something truly wrong. This has been the most challenging thing I have ever been through. I am so determined to get better for my children and husband, not just for myself.

I felt so out of control and I didn't fully agree with the panic disorder

11

diagnosis. There was obviously something going on with my hormones and my liver enlargement. The chiropractor felt that the birth control was still in my system and I needed help detoxing it out of me. He suggested that I try CBD oil to curb the anxiety, not anti-anxiety medicine. I have started a mild detox, but the last few days my emotions and hormones have been so crazy. I feel, too, like this benzo I am taking is making me worse. When I take it I feel sleepy but then later my anxiety or episodes are worse. I don't seem to respond well to medications.

I am now struggling to do my normal simple tasks. I am detoxing through my chiropractor by changing my diet and supporting my liver with milk thistle. I want this out of my body. I don't want to be on medications just to live when I was not like this before. *I want to fix the cause.* Please God, let me win and fix this . . .

I have been told these things can happen to you after having babies. Your body can no longer tolerate certain birth controls. In the past I have had mild social anxiety or anxiousness when the kids cry often, get sick, or the house is really messy . . . *but nothing like this.* When I used an IUD after having Eliot, I was having more depressed feelings so I had it removed and then the feelings resolved.

After this episode, a friend spoke with me and suggested that maybe I needed to go back to college. She thought maybe being a stay-at-home mom had worn me down. I feel she thinks it's more emotional, but it's not like that. I am *happy* being a stay-at-home mom. This is what I want in my life. This is my dream. *I am living my dream.*

* * *

I was alone in the country with my boys when the extreme episodes were happening. Sometimes I called my mom and she would drive over. I felt *safer* when she was here with me. I wasn't so much worried about dying but my biggest *fear* was my children seeing it happen. If I died while I was alone with my boys they would be unable to call for help.

There were several times when I called the ambulance for this reason. I would start to experience an episode and when my peripheral vision would suddenly go out I would call. My four-year-old son would hide behind the chair when they arrived . . . I will always be haunted by the *fear* in his eyes.

The paramedics in the ambulance were always so kind to me. I remember us discussing what could be happening. One man specifically said that he used to have extreme migraine episodes where he would lose his vision and they found out later that pork was causing it. *That's odd . . . maybe it is food related for me, but I hardly ever eat pork . . .*

* * *

I often experienced stroke- or seizure-type episodes . . . I even felt like my hearing was going out. Everything sounded muffled. My husband would often notice me making sounds with my hands over each ear to make sure they sounded the same. Sometimes they didn't. *Am I going deaf? Am I losing my vision? Why does my vision black out on and off? Am I really losing my mind?*

I began to experience symptoms of heart race while folding my laundry or from just going up the stairs. I had air hunger all of the time. My heart raced and sometimes I felt like my throat was going to close up. I started getting a lot of eye floaters. I didn't have any eye floaters before this. During episodes they burst out all over my vision. *Am I going blind?*

* * *

Terri has had to stay with us this last week and she leaves on Friday. I am so *grateful* she is here. I feel safer when someone is here with me. It puts my mind at ease knowing someone else is here with my children if I have another episode. I don't want her to leave . . . I still can't control overstimulation. It causes everything to go wacky with my mind and nerves and I get very weak and faint. I am still doing this detox with my chiropractor, so I *hope* things change soon. I see my chiropractor again on Thursday.

On Sunday we went into town and that did not go well. The noise and fast movements during church caused my body and mind to go into overdrive. I felt tremors all over and just felt like I was being hooked up to an electrical current, as if my body were plugged into something and I just feel a pulse. *I can't do normal things anymore and it's scary . . .*

February 4, 2019: Today went well, but the evening did not. I got overtired and started to experience tremors and anxiety all over. I just want to be normal.

When I research what is going on with me, it all points to a hormonal imbalance which started after the birth control was introduced into my body. I often read things, too, about Lyme disease or environmental factors like mold causing issues with hormones. It was set off after the birth control, but maybe I have an underlying factor?

I am on day 6 of a detox, and it has not been easy at all. The food hasn't been the problem, but the emotional, mental, and physical side effects have been. I had a breakdown Sunday night. Thoughts of maybe I should go on the antianxiety medication like the doctor recommended . . .

But I don't want to just *mask* my symptoms, I want to *fix* them. I will be starting some vitamins and a probiotic after detoxing. Please let this work.

My symptoms come like *waves*, like I'm helpless in the ocean and I cannot stop the *waves* from jolting me around and pulling me underwater.

2

Why Won't Anyone Believe Me?

June 25 2019,

T he last few months of my life have been a blur, ridden with spells of crippling anxiety, panic attacks, heart palpitations, night sweats, difficulty breathing, aura migraines, headaches, hot flashes, brain fog, dizziness, confusion, tingling/vibration in feet, tremors, mood swings, and loss of self. All because of a hormone imbalance? An imbalance caused by years of birth control depleting my natural hormones, causing anovulatory cycles? That is what I am being told now . . .

My body feels as if I am fighting an infection too. I even feel like I am having recurring fevers at times. I'm not sure if the birth control would have caused these symptoms because I was having mild forms of these symptoms before the birth control was introduced into my body, but it *definitely* seems to have triggered the more crippling issues. A lot of my issues are hormonal, but food is becoming more of an issue too. I have been struggling with stomach pain for several years now, but the pain can be so unbearable at times. I can't figure out what food is doing it. A lot of times my extreme reactions will occur after eating a lot of yeasts, sugars, grains, or beef.

The tipping point was the combination birth control pill that I started in December. *It had to be . . .* I was normal before that, aside from my stomach issues and feeling like I was fighting something all the time. I've been told my adrenals were fatigued and progesterone is most likely depleted . . . I'm trying to get the right tests to prove it, but my new primary seemed bewildered when it came to hormones.

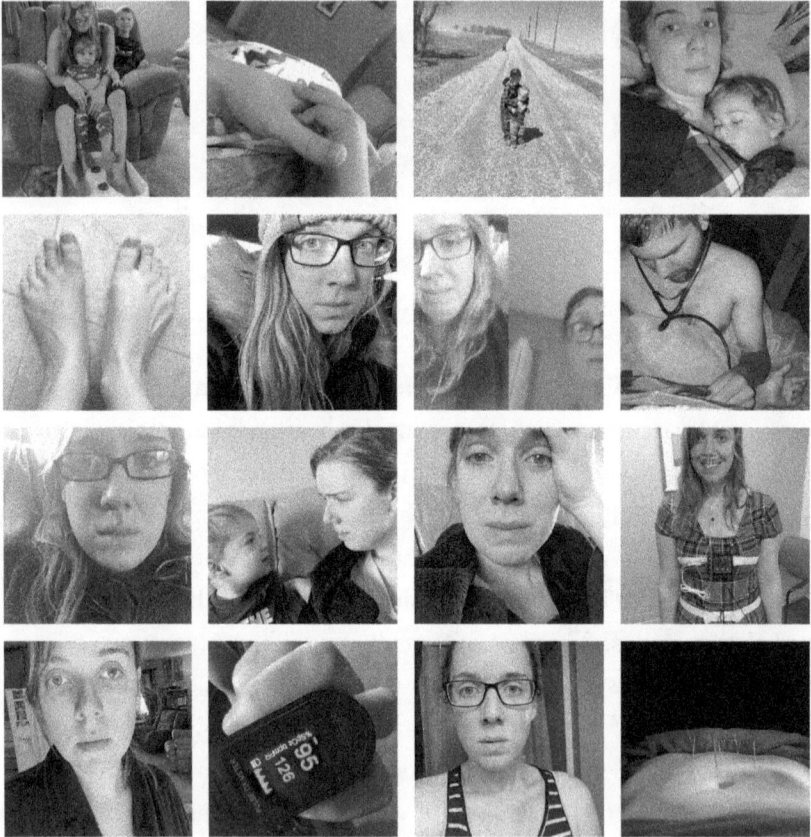

I can't even push my kids down the gravel road in the stroller anymore . . . what is happening to me?

At the end of February I changed to a female primary care provider because I thought maybe she would understand hormones better. She didn't seem to. I was so desperate for relief and told her I had so much trouble on the first benzo. I also mentioned when I tried to go on the SSRI, I ended up calling the ambulance the same day because of a terrible episode where I had dots all over my vision and briefly lost my peripheral sight. I don't even know if it was related to the SSRI but now I'm scared to take anything.

February 8, 2019: I had to call 911 today, I kept having attacks after I took my antidepressant. I just want to be normal. I don't want to feel this way anymore . . .

I need something, *anything*, to help me to not have episodes so often when I am home alone with my kids. I had to call the ambulance several times when I had increased episodes and loss of vision. The only thing that doctors think is going on with me is *anxiety*.

The paramedics thought I was experiencing aura migraines or seizures. Sometimes I feel like I am having seizures. Every time I have had to go into the ER they are rude to me and *anxiety* is stamped all over my chart. How can lifting my arms to make my bed cause me *"anxiety"*? My heart freaks out. I am walking up the stairs and can't breathe and my heart rate is very high. I've seen a lot of doctors on and off, desperate for someone to help me . . . but everyone blames it on anxiety alone. This doesn't seem like anxiety, but I don't know what else to do but try their recommendations and go on an anxiety medication. I can't keep calling my mom and terrifying my husband every day. I don't have enough help out here. I am alone for the majority of time with my young children. *No one seems to understand what is going on, including me.*

* * *

Russell hides behind the couch crying when the ambulance comes. He is only four. He is so *scared*. I usually *hide* what is going on with me from him, but one day I was having an episode in the kitchen and our eyes met when he was in the living room and he just *knew*. I called the ambulance and had to lie on the floor with my kids until the paramedics came. Russell was *scared*, so I comforted him and reassured him that *everything was going to be okay*, even though I felt like I was going to die. I had my phone on me because I had just gotten off the phone with the ambulance and my husband. I turned my camera on, hoping to catch the episode so that maybe if something obvious happened someone could figure out what was going on with me. I never did show anyone the video—not even my husband—because I was embarrassed and ashamed. While recording I was *afraid . . . at least* if I *died* the paramedics would know what happened to me.

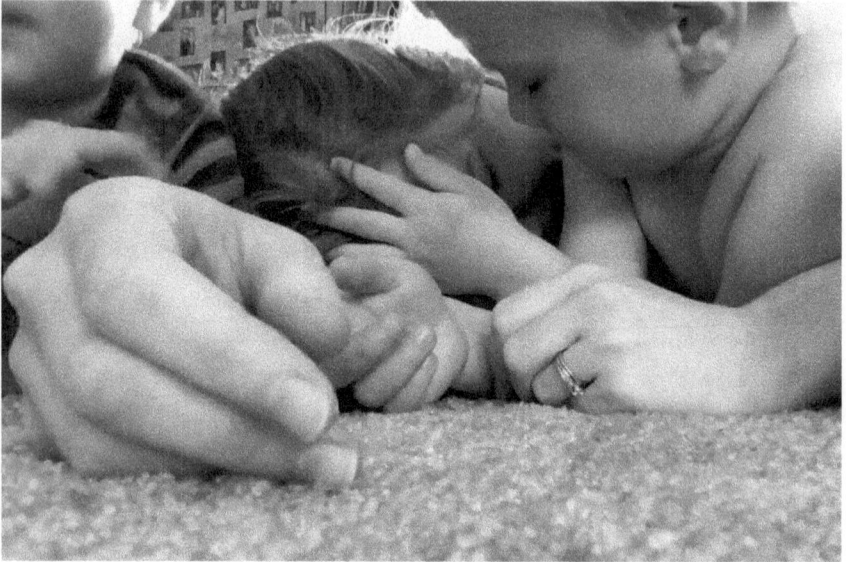

My job as a mother was to protect my children from the scary things in life . . . I had failed.

I couldn't have this happen again when I was alone in the country with my two children. After this episode I asked my new female primary care provider to put me on something that would be easy to wean off of later. I didn't want to be on something long-term if this sudden panic disorder was a result of a hormone balance from birth control. Eventually my hormones would balance . . .

My primary doctor told me she understood my concerns and when she held my hand and suggested a SNRI (*serotonin-norepinephrine reuptake inhibitors, are a class of drugs used to treat depression, anxiety, and other conditions)* as an easier alternative to the first one I tried. I accepted it. I didn't even want to research it and just put my *trust* in her. I didn't want to go on this medication but felt I had *no choice* as this seemed to be the only option for treatment that anyone could offer me. I am *alone* in the country with my children and I cannot continue to have these episodes while trying to care for them.

I knew that if I researched the medication that was being offered to me I would probably be too afraid to try it. And I needed to stop having episodes at home alone. No one is here. I am alone with my kids. *What am I supposed to do?*

February 9, 2019: All I want to do is lie in bed today. I just want to be better. We will be staying with Mom the first half of this week. I can't be alone with the kids.

I ended up having to stay with my mom in town for a couple of weeks while I was trying to allow my body to tolerate this medication. We didn't want me to end up being stuck out in the country alone again in a snowstorm or experience side effects with no one to help me. When I started the SNRI I felt a lot worse. So bad, in fact, that I even started to experience serious thoughts of ending my life. I had never had thoughts like this before. *Was this the drug?* I remember while I was at my mom's I looked at my pill compartment and thought *what the hell happened? Why is my body failing me? I don't want to be on all these pills.*

After dealing with these increased symptoms, I caved and looked up possible side effects that could explain what I was feeling. I was experiencing all the worst ones listed . . . I decided to call my doctor and tell her.

The doctor wanted me to stay on the medication longer because I could *still* adjust and as I *continued* to spiral downward I experienced increased loss of self while feeling pressured to swallow the pills. I began to experience extreme rage episodes. I felt violent at times and then would cry as I went over a *wave* of the emotion. I would tell myself *this isn't you, hold on to who you are.* I called Terri once in a desperate state because I felt very pressured to stay on the medication. I didn't know who to go to, and my mom and husband were not sure what I should do.

I couldn't stay at my mom's apartment *forever* because of rules concerning her lease, so after a couple more weeks I had to go home. When I had to leave I didn't feel ready at all to be *alone* . . .

But I was. I remember crying a lot and feeling terrified to be *alone* out there with my children. If I wasn't losing my mind before I definitely was now because of this medication.

* * *

Recently, I had my hormones checked using a saliva test suggested to me by a hormone specialist. I had to wait a few months to see her with the results but I could at least get the labs done. Every time I had my levels checked through blood work with gynecology, they said they were *normal*. I monitored a few months of my cycles and saw a pattern each month and each day depending on if it was either before or during a period or before or during ovulation. These times are when the worst episodes are occurring, and when I am having a period I am waking up in the night with heart rates in the 180s and fainting episodes. It's almost like I am anemic . . . . I had a doctor check my iron levels, but she said they are *normal*.

This has been emotional and physical hell for me. I just want to *always* be normal again. Not normal for only a few weeks then back to HELL. It has been so hard being an active mother to my sweet boys. I hide so much from everyone. Russell is four and Eliot is one.

I honestly don't know how I got through those few months of a sudden onset of *"panic attack episodes,"* trying a new medication that made me want to end my life, and then later weaning off the drug and experiencing terrible side effects.

The doctors I have seen have made everything worse throughout this. They fight me on every suggestion I make, and they don't think anything is related to my hormone fluctuations or period cycles. Even if they do agree to do a test, they degrade me first.

Eventually, because of this, I started to see alternative naturopaths

20

because the medical doctors were either failing to help me or constantly gaslighting my symptoms. *Why didn't anyone believe me?*

* * *

I had to wait several weeks to get the saliva hormone test results back and see a hormone specialist, so I started to see an acupuncturist in the meantime for hormone balancing. He was very surprised that my doctor put me on this SNRI as an easier choice. He said it is one of the hardest anti-anxiety drugs he has ever seen people try to get off of and he called their experience an *"EXORCISM."*

I asked my doctor to put me on something that would be easy to wean off of later . . . and she chose this. Disappointment was an understatement. *Can I trust any doctor?*

My acupuncturist gives me *hope* and has helped me so much. He also helped me in discovering that I had serotonin syndrome. I was later checked properly with a neurologist, and it was confirmed based on symptoms and a 24-hour urine test. It was then confirmed that I had developed serotonin syndrome from the drug interactions. I was on the lowest dose of an SNRI and a benzo, and I only took 1/4 of the benzo pill every few days. These were prescription drugs in a combination known by my doctor. *And they just kept telling me to try and stay on it and I would get better.* If this is what it is like for people going on these drugs, they should *not* be expected to just go home while adjusting and taking care of small children.

Never before in my life had I experienced this. I felt pressured to stay on these drugs by my medical doctors. When I realized it was for sure the medication making me worse I began weaning off of it because every day was a *nightmare.* I had terrible withdrawal symptoms as I tried to wean off of the SNRI and the benzo. These drugs never took away the symptoms, but they would make me tired enough to sleep. Then later, when the sleepiness wore off, I would have worse anxiety attacks. I felt if I stayed on the medications I would end up ending my life. I experienced brain zaps, terror, anxiety, extreme rage, depression, brain fog, nausea, diarrhea, and a racing heart. The medication acted as a stimulant to my anxiety. It was absolutely horrible.

My acupuncturist helped me as much as he could while I was weaning myself off of the SNRI. He is very smart and offers so many suggestions. He feels I may be experiencing adrenal fatigue too. I feel that we are finally on a path to balancing my hormones now. We went over my saliva results since I could not get in with the hormone specialist for a few months yet. My progesterone was depleted, estrogen low normal, and testosterone depleted. In the beginning of all of this I was in constant fight or flight. Since then, every symptom follows my cycle and fluctuating hormones. We are going to do acupuncture for hormone balancing and bio-identical progesterone cream to see how I do. I still believe my acupuncturist *saved my life* after discovering the serotonin syndrome. Once I was able to get off of the drugs, the severe suicidal thoughts and increased rage ended.

* * *

Tonight I feel almost normal but then the two weeks before ovulation were hell. I had a 16-day period with dark heavy clots. I was covered in fog, confused, heart palpitations, weak, faint, dizzy, nauseous, night sweats, hot flashes, migraines or headaches all day for two weeks. Hell. I'm going to look back at my last three cycles. Last month I began a progesterone cream and it worked amazing. I felt almost normal for three weeks until right before my period. I had some heart palpitations and breathlessness, then it got better again for a week while I had my period but it turned into hell the longer my period lasted and the closer I got to ovulation. My periods are so long and I bleed a lot. I can't believe I am not anemic.

Thank God for my chiropractor and acupuncturist.

I plan to keep track of my cycle a little closer and when I start estrogen cream in a week or so we will see how I do. *I talked to God.* I lay in bed and listened for a long time. Two words popped into my head. He told me *Fear* and *Trust*. Sometimes I feel like God has abandoned me. Sometimes I want to blame him for what is happening to me. I picture God like a mean figure hovering over an anthill with a magnifying glass, slowly burning them. But I am the ant. This is the first night I was able to talk to God without feeling that *anger*. I can't blame God for what is happening to me . . .

* * *

I finally got in with the hormone specialist. It took several months, but I made it. She said my thyroid was on the verge of hypothyroidism, but it fluctuates so much that I can't be medicated. She feels that the cause of this is estrogen dominance. She says I have adrenal fatigue, too, just like my acupuncturist thought. She looked at the brand of progesterone cream I was on and said that should be okay for now but she also put me on a testosterone cream. The biggest puzzle is no one seems to know why my hormones are so out of whack. The birth control may have triggered something, but there could be something more affecting my hormones. My acupuncturist said this last time . . . *your hormones are all so depleted . . . but why?* Something caused all of these hormones to deplete. The hormone specialist suggested I do more therapies to help with detox.

When I take a detox bath, I scream to myself . . . *get out of me . . .* I don't even know what I am screaming at.

* * *

Between specialists I also saw a gastroenterologist. We did an upper endoscope. They called about two weeks later and told me I have intestinal metaplasia. They said it is *precancer* of the stomach . . . what occurs as the cells start to change. *Cancer* was all I heard. I wrote it down and they told me it was about a two-month wait to see my gastroenterologist to discuss my results. *Two months.* I left home after that feeling very worried. I went to my mom's and started crying because I was diagnosed with precancer. My entire body shook when I told her the news.

They prescribed me a medication but I never took it. Instead, I researched how to change my diet and have been eating very clean and juicing celery juice every morning. When I was finally able to see my gastroenterologist, he felt like the diet change was a good idea and he was pretty calm about my diagnosis. He said it can be reversible and we will do a repeat upper endoscope in a year. But it *still* scared me . . . I felt like at least maybe now I knew why I had been having gut issues for all those years. I don't really know the *cause*, but I do know that the intestinal metaplasia is a result of inflammation.

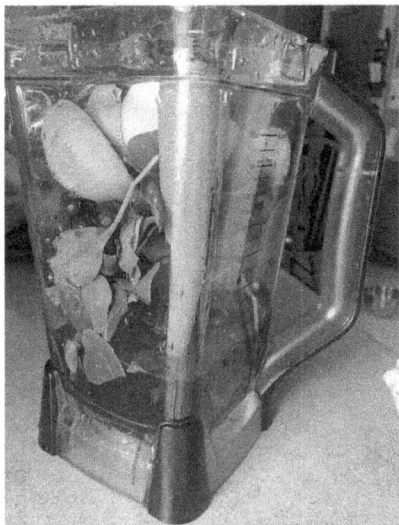

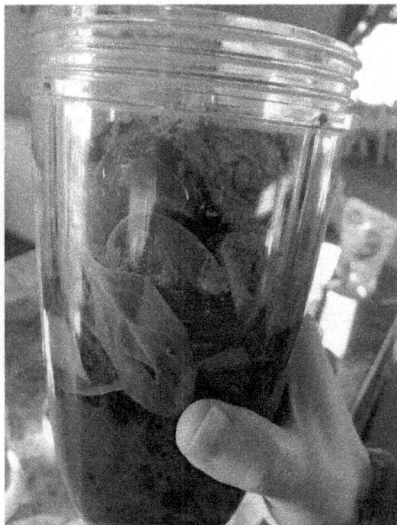

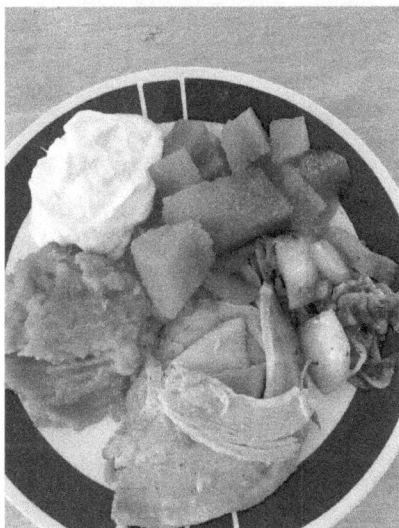

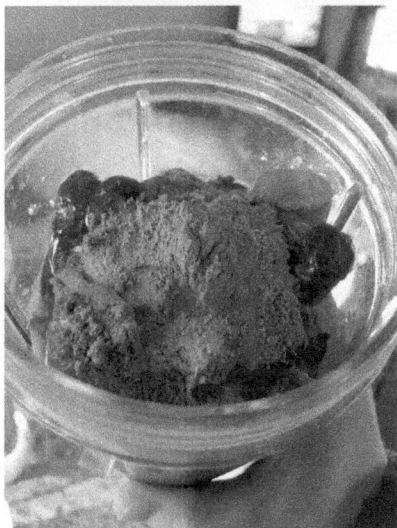

Let food be thy medicine . . .

I saw a neurologist who did a 24-hour urine test for catecholamines and metanephrines, and he said there were some signs that I may have something going on with my pituitary gland. He also did a test for seizures and said the test does not rule out seizures entirely, but it could show if I am having one right now. I also saw a few gynecologists who were of little help. I waited months to see these doctors. I was very surprised to see how little they seemed to understand hormone levels.

I am waiting to get in to see an endocrinologist, but they are six to eight months out. My acupuncturist, too, thinks the pituitary concerns need to be evaluated. I have been doing a lot of research on my own time and I keep coming across mold illness or Lyme disease as a potential cause. When I bring in my paperwork to local doctors, they seem flabbergasted by the idea and claim it is not related and don't want to test me for Lyme disease. I have had several tick bites in my life and have always struggled with illness and chronic stomach issues.

I grew up in a moldy home, but I really *hope* there is no mold in the house we are at now. We did a high-quality air test when we moved in, and it came back safe. Tim also checked all of the ductwork and there is no mold to be seen. This all has me very concerned as I don't know what kind of doctors can help me. After I go to my regular doctor, I have to wait weeks to see different specialists and most of them send me to a different specialist because my symptoms are systemic multi-body issues. No one can figure it out. No one looks at the body as a whole. Every body part is broken up into different specialties, making it take forever to see the correct doctor.

I cannot even escape my suffering with sleep. When I try to nap I wake up with high heart rates and feeling as if my throat is closing up. The same thing happens to me at night. One specific chiropractor I saw asked me what I'm thinking about before going to bed. I tell him it's nothing that would cause me this. I feel like he doesn't *believe* me. He experienced issues like this from stress-related worries years ago. Mine is *different*. I am not doing this with my *mind* or from *worries*. This is *really* happening to me and I don't know why.

I am starting to have difficulty being out in the sun too. My heart races when I pick green beans and I feel so dizzy. This doesn't make sense. I am 28 years old and I feel like I am *slowly dying*. My kids love being out in the country, but it is becoming impossible. My husband is losing weight from all of the stress. His anxiety is heightened because of everything going on

with me. We are so alone out here and don't know what to do . . .
Does God even hear my cries?

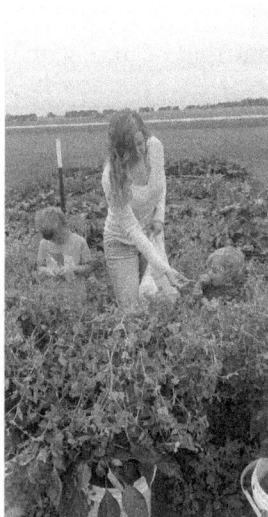

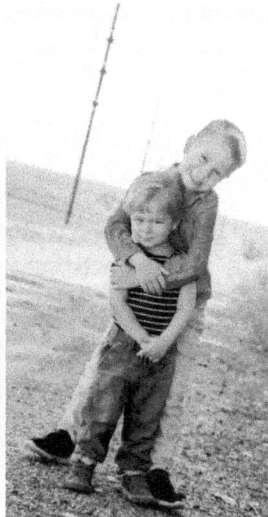

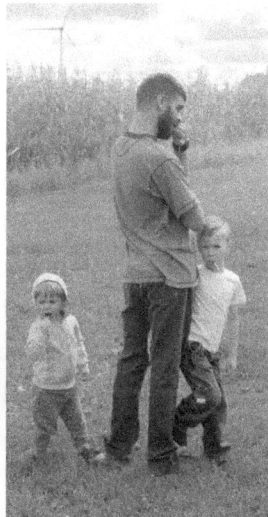

*Living in the country became a burden . . . we could hardly keep our heads
above water while the waves of hardship kept crashing down on us . . .*

Tim gets frustrated because my cognition is so off. I know he doesn't
mean to, but at times he can be so *insensitive*. I am really *struggling*. I have
so much pain and inflammation in my head and behind my eyes. I can't
understand it either. I don't blame Tim. *No one knows what is wrong with me.*
But I feel very *alone* and the only person who will troubleshoot with me is
my acupuncturist. I feel safe being able to go to him for acupuncture and
run different ideas past him. He is very helpful. When I bring up things
to my husband, my mom, or other family members, they just seem very
overwhelmed and sometimes I don't know if *they even believe me*. This is
very hard and I don't know what to do.

Sometimes I feel such rage surrounding my situation. I feel like I am the
only one trying to figure out what the hell is wrong with me and when
I bring things up everyone wants to run away from it and hide. I know

27

this is stressful and overwhelming but imagine living it. Just imagine for one second living in this condition. I am trying to get my life back and figure out what is wrong with me because doctors can't. I am strong and determined despite these uncontrollable attacks to my body. I will not give up. I will find my answers even if I am the only one that I can rely on to find them.

* * *

Sometimes I worry that Tim will grow tired of all of this and leave me. Who would want to keep living in this state over and over again with a wife that has health issues that no one can diagnose? He is so stressed because of me and I feel like a *burden* most of the time. I still keep up with most things, but my mom has had to come and help me with laundry and other tasks. I am losing my ability to do them. My body is slowly failing me and there is nothing I can do to stop it.

When we try to drive anywhere my body goes into fits. When I go into a loud room I feel like I'm in a tunnel while extremely drunk. I feel like I'm tipping over when I walk, as if I am in a state of drunkenness all of the time. When I hear too many noises I get tremors and feel like I am having seizures or something. *This is not normal.* Something is seriously wrong with me.

* * *

When I go to these doctors I downplay my symptoms. I have learned that if I act a certain way or look a certain way they will make *assumptions*. If I present with my real level of pain or suffering I am labeled as *attention-seeking*. Because I am a woman, a lot of my symptoms are *blamed* on that fact alone. If I say I am scared they will write *anxiety* on my chart. If I don't look nice enough I will be labeled as *depressed*. If I look too nice they won't *believe* that I am sick. If I try to discuss ideas that I have researched they get *upset*. If I cry I am *frantic*. Because of this, I meticulously fretted over if

28

my appearance was okay before seeing a doctor and I worried the entire time if I said the *wrong* thing or *acted* the wrong way . . .

If I had any anxiety it was because of how the doctor treated me.

I stopped reading the doctor reports after awhile because I couldn't handle the things that they would write down in my chart. Most people who know me would know that none of those things were true . . .

When you are dealing with chronic issues that make the doctors stumped, they don't like it when you offer suggestions. Sometimes I feel that they would rather I acted dumb with no insight as to what is wrong with me. I feel like my determination to find my answers upsets many of them. I feel like my persistence and drive intimidates them. Which is silly . . . I am not intimidating at all.

I feel that my stubbornness and drive to find my answers and not accept lazy diagnoses intimidates a lot of people.

I have two small children to take care of and I can't even push them down the gravel road in the stroller anymore. I have to be determined and persistent because my body is gradually failing me. I am slowly deteriorating and no one can help me. No one knows what is wrong. I have ideas that go dismissed. Over time, the mention of mold or Lyme disease seemed so off of everyone's radar that I decided to not even try to bring it up anymore. *I don't know what to do.*

Some doctors are kind, but I tread carefully around every one of them now because of my negative experiences.

* * *

A friend's dad called us and told us it could be because we are living on a wind farm. So now I am looking into that and I have no idea anymore. Between this and the mold idea . . . it all sounds ridiculous. Even if it was causing my issues, doctors wouldn't believe it. I even tried to stay out of my home again to see how I felt. I didn't feel much different. I still had episodes. It was mostly just nice not being alone in the country anymore with my babies. It's becoming so scary and impossible living here. How does someone just go from being normal one day to debilitatingly ill the next? And no one can figure it out . . . Tim wants me to go to the Mayo Clinic in Minnesota. He had a good experience at Mayo years ago. We are going to see if my neurologist can refer me. I still don't know if Mayo can help me. I feel like mold/Lyme is far off my husband's radar, too, and I don't know if Mayo can help if it's an issue like this. But I have *hope* . . .

* * *

Cycle monitor:

May 3: Period starts. So irritable before this period, horrible.

Day 4: Bled through 3 cups in 1 hour. Faint, nausea. Panic. High anxiety AM.

May 12: Period ends. Start progesterone cream. Woke up estrogen: migraine, hot flashes, nausea (got better after 3 days then felt great until some heart palpitations and brain fog before next period).

June 2: Period. Felt good until day 10 of period.

Bled: 16 days Ovulation: cycle was terrible days 17-21. Faint, dizzy, weak, heart palpitations, sick, migraine, constant feet vibrations, crying spells, and headache. The long period and symptoms could indicate low estrogen - went off DIM. Tremors, shakes, panic, AM but mostly 10:20 PM or 1 AM.

Day 22 of June: Felt better but not 100%.

Saw acupuncturist for acupuncture on day 24. Felt almost normal by midday day 25.

August 19, 2019

My boys: "I wasn't able to be there with you at the zoo. I couldn't see your eyes light up to watch the fireworks. I couldn't swim next to you on the day we went to the pool. Too many days were spent bedridden, alone in my room. I couldn't be the mother I wanted to be and it broke my heart in two. I wanted to have more children but two will have to do. All that I want in this life is to enjoy each day with you. I may not always look sick but I have stayed quiet long enough. I hope that I can find the answer that seems so far out of reach. I hope that I can be the mother that I was instead of the shadow of the mother I had become."

I have been sick since December, but I have had issues with periods since I was thirteen. When I feel the worst I have severe hot flashes, full body shivers and trembles, severe leg pain and uterine pain that radiates into my upper abdomen. I often feel very dizzy and faint. Everything is enhanced. This happened again during the week when I was supposed to ovulate and did not. Two days ago, I had a migraine so severe that I lost peripheral vision temporarily. I felt faint, scared, and I had to call the ambulance again. I didn't call because I had anxiety but because I was afraid for my children if I lost my sight or fainted. What would they do? This has been so hard for Russell and I see it in his eyes. Not knowing what is causing your symptoms is very scary. This happens during the same time frame every month and I refuse to put a blanket on my symptoms like I have done in the past. It's time to find out what is wrong with me and how to fix it, even if that means a full hysterectomy at age 29 and the hard truth as a result: no more children. My issues must be hormonal. I have 10–16 day periods and they're so heavy. I feel like I'm going to die when I get them. I feel like I'm bleeding to death. I just found out that my uterus is prolapsing, which is a shock to the doctor as I did not have a lot of strain during deliveries. They are suspecting endometriosis . . . I am starting to wonder if I'm having ovarian failure. Something is wrong with my body and making my hormones unbalanced. Unfortunately, the only way to diagnose a possible cause is to have surgery. I am preparing for this mentally but still don't know when that will happen.

I just finished blood work this month and am told that although my hormones are in range my ratio is not balanced, making me estrogen-dominant, but my estrogen is also on the low side when it should be higher. I may need to start additional hormone therapy, but I won't know until I get someone to look at it that knows how to properly read them. It's hard for me to share personal things like this, but I need people to understand that just because someone looks good on the outside when you see them, it does not mean they are okay all of the time. These issues need to be talked about more. Women should not have to suffer in silence and be made to feel that it's "all in their head." Sixteen-day periods are not normal, feeling faint often is not normal, missed periods are not normal, birth control does not fix the underlying problem, and anxiety is not the cause of everything! It is not "all in your head." You are not going crazy. Listen to your body. Keep fighting. Stay strong. Ask for help. Pray. I go to Mayo in two weeks. Until then I expect to get sicker, as I always do. I get an internal ultrasound again to check my ovaries and uterus and I also see a functional medicine doctor soon for my hormones as I have not had any help through my regular doctors. I'm very hopeful Mayo can diagnose the root cause so that I will be able to move past all of this with the right treatment.

3

I Had to Keep Living

December 2, 2019

Today a dear friend asked me if I had been journaling my experience since I went to Mayo. My answer was *no. I have wanted to push everything into a deep dark hole in my past so that I can bury the pain.* So much has happened since the time I last wrote.

I was accepted to Mayo and while there I was diagnosed with PCOS (polycystic ovary syndrome), aura migraine, suspected early stages of hypothyroidism and POTS (postural orthostatic tachycardia syndrome). The definition of a *syndrome* is this: *A group of signs and symptoms that are known to go together but don't have a clear cause, course, or treatment plan.* The PCOS diagnosis has been confusing for me because none of my blood tests show common markers for PCOS and I was told that my ovarian cysts have not been common PCOS cysts.

In the past, I was told by my hormone specialist that these cysts are caused by high estrogen and low progesterone. Estrogen is a grower and, as much as the medical establishment fails to understand hormones, my levels are unbalanced. I am experiencing everything associated with a hormone imbalance including PMDD (premenstrual dysphoric disorder), which was later diagnosed by my second local endocrinologist whom I found after the first one failed.

"We don't look at progesterone when testing hormones. We find it unimportant unless you are trying to get pregnant."

This was the same concept repeated by many gynecologists.

Progesterone *is very* important and I have had low progesterone for a very long time now.

Prior to attending Mayo, I saw several different specialists and had an at-home and in-hospital sleep study done, an echocardiogram, and a week-long Holter monitor for my heart. These tests were sent to Mayo for review. There was enough evidence from those tests alone showing signs of POTS episodes, but it was missed for an *entire year*.

One of my highest heart rates was 185, *while sleeping*.

The doctor had to inappropriately add, "Unless you are doing something *else* in the middle of the night, this is *not* normal . . . " He ended his statement with a squeeze to my leg. *Something serious is happening to me and I am suffering daily and he thinks it's okay to make a sex joke?* I was really hurt by this. I was so taken aback that I didn't even respond.

I'm assuming these nightly episodes were before or during a period as I marked my nightly episodes on the calendar and they always fell within those time frames.

* * *

Our summer was complete madness. My symptoms began to worsen in some ways and get better in others. I wasn't stricken every day with panic attacks, but I began to experience dizziness, heat sensitivity, and a racing heart while doing simple tasks like going up the stairs or lifting my arms to make my bed. Getting up out of bed became an amazing feat and even light exercise became impossible as I would gag and wretch every time I attempted it. My bleeding and migraines worsened and I developed large ovarian cysts that were apparently there since at least early March. But I only found this out later because the medical establishment failed to tell me that these cysts were showing up on my scans.

Instead they told me, *"Everything is normal, go on an anti-anxiety med . . .*

"

Again and again.

The mental anguish was unbearable. My periods became 10–16 days long with heavy bleeding. My migraines became so crippling, to the point where I would become so confused, could hardly form words, and would lose my vision at random . . .

. . . *but I just had to keep living every day.* I had to care for my four- and one-year-old when I could hardly care for myself. Some days were tolerable but the bad ones were terrible. My mom and Terri helped me when they could and my husband would go to work with severe anxiety every day, worrying about what might happen while he was gone. He worried often that he would wake up in the morning and find me dead. The mental anguish tore him apart because he was a fixer, he had always fixed everything for me before . . . but he could not fix what was wrong with me. With all the medical doctors saying it was anxiety, what could we do? I think he was torn over this also because he didn't understand what was going on with me . . . I'm sure he wondered off and on if it *was* all anxiety.

I slowly began to loose my ability to drive and became trapped in an endless nightmare with *waves* of symptoms drowning me every day.

As the summer months progressed I began to develop episodes of brief full-body shivering and tremors. I would become so freezing cold and so sick, as if I were about to throw up but never could. I am still sick. But we are going to figure this out.

* * *

Prior to being accepted to Mayo, my neurologist was unsure if I could get in. There is a referral process and a lot of cases are denied. Because of this concern, he pushed for me to get in with a local endocrinologist as there was an opening sooner than expected. I thought this doctor was going to be my *savior* . . .

Living in my condition with a suspected pituitary or adrenal disease and having to care for my children was not ideal. I was so *grateful* to get in with someone who could help me . . . *finally*. An endocrinologist could do the right tests for my hormones and rule out a pituitary disease or adrenal failure.

The endocrinologist listened to me somewhat and complimented me on my appearance. "Well, you look in great health."

I continued to express my health concerns, but he stopped me as he read my chart and pointed out that I had been seeing the local hormonal specialist. I was thinking maybe he would want to discuss what we had found out concerning my hormones, but he started to talk very badly about her instead. I was confused when he asked me what I thought of her. *What does this have to do with my health concerns?*

He ranted on about her. He called her a *zealot* and a *quack*. He also said if I continued to see her he would *not* see me anymore and he was embarrassed to live in the same town as her.

I was shocked and very taken aback by his words. *"Keep this between us . . . and don't see her again. Only then will I be happy to run some of these labs for you."*

Oddly, I couldn't help but notice that her facility was a lot nicer than his. Later I found out that a lot of her patients *used to be his too . . .*

I didn't say much to defend my hormone specialist because I was still hoping this man could help me with some of the labs . . . he was the only local endocrinologist available in an 8-month time frame. I felt like I had to tread carefully around how I responded and didn't know what I would do if I had to wait several months to see someone else.

I redirected the conversation back to my health concerns and by the end of our conversation he told me that he knew what this was. He flipped through my paperwork and tapped on it while repeatedly saying *I know what this is.*

He patted my leg reassuringly and kept saying, "I know what this is. I will be right back."

He left dramatically and I was so relieved that we may have an answer.

He came back in and very seriously said to me, "You need to see a psychiatric specialist."

I didn't know what to say but I went numb all over. Tim was crying. I don't think that I cried much.

This doctor affected me in a way that I cannot explain. I knew he was wrong, but at that time he was my last *hope* for some kind of help in a reasonable time frame. He told me if I went to Mayo they would find *nothing*. He told me repeatedly that I had a million dollar work up done *already*.

I felt defeated and lost and alone in my battle. He asked me a lot of questions about family history.

This was when my husband stammered, "Well . . . her mom did go to mental facilities on and off when she was growing up."

I could tell his reply was questionable too.

"But she was abused," I said. "And I have never had any issues ever before in my entire life. I'm having heart rate issues when I'm going up the stairs. I can't go on walks anymore and the heat makes me sick too . . . I almost throw up or pass out when I stand up in the morning or while showering . . ."

But in my mind I kept thinking *Maybe this doctor is right. Maybe I am just going crazy.* And I feel my husband was battling with the same internal thoughts as I was . . . neither of us really *believed* he was right, but he was an endocrinologist. *He should know more than we do* . . . and no one else could give us any other answer besides *anxiety*.

I would compare my experience to when you are being interrogated for a crime that you did not commit and everyone coming in keeps repeating the same thing over and over again and telling you what you have done. Even if you are *innocent,* you start to *believe* it.

It's a form of mental torture.

The endocrinologist agreed to run a few labs for me to take along if I got in with Mayo, but not without repeating first that I probably *wouldn't* get in and if I did they probably wouldn't find *anything*. We left with him *repeating* that I really needed a psychiatric evaluation.

My husband and I both felt very defeated. Tears were streaming down our faces with this reality that we had to go back home with no help . . . and maybe I *was* going *crazy*.

But then as soon as we drove off my husband wiped his tears and said, "No . . . this doesn't make sense. It doesn't explain your 16-day periods and a lot of your symptoms. We are going to Mayo. Call your neurologist and tell him what happened."

A glimmer of fight crept back into him and rubbed off on me. I agreed. I called my neurologist and told them what had happened. They apologized repeatedly and said they were worried about this, but he was the only local endocrinologist available and they were hoping he could help me sooner. They said they would never refer future patients to this clinic and went on to say that some older doctors are just set in their ways and very unprofessional when it comes to competitors.

Later, I was informed by other providers who practiced under him that he treated nurses in residency very poorly. I now know that he was an endocrinologist stuck in old ways, unwilling to learn anything new, and *jealous* of the local hormone specialist who got all of his patients and had a nicer facility than him . . . but at the time it still affected me deeply. I went home after that and felt very dead inside, knowing that I would have to wait months for a different referral.

* * *

The only thing I could do to lift my spirits in the meantime was to see my acupuncturist. He was so angry when I told him what happened . . .

I thought he was going to burst. He suggested I complete the psychiatric evaluation just to prove him wrong. I did call in for a psychiatric evaluation, but then my neurologist called and said I was accepted at Mayo.

The neurologist must have worked some magic out of remorse because of what I experienced. Since it *was* his referral, I'm sure he felt bad. I never felt upset at my neurologist, though. He was a good doctor. He got us in, in just a few weeks' time frame rather than a few months. I was so *grateful*. I canceled the psychiatric evaluation because *I was going to Mayo* . . . and *despite* what the endocrinologist said, *I knew they would find something.* I would prove him wrong at Mayo.

I was seeing a therapist locally, too, because of what I had been going through. This was the first time in my life that I had seen a therapist. She told me that *none* of my issues pointed to psychiatric and she pushed me to keep advocating for myself and go to Mayo.

In her words: "The health issues you are experiencing would give anyone anxiety, but it is *not* anxiety causing them. This is a normal human response."

I often told her that I didn't have anxiety or depression until after doctors treated me the way they did. I went home over and over again with little help or acknowledgment that something was wrong and I had to live my life in trauma and pain knowing this . . . and being told repeatedly that this *was all in my head.*

My therapist told me, "Who wouldn't feel anxious when going through this?"

So many doctors say *It's all in your head. It's all in your head. It's all in your head . . .*

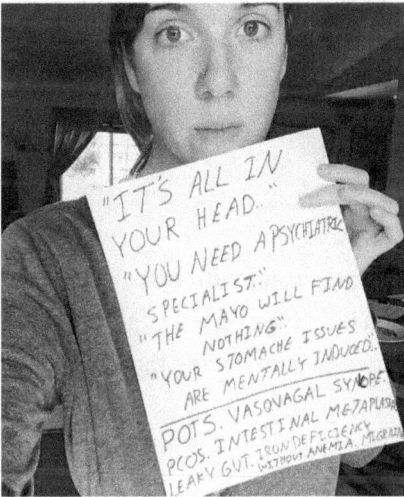

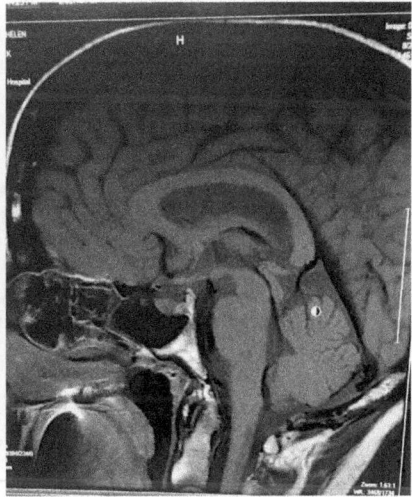

You need to see a psychiatric specialist . . . Mayo will find nothing. Have you ever considered that it may all be in your head?

This experience still affected me. I was over the moon about being accepted to Mayo, but then the reality struck that I still had to go home and suffer every day while trying to raise my children until I could get in. At least it was a few weeks rather than a few months, but it was still a hard reality and the words of the endocrinologist echoed in my head.

I called a longtime friend from high school shortly after my failed endocrinologist appointment. She was able to comfort me and help reassure me that I wasn't crazy. Knowing the doctor from nursing residency, she expressed how terrible he was to everyone and convinced me that I needed to pursue Mayo.

I was so hopeful by this time, though, that I would have an answer and a treatment option to help me so that I could take care of my children normally. If I had an answer, and treatment options, I could also be present at Kara's wedding in Texas.

After this failure of an appointment, and the fact that I had to go to Mayo, I called Kara and told her that I could not make it to her wedding. *I was supposed to be her maid of honor.* I cried on the phone with her. I told her that we just didn't know what was wrong with me and that we had to go to Mayo. I was so sorry. *I still am.* I was worried that she wouldn't understand or believe me.

This health crisis took so much from me and now I was heartbroken that I was going to miss her wedding.

* * *

I cried for a long time after getting off the phone with her. When I got home I just went to my room and sat for a long time on the edge of my bed . . . *hopeless.* Everything in the world seemed to stop during those moments. I felt so empty inside . . . defeated.

The doctor's words kept repeating in my head . . . "*You need a psychiatric evaluation . . . Mayo will find nothing.*"

I remember lying down and just gazing emptily at the pictures on my walls. I looked at the light in my eyes in the photos and turned to look at myself in the mirror. All I could see was that the light had gone out. *How could I lose my health like this?* My mom was very angry about what the doctor had said to me. I could tell she wanted to drive right up there and tell him a thing or two. Terri was there as well and both of them had to convince me that I was *not* going *crazy*.

* * *

In the days following, I felt completely gone emotionally. What I was experiencing repeatedly with doctors was a form of mental torture that I did not even know could exist. I always thought doctors helped people . . . not turned them away. I always pictured all doctors to be good. But I was learning that that is not always the reality.

I thought that medical mysteries like this were how they represented them on a TV series like *House*. A full team of doctors would be at your side, trying to diagnose your condition and help you. But this was far from the reality of what I was experiencing. How very disappointing it was to realize this was not the case.

I did not know what to do anymore in between then and going to Mayo. I was worried I would have similar experiences at Mayo and I was very distressed and began to just *wish I would die*. I didn't know if I could handle anymore hits like this. I knew something was wrong with my body and I felt like I was fighting an infection all of the time.

The biggest help for me was going to my acupuncturist and doing acupuncture. I felt safe there. He helped light a fire back inside of me without even knowing it, and this helped me to keep fighting. He does not know this, but he saved me from giving up more times than I want to admit.

* * *

A psychiatric disorder does not cause 16-day periods, cysts, acne, hot flashes, and the severe dizziness and heart rate when trying to do simple tasks. As I continued to experience the debilitating symptoms, I would often look at myself in the mirror and ask myself *Am I okay?* This became a common occurrence.

I was becoming nauseous all of the time too . . . especially after my periods. Before my periods, a lot of my symptoms increased for some reason. I would get more irritable, with severe aura migraines, confusion, and dissociation.

The first time I began to experience depression and hopelessness was after the appointment with this endocrinologist. The reason I was there was because my catecholamines and metanephrines were elevated, indicating a possible neuroendocrine tumor . . . and instead he did nothing but pick at my other provider and gaslight me.

Later I had a full-body CT scan to look at my adrenal glands and to recheck the nodules in my lungs.

* * *

Tim and I had so much worry about all of this. I don't know how we got through it. It was like we were living in a constant state of *fear*, clouded with worry and anxiety over what would happen next with my episodes. We just survived but we were really *drowning*.

We did the best we could to try and have normal days with our children, but the unknown was so hard. Our children were so happy living here, but my husband and I could barely stay above these uncontrolled *waves* of worry over the unknown.

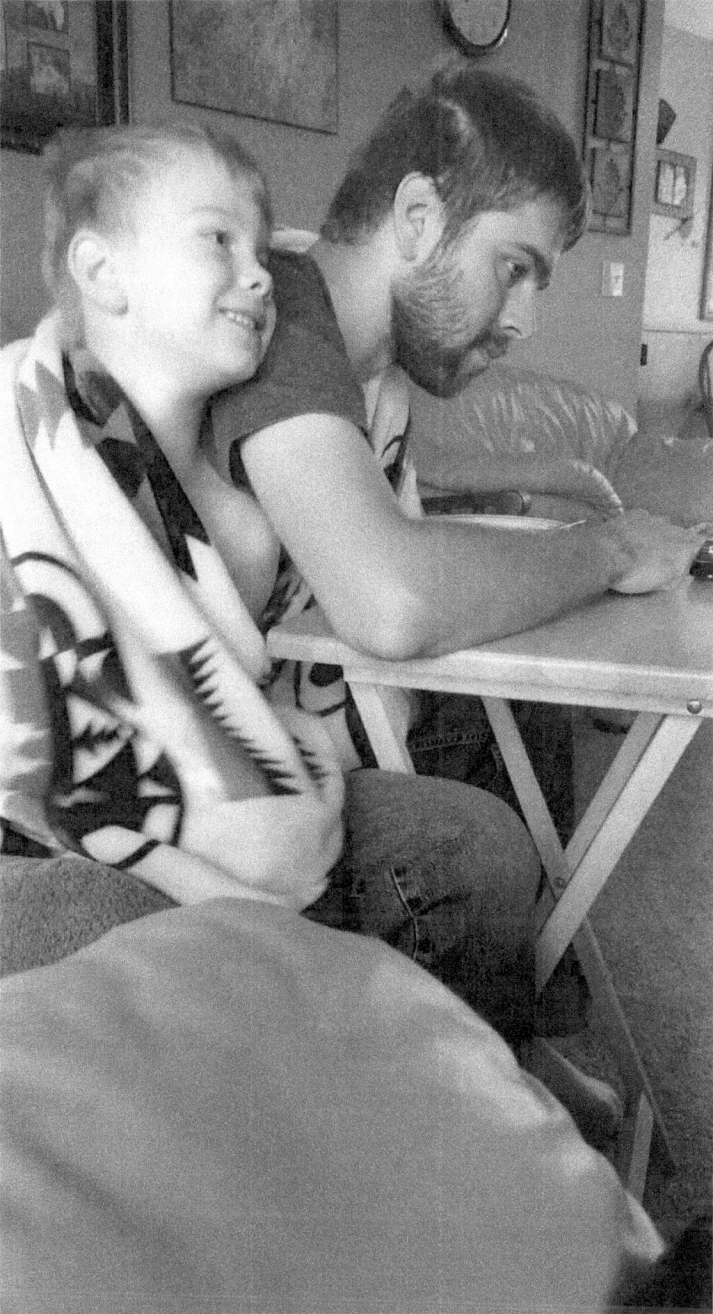

While my son was living his best life in the country, we were not really living . . .
we were drowning.

43

We sheltered most of it from our children and tried to find care for them during appointments, but sometimes we had to take them with us. Russell would listen intently when we did.

They found nothing in my CT scan, no signs of an adrenal tumor, *thankfully*. But it still left us with no answers. I had a repeat MRI of my pituitary gland after much struggle in deciding if I should do the gadolinium again (that's a rare heavy metal used in MRI scans). Because of my last reaction, we were very hesitant to use the contrast again. The neurologist agreed that we would *not* do the gadolinium, *but* we would *compare* this MRI scan to the previous MRI scan that was done with gadolinium. Then I would test my adrenal function at Mayo.

* * *

My husband and I spent a week at Mayo. My children cried when I left, and I remember watching them play in the snow with Grandma as we drove off. By this time they were laughing as they threw snowballs at each other, and I wished my body would allow me to do that with them again. *They were safe, no longer in tears, I was good to go.*

I was able to tolerate part of the long drive to Mayo, but I would get heart rate flares off and on. I felt dizzy often and foggy.

I was very relieved to find that the doctors I saw while at Mayo were all very nice. You could tell they saw a lot of complicated health cases. I really do feel that they meant well. The endocrinologist was a pleasant surprise, especially because of my last experience with the local endocrinologist. She was very kind to me and was sure we would find *something*. Right away she diagnosed me with early stages of hypothyroidism and PCOS. I saw a neurologist after that, and he diagnosed the aura migraines. I felt at first that things were going very well and it was a pleasant surprise that you could get in with one specialist after another. You would have had to wait months in between to see specialists normally.

A big thing I noticed was how much they relied on each other for treatment diagnoses and treatment options. Not one doctor viewed the body as a whole and they would have to run options for treatment by the other specialists first to see if they would affect other diagnoses or body parts. For example, I was suggested birth control as possibly helping my periods, but then she sent me over to neurology who said the type of migraines I had may respond *worse* to birth control. I liked how they approached this. Back at home, when a specialist suggested a form of treatment they never ran it past another specialist first as to how it would affect other systems.

* * *

In the mornings, my husband and I would get up early and ride the bus from our hotel to Mayo. I remember meeting a pregnant woman with a brain tumor. I still think of her often and *hope* she is healed now. It was nice to be with my husband and not have a crippling worry of something happening while I was alone with our children. I began to feel more comfortable, too, while I was there because none of the doctors treated me like I was crazy.

Our trip to Mayo wasn't like old times, like the fun we had on our trip to D.C. This was much different, with scary circumstances, but we were *grateful* to be together and he stuck close to me throughout the entire experience.

We took our scans to Mayo. There was a slight indication of a microadenoma of the pituitary gland, but when the endocrinologist and neurologist reviewed my images they said it was a coincidental finding and would not cause any problems associated with pituitary disease or adrenal insufficiency. It was benign, and we proceeded to do some tests of the adrenals and hormones to ensure that.

My doctors ordered another MRI on one of their stronger machines. They were not concerned in the slightest that I could not have gadolinium as they had other patients who could not have this contrast. They just said it needed to be done on a T3 machine. There are times when I still wonder if we made the right choice by declining the gadolinium, but they assured me that with their machine and other testing we would not need it. They tested for first and secondary adrenal insufficiency and they were both negative.

On the fourth day, we had some tests to run concerning my cysts and ovaries. Prior to going to Mayo, I had two very large cysts show up on my ovaries and they wanted to reevaluate them. Those were suspected to be what was causing my *"liver pain."* The pain always radiated up into my liver. I had to do an internal ultrasound at Mayo. Prepping for the test was difficult as I had to drink a gallon of water in under an hour. Halfway through drinking the water, all of a sudden I experienced a sharp pain in my lower right pelvic area. My heart started to race and I felt very nauseated and shaky. My husband looked worriedly at me and suggested I walk up and down the halls to try and calm my heart rate. We were worried I may have to miss the test since we were leaving the next day. My bladder was full, which made me feel even worse, but I walked around until the technician called my name. When the lab technician performed the test, she saw that one of the large ovarian cysts had burst during the test because of all of the pressure from the large water intake and another one was on its way to rupturing.

The next day I had horrible POTS symptoms. I could hardly walk without the room spinning. I was faint, breathless, and my heart was racing a lot. This was exactly what I would experience when I had heart rate episodes in the country. *How many times did I have cysts burst in the past, causing these symptoms, and I didn't even know it?*

* * *

I had a good experience, for the most part, at Mayo until I was diagnosed with POTS. They put me on a tilt table after my cyst burst the next morning and they based the diagnosis on my heart rate increase alone. *But it increased right after the cyst ruptured . . .*

My autonomic test was otherwise normal. They sent me home with paperwork for a diagnosis of POTS/dysautonomia and a treatment plan of more salt, water, and compression socks. I was under the impression at first that I would go back for more testing the following week. But I was wrong.

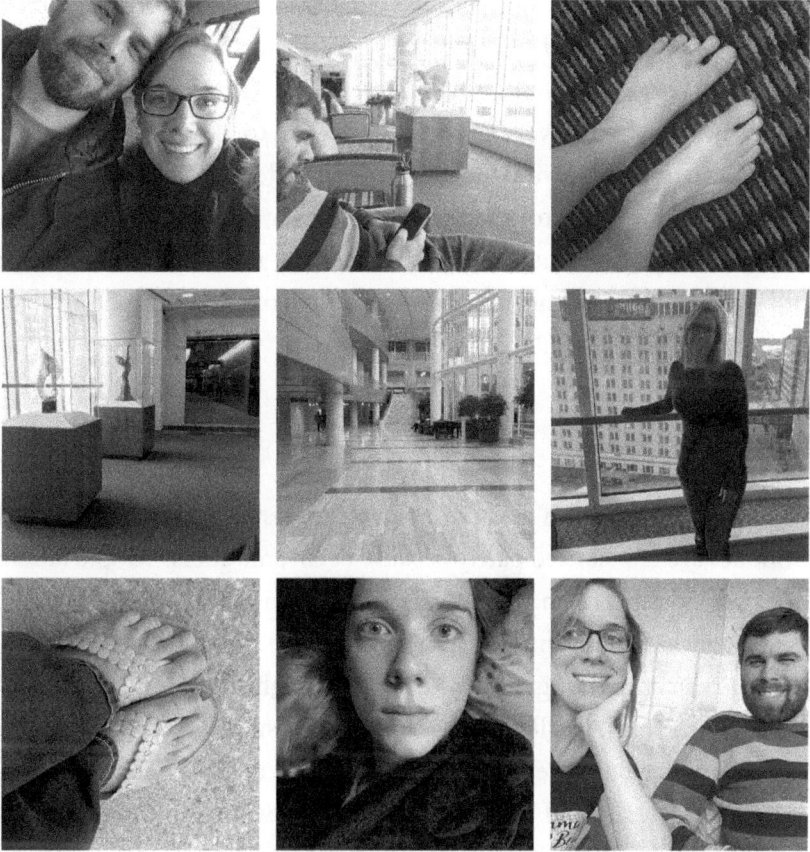

After all of our tests at Mayo, I remember going to Walmart with Tim and picking out my compression socks thinking . . . can it really be this easy? It wasn't . . .

When I met with the many specialists at Mayo, I expressed my concerns of always *feeling like I was fighting an infection.* I felt I needed more evaluation in this area. I even brought along some research paperwork requesting to look into some environmental conditions like CIRS (chronic inflammatory response syndrome) from mold factors or Lyme disease. I read a lot on how difficult it was to diagnose both and how both could affect hormones.

The concerns were mostly brushed aside, so over time I tucked the papers back into my binder because what was the point? Birth control was suggested on and off as a treatment for my heavy periods and other symptoms. *Yeah . . . because going on birth control went so well last time.* The options I was left with were to try birth control to treat PCOS even with the concern of it increasing the migraine episodes. The other suggestion was to have an exploratory surgery to look for endometriosis. I didn't think that suggestion was a bad idea because my mom had endometriosis. But I was unwilling to fling my body back into panic attack mode by trying another birth control pill.

* * *

From my own research and understanding, I strongly believe that my hormones are imbalanced partly because of chronic gut issues and adrenal fatigue, or possibly from an underlying infection.

The medical establishment doesn't seem to see the connection with any of these concerns though. Maybe they are right and I am just being a difficult patient. But it all fits so well with my issues. The cysts and mood fluctuations can be caused by high estrogen and heavy bleeding.

After the diagnosis of POTS, I felt like they wanted to close my case. *No further study.* When I asked for further testing, I was denied for the moment. It wasn't the fault of the medical specialists I saw, but because of the way the system was set up. I felt like I didn't have enough looked into at Mayo. The infection idea was a big concern of mine, but I also had a concern that a CFS (cerebrospinal fluid) leak could be a possibility.

After my spinal tap and MRI, my condition worsened and I was unsure which caused the regression. POTS can sometimes be linked to leaks of the spinal fluid as a result of a spinal tap, and I was hoping to be evaluated for that at Mayo as well. It could explain a lot of my symptoms.

When I got home, I felt like my family had some relief in me being diagnosed with POTS. For me, it just kept my concerns persisting because I knew that it was a syndrome and something had to be causing it. You don't just develop POTS for no reason. Compression socks and salt water were not improving my quality of life.

* * *

I started to work with a craniosacral therapist to try and improve my migraine symptoms. During her light adjustments I would notice that my heart rate would fluctuate. I told her about my epidural injury after having Eliot and my recent diagnosis of POTS. I expressed concerns that maybe something structural was causing this because of past issues. I expressed my concerns over the other potential factors as well. I would feel such relief of the pressure in my head after her adjustments, and for a time my migraines were better. She was curious about the possibility that it could be structural, but because I was denied more studies through Mayo, I felt pretty stuck on what to do.

I gathered my paperwork and scans and sent them off to a top neurosurgeon in Arizona to get a second opinion and evaluate for a probable CFS leak. CFS leaks can cause POTS, but so can a lot of other factors. The neurosurgeon was very kind to me and he didn't see any signs of a leak, so I closed the chapter on that concern.

In his words, "I wouldn't do further testing and put heavy metals back into your brain."

I was surprised he said that, because I didn't elaborate much on my previous experience with gadolinium.

* * *

Later, because of my continued symptoms, denial for further studies at Mayo, and uncertainty on the POTS diagnosis, I saw another cardiologist. I visited with the cardiologist's practitioner first, and I expressed my concerns toward feeling that I was dealing with more than just POTS.

Initially, he pushed my words to the side and his mannerisms were very confident in my POTS diagnosis *because* it was diagnosed at Mayo. As soon as he looked at the diagnostic sheet, though, he froze and got a puzzled look on his face. His demeanor and tone of voice completely changed. He seemed confused at my diagnostic sheet because all that had changed on the autonomic test was heart rate alone, everything else was normal.

"Yes," I said with a sigh of relief, "and I had an ovarian cyst rupture the day before. That's what caused the episode right before I was placed on the tilt table."

I expressed with him that I felt I was dealing with an iron deficiency related issue and possibly an infection of some sort. He left the room and went to speak with the cardiologist. When he returned, he still seemed confused, but he said that even with the other normal findings the heart rate increase should be diagnostic enough for POTS. After reviewing my records from Mayo, he didn't seem convinced that I even had POTS, but we went over my recent echocardiogram, which was normal anyway.

He did help me with referrals to infectious disease and internal medicine. But again, I left feeling like we got nowhere.

A few months after Mayo, and after the cardiologist visit, I did see an internal medicine doctor and an infectious disease doctor locally. I decided to explore the possibility of an infection or Lyme disease causing this. I took in the same sheet that I had brought to Mayo concerning Lyme disease or a possible environmental illness.

The first doctor asked my husband to leave the room. He looked at me very seriously and asked me if I was being harmed at home. I told him no. He then asked me if I had slept with any other people or was concerned if my husband had. I said no again and he proceeded with a couple of tests for sexually transmitted diseases anyway and sent me on my way. *That was odd. Do I look the type?*

The infectious disease doctor did test me for Lyme disease and EBV (Epstein-Barr virus) like I had asked. Both were negative. I had come across a syndrome online called alpha-gal syndrome (a meat allergy) . . . but this is said to be caused by a tick bite. With my *negative* Lyme disease results, no doctor will look into it as a possibility . . . even when I saw an allergist later. He was not very helpful with the concerns of it being related to mold and did not seem very keen on evaluating me for a beef allergy. *So now what?*

In his words: "I would just stick with the diagnosis Mayo gave you of POTS and move on."

* * *

The entire first year of my health decline was very challenging. I felt often like I had to battle every doctor along this path to get a POTS diagnosis alone. There were a few good doctors, which I was *grateful* for, but the ones that were not made me feel ignored and insulted. *I know my body.* I was not sick like this before. This was finally proved through a POTS diagnosis.

But something happened to me to cause this syndrome. We decided to seek alternative care through a functional medicine doctor to discover the underlying cause. We had to leave our home. Our beautiful home in the country. *My dream gone.* I couldn't stay out there alone with my two children anymore with the health conditions I was facing with POTS. If we wanted to afford alternative care this was the only way.

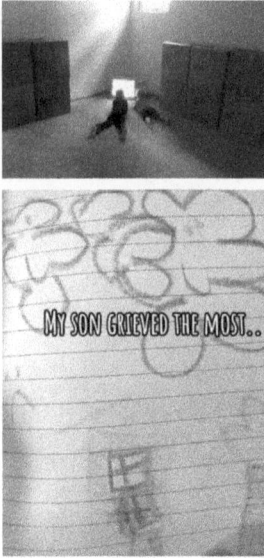

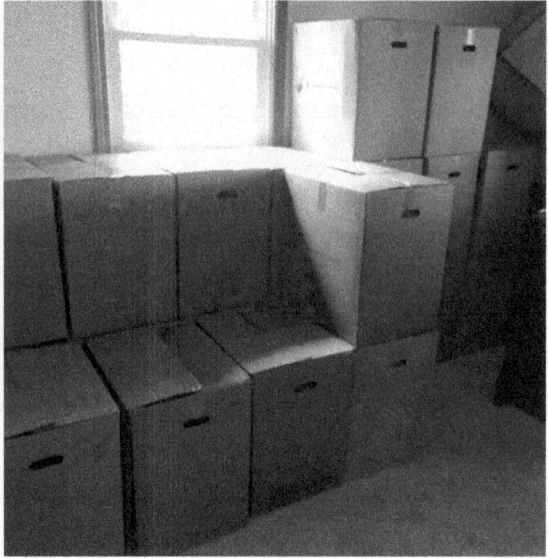

My son grieved the most . . .

I don't know how I found the *strength* to pack the boxes. I did have help on and off but I did a lot on my own. I always had this concern in the back of my head that if I did have a mold illness, what if there was an exposure here and we were just taking all of the mycotoxins with us. These ideas would flash into my head because of months of researching the Shoemaker Protocol for mold. The guidelines were extreme: mold avoidance, replacing every item in your house that was exposed to the mold, and ensuring your new home does not have any. *It seemed entirely impossible.* I even thought maybe we could wash everything down somehow before moving it into our new home, just in case. But I didn't even know if this was what I was dealing with.

Any time I would bring up these concerns to my husband, I did it in a very careful manner because I knew how ridiculous and impossible it all sounded. I didn't even know if this was my problem. But the possibility of it being a concern was overwhelming.

* * *

Selling our home was a hard decision, but I am still so sick and need help often. I need to be closer to my mom and closer to Tim and town. I felt emotionally dead inside when we moved. We moved shortly after getting home from Mayo.

We moved with a surgery date set for the following month, following the advice from the Mayo endocrinologist to go through with the surgery to look for endometriosis. I had wanted to do the surgery at Mayo but was too sick again for travel. Our plan, if they didn't see anything during surgery, was to proceed with functional medicine care. I had just gotten back from Mayo and was the sickest I have ever been physically and emotionally.

A part of me was *grateful* that we had some form of diagnosis. I was gaslit for an entire year and was told repeatedly that I just had a panic disorder and anxiety. When I was diagnosed with POTS I felt relief at first, but when I realized it was a syndrome it made me want to find the underlying factors even more. I felt that I was left with a blanket diagnosis . . . a syndrome . . . with few suggestions for therapy and no direction moving forward . . . I was determined, stubborn, and resilient the entire first year and I wasn't going to stop now. I knew there was something causing this syndrome and *I was going to find out what.*

* * *

When I was home, I was still recovering from the hemorrhagic cysts. I was stuck in a horrible fog from lack of oxygen to my brain and felt very sad about my declining health.

Somehow, I had to hold it together and help my five-year-old son, who was going through very hard emotions himself. *Mommy is sick and we are leaving our home. The yellow house. "The village."* He did not want to move. He did not want to talk about my upcoming surgery. *Fear*, worry, and not understanding was all that I could see in his eyes. He began to have bad dreams about a *black fox* while I was at Mayo. When we came home he just cried and cried . . . never wanting to let me go. As I lay next to him, I wondered if I was going to die that night.

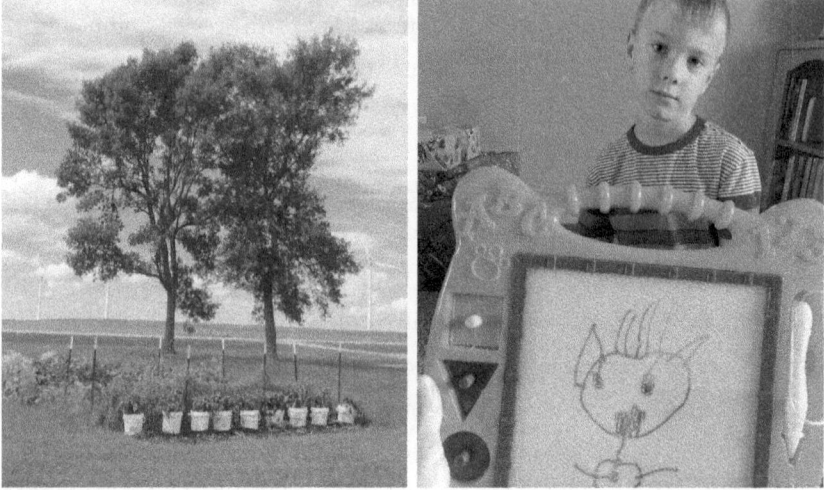

I am so sorry.

We didn't know if we should bring Russell back to the empty acreage on closing day, but we wanted him to have some sort of closure. When we said goodbye to our home our sweet Russell stood in the big window and looked at the emptiness around him. I will never forget his face.

The loss . . . hopelessness . . . sadness. "Momma," he cried as he stood in the window.

I put my arms around him in a comforting embrace. We both cried as *his life and my dreams crashed all around us.* I just felt such sadness and guilt and anger. We were leaving because of me. I got sick. I couldn't do this all alone anymore. We couldn't. Dad was sick, too, from all of the stress but he didn't show it. The anxiety of having his sick wife home alone in the country was more than he could bear. We didn't have a village of people to help us. Some neighbors questioned what was wrong, but with our only suggestion from the doctors being a panic disorder at the time, they were at a loss of how to help us. Family was not close. The burden of me, plus keeping up with work and everything that needed to be done at home, was overwhelming. Especially the hard winters.

We placed a camera in Russell's hands and he felt very relieved to run around and take pictures of our home to keep as memories. It was the only way I felt he could cope and it did work for the rest of the time spent there. Tim and I had held it together for so long, but in one of the images you could see us in the background in an embrace, sobbing. We could no longer hold it together on that day. I deleted that image as even I, a photographer who captures everything, did not want to remember it.

I am sorry, Russell.

I wish that I could change things for you. I am trying and fighting so hard to get better. I hope that someday you can understand and forgive me. I hope that your childhood is just as magical as I dreamt it would be with our home in the country.

Living in the country was hard even when I wasn't sick, but I always knew it would get better. I did not want to leave. I lost my home too. I lost my health. I lost my identity. I lost our dreams. That was my dream home—my family dream—and I will always see you playing in that big beautiful yard. Playing with the cats and the ducks and with our Annabelle and the freedom that you had with a country childhood. It was taken from all of us.

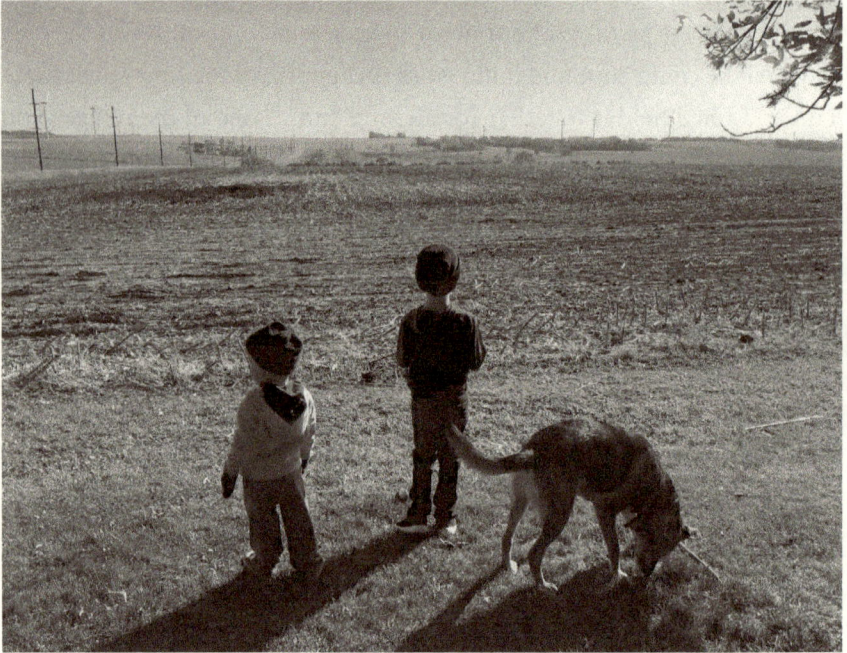

I am sorry that was taken from you . . .

After Mayo and the other failed appointments, I sadly lined up the exploratory surgery to see if I had endometriosis. As a last resort, to avoid getting cut up in my condition, someone had heard of a chiropractor that had helped heal a lot of chronic issues in a small town near us. I went to him in a desperate state . . . he seemed nice enough. He was the assistant to the owner of the clinic.

I was with Terri and our kids that day, and we went to the park for an hour while he looked over all of my paperwork. I watched the kids run around through the leaves with smiles on their faces. I couldn't really do much . . . I couldn't be active with them . . . but at least I was there. This was the first time I had really seen Russell smile like that again since we moved.

When we went back to the clinic, he did some iodine testing and then lastly performed some energy test. He was sure all of my issues were being caused by an internal staph *infection* and it was in my liver, kidneys, lungs,

56

and heart. *He was surprised I was alive with how bad he felt the staph infection had spread.*

This was terrifying to me. All I really heard was *infection* and with the Lyme disease test coming back negative maybe this was really what was causing me to have symptoms associated with an underlying *infection.* When I left his office I had a bag full of supplements that cost me about 400 dollars. I didn't even know if I should have the surgery anymore. His voice repeated in my head . . . *surely if you do have the surgery the infection may move to your heart. The surgery may kill you . . .*

I tried his suggestions for several weeks but continued to have debilitating issues. As my surgery date drew closer, the assistant's words kept repeating in my head over and over again and I was worried I may die during surgery. It was very difficult for me because most of my previous experiences with doctors were so negative and my experiences with chiropractors were so positive. It was very difficult for me to follow through with the surgery. But I trusted my surgeon. He delivered both of my babies and was always so wonderful to me. During my appointment with my surgeon, he told me that he had read a book about how a woman was put in a mental facility and later they found it was because of a severe hormone imbalance. He also understood so much about the gut microbiome and suggested if we don't find anything with the surgery to focus more at trying to fix the gut microbiome with a different specialist. I trusted that he would take good care of me and he had performed many endometriosis surgeries in the past. But in my condition getting cut open was still terrifying and the assistant's words still rang in my head repeatedly.

* * *

The morning of my surgery I stopped in my babies' room before going off to get cut open. I didn't know what the hell I was doing, but I knew that there was a strong likelihood that I had endometriosis and a small likelihood that I had an internal staph infection. My mom had endometriosis and had a full hysterectomy in her 30s, and her health struggles were similar to my own. She had cysts that grew to the size of a small football often and heavy bleeding. *Wouldn't a severe staph infection show up on my labs too?* I looked at Russell and Eliot sleeping so peacefully. *Time stood still.* I was very scared and prayed to God to let me live and let me beat this. I wanted to live.

* * *

Russell,

You still say to me, "Mommy I wish Jesus could come down and touch you so you can get better."

My heart . . . I love you, Russell. Your kind heart. When I went in for the surgery I didn't know if I would come out. The chiropractor's words were still in my head that *I might die during this surgery.* I was so sick too. I didn't know how a person could feel so close to death, but no one can do anything and I looked normal on the outside.

* * *

I remember looking up at the bright lights before being put under and praying silently that I wouldn't die. Surgery was pretty uneventful. My gynecologist surgeon said that all he could find was old scar tissue from an old internal infection indicating inflammation. He saw no signs of a current infection and no signs of endometriosis. He cut out the scar tissue.

I didn't do well after the surgery. My air hunger increased and my heart rate was all over the place. I was so breathless, had increased vertigo, dizziness, nausea, and my brain felt on fire. My oxygen levels also kept dropping. My oxygen kept dipping on and off into the 80s. My heart rate was often at 155 bpm when I was just standing. The severe vertigo was as if I had had a bad night drinking. I felt like I was severely anemic but when they checked my levels they said they were fine. This only caused the words of the chiropractor to come back into my head . . . *I must have had a staph infection and now it's going straight to my heart.*

The surgery took place right before my period and the stress on my body delayed my cycle. I felt like I was stuck in the worst time of my hormonal shift. I went to urgent care once for fluids and spent a lot of time with my acupuncturist, doing therapy, or on the phone with nurses concerning my increased symptoms. My vision was double, but I didn't say anything right away because I worried they would blame it on *anxiety*. At first I thought I was *really deteriorating*, but when I finally called my nurse I was told it was a side effect of the nausea patch that was put on me during surgery. Once I removed the patch the symptoms went away over time, *thank God*. Russell did not want to look at my tiny surgery wounds.

Eliot would say, "Awwww, owie," and he hugged and kissed me.

Russell was afraid.

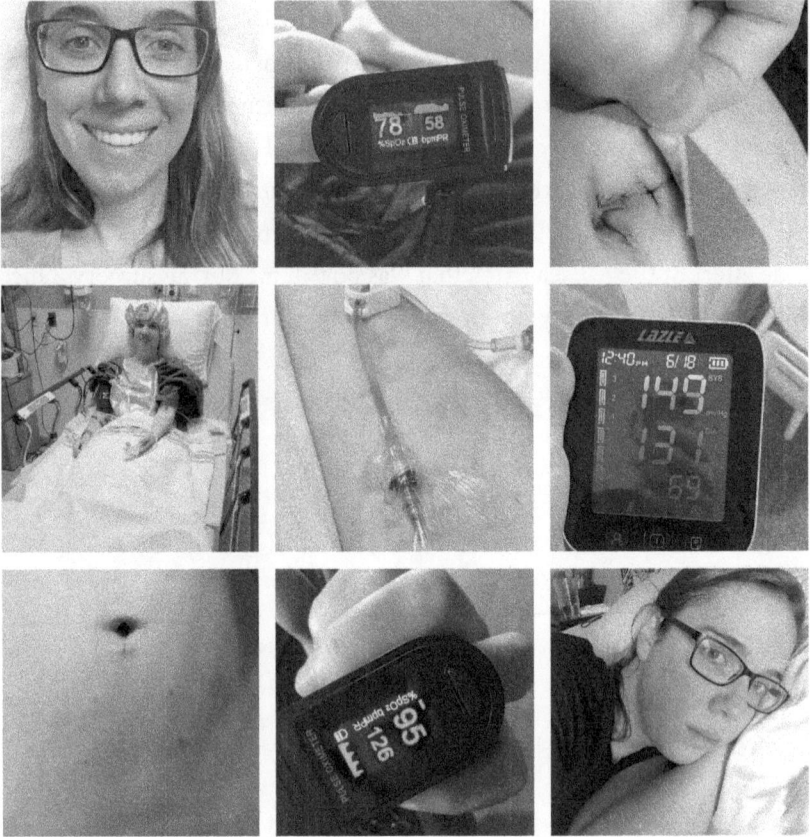

I felt much worse after the surgery . . . the words kept repeating in my head "you have an internal staph infection and it could go straight to your heart . . . "

One of the reasons we sold our house was because we knew we were going to need a functional medicine doctor if the surgery was unable to help me. One of my friends was able to reverse her POTS condition with a doctor out of state. I chose the same doctor because locally it would take at least six months and I could get in with her in just two.

My first appointment with her went well. She ran a bunch of tests, most of which were covered by insurance. She was very reassuring, and over time it felt as if I were talking to a good friend as well as a doctor. She reminded me a lot of my acupuncturist and displayed the same determination as he did. I liked her drive and could tell she was very passionate. Sometimes it was hard for me to get my thoughts out and she was often very rushed during appointments because she had so many sick patients that needed her. I never was upset at her, it was just difficult to communicate with her and I believe this is because she was out of state. Over time, she did see this as a problem, too, and we were able to slow the pace down during my appointments.

She reviewed what I did with the hormone specialist locally and felt the hormone specialist missed a lot of things and went the easier route with a hormone imbalance and a vitamin B12 deficiency.

Later, after my labs came back, I did test positive for a mutation in the MTHFR gene. I have been told that when you have MTHFR gene mutations you lack the enzymes responsible for the conversion of folate into the active form 5-Methyltetrahydrofolate. This important reaction then is directly involved in the utilization of B12. If your vitamin B12 is not working properly because the folate metabolism isn't working properly, this causes homocysteine imbalances. Which I have. My homocysteine levels fluctuate between high to low. They were high when I first had them evaluated. High homocysteine is related to an increased risk of certain health conditions such as blood clots, heart attacks, strokes, and others. Low homocysteine is not normally as concerning but can cause some issues with the nerves. There is an optimal level that functional medicine doctors shoot for.

When I worked with the hormone specialist she put me on B12 injections. I feel she was on the right track with a B12 deficiency. Because of the low progesterone, I stayed on the progesterone cream at the time while I had my appointment with her.

My functional medicine doctor feels that since we went by the saliva hormone panel three months prior to seeing the hormone specialist, we never were on the correct hormones. She confirmed that I had estrogen dominance and a hormone imbalance. She said my progesterone was at the level of an eighty-year-old woman. *No wonder I had so much trouble getting pregnant.* Since I didn't experience any major difference with the

B12 injections, she felt that was an easy diagnosis for my previous hormone specialist at the time.

She told me my acupuncturist was on the right path with adrenal fatigue, she could see this in my labs. I was at a stage 3 for adrenal fatigue.

My functional medicine doctor thinks I have some type of underlying infection as well. I mentioned the possibility of Lyme disease or mold and she said those were her thoughts too. I even brought up the co-infection to Lyme disease, Bartonella. I had been bitten by cats before and I knew the disease could cause debilitating symptoms over time. Lastly, I mentioned the potential staph infection that was suggested to me by a chiropractor. She didn't feel this was as likely. *She knew it was something. She just wasn't sure what.* She was sure, though, that we would be able to detox any mold out of my body if that was a factor with the glutathione injections. I was prescribed these injections during the early stages of my diagnosis and have to do the injections a few times a week. I was told that glutathione is the body's master antioxidant. The liver makes it naturally, but some people don't make enough and need it to help them detox. She didn't want me to have to spend too much money on testing for mold because it would not be covered by insurance and she assured me the glutathione would take it out.

I was also diagnosed with heavy metal toxicity, the level of concern later showed up as aluminum.

She went on to say I had anemia because of my ferritin levels. My level was a 7. The ferritin is the iron storage and mine was almost depleted and was missed by medical doctors. This fit very well because of all the times I fainted during my periods and with how sick I got after the blood loss from surgery.

She was also suspicious of H. pylori, SIBO (small intestinal bacterial overgrowth), or some other virus affecting my immune system. I was also vitamin D deficient and zinc deficient. I tested positive for having had Epstein-Barr virus in the past. It is inactive now, but it could have been active as of this year. EBV can trigger a cascade of health issues.

I mentioned possible mast cell activation syndrome (MCAS) to her as well. She felt this could be a possibility but testing for it is *difficult* and she stressed that there is *always* an underlying cause and finding the cause is where we needed to start. MCAS is a condition that causes mast cells to release an inappropriate amount of chemicals into your body. This causes allergy symptoms that can be as severe as anaphylaxis, plus a wide range of other severe symptoms. In her words, the condition I was dealing with was a result of *"a perfect storm"* of events. We just needed to make sure we could find and reverse all of the underlying factors.

She feels the birth control was a *triggering* factor but *not* a cause alone. It made me remember all of the months prior to the pill where I always felt as if I were fighting an infection or illness. She said that extreme conditions like these *always* have more than one underlying cause.

I am still waiting on more testing, and she is even suspicious of a parasite causing these issues. "I have seen parasites come out of a person's eyes or nose. They've been found in the GI tract, and we have *even* found them in the brains of sick patients."

This was very scary to me.

The last thing she brought up was the fact that my health declined after surgery. She has had patients that had small internal bleeds that went undiagnosed for years. She was hoping that I wasn't still bleeding internally. She also felt that the scar tissue seen could have been the sign of a less-detectable form of endometriosis. I did not know this at the time, but she said a lot of general gynecologists performing the surgery will miss endometriosis. If so, the endometriosis and potential bleed could be a big reason for why I am dealing with increased symptoms. I really *hope* we don't have to do surgery again. She said we will try other things first and see how I do before thinking about a repeat surgery with a different surgeon.

As of now, I am diagnosed through Mayo with POTS. Through my functional medicine doctor, I am diagnosed with adrenal fatigue, estrogen dominance, heavy metal toxicity, anemia causing POTS, and a potential underlying infection causing POTS.

I believe she is right, but we need more answers. POTS is a blanket of a diagnosis and the medical field needs to find the root cause. I believe if one is able to find their individual cause and reverse it, the body can go back into a normal state.

4

This Is Not Anxiety

April 1, 2020

My mom was bitten by her cat, Eddy, a few days ago. They were outside together when a dog ran up to them. When my mom went to grab Eddy, he thought she was the dog and he bit her right on her wrist! The next day, my mom's arm was swollen and hot to the touch and she was running a fever. She went to the ER and was diagnosed with cat scratch fever and had a bad infection. *Bartonella.* I know that disease all too well because it was one that I meticulously researched because of my own chronic illness. I had cat bites in the past and developed a stretch-mark type rash not long after the bite. Bartonella can survive and lay dormant in your body. Sometimes even after treatment. I still wonder if I have it. *But not my mom . . .* she can't get sick like me. They did IV antibiotics for her and she ended up with C. diff. She had to go on antibiotics for that serious infection and is doing okay now . . . I *hope* the antibiotics were enough to eradicate the infection. I *hope* the infection doesn't persist.

* * *

She moved recently into an apartment that smells kind of moldy. When I looked at it with her, I didn't feel right while I was there. But I don't even know anymore. I just react to weird things. I asked the landlord, and of course they said there weren't any mold issues, but she didn't appear very truthful. I just want my mom to live in a healthy environment and I feel bad because when I try to see her I don't feel good in her apartment. My heart palpitations increase and I feel like I am having some type of allergic reaction.

I don't understand why my immune system overreacts to environments. Sometimes I just feel like I sound so incredibly *crazy*. But I really do feel sick when I'm there. I hope my mom gets better. I don't want her to ever have to go through anything like me.

My mom helps me almost every day. She is a light in my life. She doesn't know how much she means to me, and a lot of times just us being together acting silly and going on small walks helps pull me out of depression. I don't know what I would do without my mom.

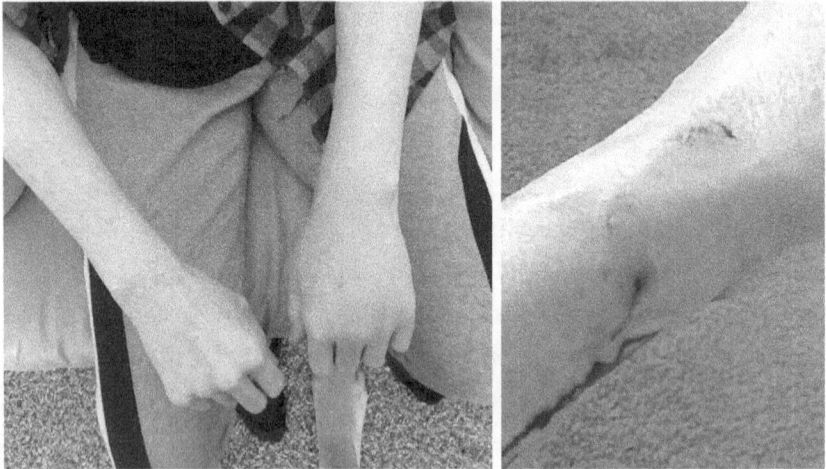

Bartonella . . .

June 16, 2020

Sometimes I feel as if my questions will never stop and my health issues will never truly be resolved. I have done so much over the last few months with functional medicine. I have okay days, but I am still having so much trouble. It's almost as if we are *missing something*.

I am constantly battling to get my iron up. I still have episodes of near fainting and heart rates in the 180s during periods. Every month when I get a few notches up in my ferritin my periods just take away all of my progress. It's upsetting because I do feel better when my ferritin stays up. I keep fighting through the pain. I keep my spirits up because my children need me.

So does Tim . . . very much. Sometimes the thought of being so needed can be such a *burden* when I need to *heal*. My mind won't stop until I heal and I feel pressure to heal fast so that I can be able to care for everyone. I know we are moving in the right direction. Iron deficiency, leaky gut, estrogen dominance. My functional medicine doctor does not think I have PCOS, but feels these issues are coming from estrogen dominance. I feel like we are doing the right things through food and supplements, but there are still times that I wonder why my body is this way. Is there a certain factor making my hormones so messed up?

About a year after we moved, the new owners of our yellow house emailed me and told me that when they remodeled the basement they found black mold and running water with open wires all under the sheetrock in our previous basement. I was very shocked when she told me this, and it made my questions go back to if it could still be mold in my body making me this way. She was not upset with us, but really felt that if we had kept living there, not knowing this, eventually a house fire may have started. It's scary to think that was undetectable under the sheetrock. There were no signs of damage from this on the outside. It was a very nice basement. But my functional medicine doctor keeps saying the glutathione will get it out if it is mold.

I had a repeat upper endoscope and the intestinal metaplasia is reversed. I have healed that condition with food. I ate very clean and juiced celery juice daily for around six months. My functional medicine doctor also put me on supplements for inflammation like aloe vera, licorice root, and turmeric. I wasn't on lots of supplements leading up to the reversal of that condition. I give most of the credit to the food I was eating. Let food be thy medicine.

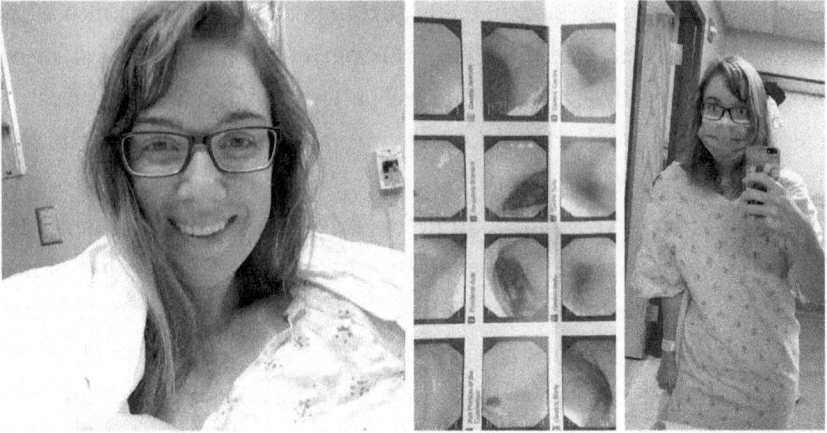

The intestinal metaplasia was reversed . . . Let food be thy medicine.

The adrenal fatigue and iron deficiency has been a constant battle . . . I went to the ER again because my heart rate shot up to 185 during a menstrual cycle and I fainted.

I was walking to the bathroom when it happened with my pulse oximeter already on my finger because of how terrible I had felt that day. When I came to, I cried out to Tim, who was in the garage. Terri was staying with us again because of my recent flare. Unfortunately, she heard me first. I felt bad for that because she had experienced trauma in her past when her husband dropped to the floor and died from a heart attack. Now here I was lying on the floor.

I remember the way my husband's hands trembled as he checked my heart rate and helped me to my feet.

"Did you hit your head?" he breathed heavily.

"I don't think so . . . " was all I could muster.

This was only the second episode that my children had witnessed and they looked terrified.

Tim and Terri took me in to the ER. This was the first time my husband spoke up to a doctor.

He was shaking when he told them, "I don't want to hear anyone saying this is anxiety. Something is seriously wrong with my wife and if we don't figure out a way to help her she is going to die!"

They took things much more seriously after that. My husband has never had the best self-image . . . he always thought he was too small . . . or didn't have enough muscle . . . but when he gets that fire in his eyes people take him seriously.

The doctor had me walk the halls and the nurses kept pointing out how much my heart rate would skyrocket just from standing. The doctor looked at my old reports and saw signs in my past heart monitors of SVT (supraventricular tachycardia) episodes. He said this needed to be reevaluated. He felt I should be pursuing this more than the POTS diagnosis because sometimes an ablation can fix it. I was signed up for a stress test shortly after this event.

I often wonder what everyone thinks of me going to the ER over and over again. Does my mom believe me? Does Terri? Do my sisters? Do my friends? Does my husband? I feel so isolated in this experience because no one can understand and I would never want them to. *Because then that would mean that they are living in hell like me.*

* * *

During my stress test, Tim and I were not very impressed with the doctor who was examining me. She was on her cell phone a lot and seemed very arrogant. When I was running on the treadmill, my blood pressure suddenly dropped and she told me to stop.

She stopped me very dramatically. "We got it, we got it!" She elaborated, "We know what is wrong. It is just that your autonomic nervous system isn't *mature* yet."

She told me it would fix itself over time. She said I was a tall girl and the vasovagal response may improve with beta blockers. *But my blood pressure was so low . . .* I asked her if this could be from an iron deficiency. She said it was very possible but that I was a tall girl and my autonomic nervous system was just underdeveloped. I felt like this was *not likely . . .* I was a 29-year-old woman and my autonomic nervous system worked perfectly fine before.

I began to *trust* doctors' opinions less and less. I felt like they didn't even know what they were talking about and were just guessing.

This was the first time I was offered a beta blocker as treatment. I filled the prescription but never took it. My blood pressure was always so low. *Couldn't this make me feel worse even if it did slow my heart rate?* I would notice improvement with my heart rate, too, when I would get my iron up. I would also notice improvement when avoiding certain foods. I still had the episodes, but they occurred mainly during my periods and I was determined to fix the cause. If I went on the medication now, I would never know if the iron deficiency was the real problem or if it's food . . . or something else.

* * *

I still cannot do a lot. My body is weak. My anxiety has been much less and the *"panic attacks"* are more a thing of the past. I still get some mood shifts and sometimes tunnel vision with my hormone shifts. The migraines and pressure behind my eyes still scare me. The worst anxiety I feel is when I bleed heavily during my period . . . this is pretty common with iron deficiency.

I get blood pressure drops, heart palpitations, breathlessness, confusion, heart race, etc. Those symptoms are debilitating, and the buzzing in my feet and tremors are worrisome and become so irritating. If I get hot or do simple physical activity it gets worse. I can't go on walks anymore without feeling like I am going to drop dead. It's hard.

A doctor recently asked me if I am deconditioned. Well . . . I was exercising at a normal rate prior to the onset of all of this and I still get up and do the normal tasks throughout my day to day. It was night and day . . . I could do normal tasks one day and the next I could not. I don't think I put myself here by not moving around enough. I do have to stay bedridden on and off, and normally I need a nap every day, but I still move.

I just want life to return to normal. Sometimes I still wonder about my pituitary microadenoma or if I do have a secondary form of adrenal insufficiency. I am sometimes on the verge of thyroid issues but never enough to be able to go on medication. My doctors check me often for autoimmune issues, which are always negative.

I just take things as easy as I can . . .

I would love to go on adventures again with my children and not be in this never-ending cycle. I wish I were having more improvements with getting my iron up, but it's just not happening.

I have had some improvement through my functional medicine doctor. My stomach feels a lot better . . . but I regress with every menstrual cycle.

* * *

We are in a pandemic right now from the coronavirus. The weird thing is that COVID sounds so much like the chronic illnesses that I am dealing with now: POTS and dysautonomia. Life has changed for a lot of people but because of my chronic illness it has pretty much stayed the same for me. Isolation is what I have felt for several years now.

Tim has been doing these hot and cold showers to help keep his immune system strong. He is considered an essential worker and has to go to work every day. He is concerned about bringing it home to me in my condition. His coworkers laugh when he tells them what he has been doing, but I feel they would do the same if their loved one was in my condition. We don't really tell many people how sick I am.

June 24, 2020

I met my neighbor yesterday. She was standing outside and I said hi to her. She told me she was sorry, but she was struggling with a migraine. I let her know that I understood as I get those often too. It seemed that this allowed her to feel comfortable enough to talk with me.

She told me about how for years she had undiagnosed Lyme disease. She found out much later through a Lyme-literate doctor out of Minnesota who was now retired. I told her that Lyme disease is a suspicion for myself and I *hope* that I am working with the right type of doctor.

She told me what she had to do to get better and that her son also had the infection. They both struggled for many years before having improvement. She still struggles with body pain and migraines and wonders if the Lyme is still affecting her.

She expressed, with deep sadness, how her friend had Lyme disease and it went to her heart. While she was playing in the yard with her two-year-old she suddenly died from heart failure. I thought of all of the episodes I had that felt like heart attacks. I thought about all of the times I was terrified I would die when I was alone with my children.

It is ironic to me how we lost our home in the country just to move next to someone who may be the person that opens up a gateway of possibility in discovering the underlying cause to my illness. Because of her willingness to share her experience, it could help me with my own. I *hope* I am making the right choice with my functional medicine doctor. She does suspect Lyme disease but says her other patients get better when targeting the other infections. I *hope* she is right.

June 25, 2020

I'm watching Russell and Eliot play with a little neighbor boy. They have so much fun together but, unfortunately, they will be moving. Russell is still not very adjusted to where we are living. I know when Tim gets the playhouse up that will help. We had such a beautiful yard in the country, full of trees. Our yard right now has nothing in it. Not even a tree. It's just a square. Russell still talks about how we used to go on walks down the gravel road. Even if we had a gravel road here, I wouldn't be able to go on long walks like we used to.

I feel that a big part of what Russell is grieving is *not the house alone but the loss of his mother's health.* I am trying to make this new place feel like home for him. I am trying to heal me and heal him too.

* * *

Russell and his friend like to ride these little race cars around the yard. They have also been playing in our new playhouse since Tim got that set up. They needed something to bring them joy in our empty yard. The boys are enjoying homeschooling. I didn't think I would be able to continue, with my health concerns, but then COVID hit and we didn't really have any other choice.

June 26, 2020

Today is a beautiful Friday. I finished up our second week of homeschooling. I use a Christian-based program. I think it's going well considering I am sick every day.

Russell told me today that, "Jesus is the light of the world."

Sometimes the lessons help me more than they do him. Tears filled my eyes while we completed the lesson on *perseverance.* It related so much to my own situation. Russell tells me that he loves doing school with me. We baked banana bread while Eliot played with Play-Doh.

Russell said, "Best day ever!"

It was cute seeing his face brighten and his dimples show up with his sweet smile. It's so hard to do these tasks but I do it for them.

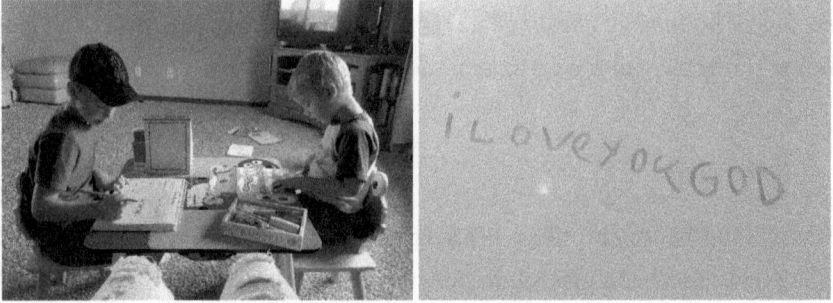

Since I started homeschooling my boys, Russell talks more about God and he sings to him every night . . .

Eliot liked the banana bread and he was being so goofy. He kept looking above himself laughing hysterically. I entertained the idea that it was either Grandpa Bert or Jesus making funny faces at him. It was sweet.

Eliot's third birthday is coming up. His cake will have 101 Dalmatians on it. We decided on a small gathering at a park because of the coronavirus concerns for grandparents. I really *hope* it's not too hot that day. I *hope* I am well enough that day. Everything is hard with chronic illness like this. Tim has been working a lot this week, and sometimes it feels like I never see him. He feels like he has to work a lot more hours because of the cost of the therapies and our medical debt. I feel so badly about this. Who would have thought I would have racked up the bills in this way. *I often feel like a burden to him . . .*

* * *

Russell still talks about the yellow house. I'm trying to adjust, too, to town living. Sometimes I find him drawing pictures of a yellow house. It is bright and the sun is shining. There are beautiful big trees everywhere, but he always ends his drawings with a sad face next to it. He doesn't know . . . but when I see these pictures I shut the door behind me in my room and cry.

* * *

The best part of living in town is that my mom lives just down the road and she helps me so much. A lot of days I don't tell her how I feel but just her presence and her simple acts of kindness make me want to live another day.

I have sat with her just a handful of times crying over my health. I don't tell her very often that I feel like I am going to die, but when I do, all I need is for her to just sit with me and be there. And she does. I don't know how I would manage without her.

I experience this same feeling when Terri is here and wish she were closer, but I am *grateful* for when she can stay.

I know she wishes that she were closer, too, and when we talk about it, I always agree when she usually ends the conversation with, *"At least your mom is here."*

I know that makes everyone feel much better.

I can tell that Tim feels more at ease now that we are in town too. He can finally rest more in knowing that I am not alone with our children in the country anymore.

We experienced a lot of loss because of this chronic illness, but at least we have each other. I often try to explain to Russell that it really doesn't matter where you live. *What makes a house your home are the people in it.*

5

Something Needs to Change

I have been working faithfully on my health issues by following my functional medicine doctor's protocols. I am still not having improvements on certain things. Especially the iron issues. The duration of the menstrual cycles and the stomach pain has improved, but I am still having seizure-like episodes and near-fainting spells. I never cheat on the food and Terri would attest to this as she has offered me sweets several times and I always say no.

* * *

My endocrinologist from Mayo agreed to do a test on the adrenal glands that we never completed. I wish they would have me test for more things like mast cell activation syndrome or infectious disease, but I will take what I can get for now. It will be a shorter trip this time. We are doing a thyroid ultrasound as well as the secondary adrenal insufficiency test. I am conflicted with how I feel about doing more tests, but it's difficult to stay in this condition. Part of me wants them to find something, while part of me doesn't because then I would most likely have to be medicated my entire life and I have this desire to heal because my functional medicine doctor says I can.

I feel there is a cause that is more than just what my out-of-state functional medicine doctor has found or what regular medical doctors have found. I still think about Lyme disease on and off, but my functional medicine doctor is convinced that Lyme disease is mostly just another parasite and some of her protocols would clear it. I don't know a lot about testing for Lyme disease, but I have read online that the testing is very inaccurate.

I will be going back to Mayo for a few days to complete the adrenal testing and thyroid ultrasound and if that is clear I will be able to put an end to that possibility. I want to do more testing in other areas, but certain departments won't accept my case. The possibility of finding something at Mayo with my adrenals could result in an improvement of my quality of life so I want to ensure there is nothing wrong there.

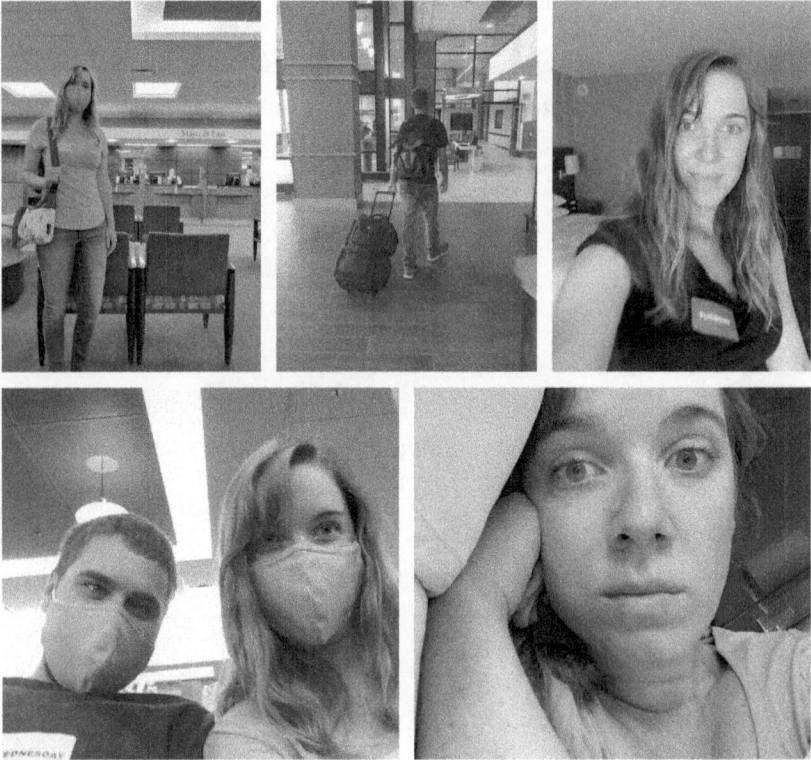

We went to Mayo again to retest my adrenal function.

My treatment right now through my functional medicine doctor has been very expensive. Somehow we manage. Some of my family worries that she is taking advantage of me. I understand their concerns as it can happen. But I don't feel that she is that way. Most of the expense comes from the food and supplements, but I have compared the cost with other similar locations and they are the same.

I am very restrictive on my food options, and it just doesn't seem to be working like it should. Even though I have good days, the bad days always come back and are still very related to my hormone shifts and periods. Sometimes I just wish I could rip my whole uterus and ovaries out . . . but then you can risk severe mental health factors from the abrupt loss of hormones, and I don't want that on top of all my other things right now.

My mom suffered with that after her ovaries were removed.

I just don't want adrenal fatigue to be misdiagnosed if I actually have adrenal insufficiency. If something is wrong with my thyroid or pituitary gland, natural methods cannot get rid of the damage. I just want to live a better life. I go a long time trying one path, but my kids are growing up. I want to be able to go on adventures again with my family and live a normal life. I want to live fully again. The hardest part is being a mother and aunt and seeing how much the children in my life are all growing right before my eyes. This illness has taken so much of my time away from them. I can't be there when I want to be and I am *forever sorry for that.*

* * *

My liver has returned to a normal size, which shows how well the glutathione injections are working for me. It's never fun getting these injections. Tim has to do them for me. I lie at the edge of the bed and wait for the burn of the needle.

I've never tried doing the injections on my own, even when I had to do the B12 injections in the past. Tim did those for me too. I remember trying to talk myself into doing them. I even had the needle in my hand once and counted, *"Three . . . two . . . one . . . "* Then I started over and recounted several times. I didn't want to burden him more, but in the end I gave up and passed the needle to my husband. I never would have thought I would be here at this time in my life, lying at the edge of my bed and getting a needle jabbed into my backside by my husband.

I have learned a lot from this experience. I will have more patience and more understanding over things I cannot control. I will be more understanding of Tim and find my own kind of happiness and enjoyment within myself. I have a lot of dreams. Sometimes I don't know if Tim believes in the underlying factors that my functional medicine doctor has diagnosed. *I don't blame him. Sometimes I question it too . . .*

I want to travel with my family. Not far, but I want to visit family members and not get stressed like I used to about the little things. I just want to enjoy life. I want to live and not just survive. I want to live life fully again. I want to go on long walks again. I want to swim. I want to dance. I want to destress and find myself again in a different way. I *hope* that I can achieve full health again. Others have. Others have healed. I have missed so much. Weddings . . . time with all sides of the family. It's hard to explain why I can't go to things.

I want to be there for my children and husband during hard times. I want to be around for my grandchildren. I want to live a life always *being there* for my loved ones . . . to love, comfort, and support them. I want to teach my children to always fight for themselves and question things. I want a long life. I want to help others going through the same experience that I have. I want to do good work. I want to live a life full of God's purpose for me.

I pray for healing so that I can live that purpose driven life.

God, please hear me. Please take away my suffering.

July 31, 2020

It is very hot today and my feet are buzzing. My POTS or thyroid or whatever the hell is wrong with me flared again last night. I ate yeast yesterday before my heart and body went nuts. I don't understand that. Heart palpitations, racing heart, freezing cold and trembling. My eyes are very dry in the mornings and I have a lot of blurry vision yet and pressure under my eyes. The eye doctor never sees anything wrong, though. I might get a second opinion. I am near ovulation so I think it's another stupid thyroid flare. I rarely keep track anymore, but sometimes it helps me emotionally if there is an explanation for why I am suffering. I don't know . . . these issues also seem to trigger after eating certain foods. It's just a miserable way to live.

I don't know why this had to happen to me. The Mayo Clinic found nothing wrong with my adrenal glands. I have just had to keep persisting with my diet and hormone balancing protocol. I debate on and off whether a surgery may help if there was endometriosis missed. I just want a normal life. I don't want to have to stress so much anymore about what I can and cannot eat or what flares this hell. Why can't it just go away? I am doing everything I am supposed to. It's been almost two years of this. *I want a normal life.* My body needs to quit misfiring. Last month the panic and depression feelings were just awful. I don't want to go through it again. It was awful up until I got my period. The migraines were horrible.

I just want to rip my uterus out, but what if that does nothing? At least it would stop these horrendous periods.

* * *

Prior to being accepted to Mayo, my neurologist had referred me to another local endocrinologist that had about a year-long wait. I debated about whether I should cancel this appointment, but I decided to keep the visit just in case I *ever* needed a local endocrinologist again. Because I knew . . . I would *never again* go back to the first local endocrinologist that I had encountered.

The new endocrinologist was very nice and went over my most recent pituitary hormone levels, which she also confirmed were normal. She definitely felt that I was experiencing PMDD (premenstrual dysphoric disorder). This condition is basically caused by a *hormone imbalance.* Not surprised. I could tell she felt very bad for me and in the end she suggested that maybe this condition is environmental. I was surprised when she said this. I had *not* brought up any of my concerns of the past with mold or Lyme disease causing this. This endocrinologist was the first medical doctor who had suggested something like this to me. I thought about the mold but said nothing.

As our visit was coming to a close, I was trying to keep it together and the words that I silently felt on and off escaped my lips. "I wish they could find *something,* like cancer . . . anything that can be treated . . . "

She looked at me very sadly and said, "No, don't say that."

"I'm sorry," I said as I wiped away a silent tear. "I don't really mean that. It's just that at least if it *was* something . . . like *cancer,* we would know what was wrong with me and doctors would *believe* me. My outcome would either be to heal or to die, not to suffer in this state with no easy answer or help for healing."

I felt very bad after I said that. I was not trying to dismiss the suffering of those who did have cancer . . . but I felt very lost. I could tell these words had a big impact on her too. I could tell she wanted to help me but did not know how. Tears filled her eyes as our appointment came to a close.

I left her office feeling *grateful* that I at least had someone nice on my team in case I ever needed her again.

* * *

I don't even know what to eat lately, and the food limitations make things very hard. I have to eat a lot of salt, too, which triggers stomachaches. My diagnoses are now: POTS, possible PCOS, adrenal fatigue, migraines, leaky gut, intestinal metaplasia (reversed), estrogen dominance, iron deficiency, subclinical thyroid issues, aluminum toxicity, zinc deficiency, and vasovagal response episodes. Other positive genetic factors are MTHFR and COMT. The COMT gene affects how the body detoxes estrogen and other environmental toxicities from the body. I have issues with heat intolerance, visual disturbances, light sensitivity, exercise intolerance, breathlessness, internal body tremors, buzzing in the extremities, heart palpitations, slow heart, racing heart, low blood pressure with high blood pressure spikes, blood sugar issues, dizziness, nausea, lightheadedness, headaches, seizure-/stroke-like episodes. I experience anxiety and depression because of these extreme symptoms. This has been going on since 2018. I used to be healthy, and I don't understand how this can happen.

I used to only have gut issues and bad period cramps . . . none of this debilitating stuff. I just want it gone and to feel present. My functional medicine doctor and I go back and forth on if a hysterectomy may help me with these fainting episodes. I have been told by many providers that they are hesitant about removing my ovaries. So am I, but I still get so many ruptured cysts. My uterus is prolapsing. My cervix is falling out . . . I tried to find a new gynecologist recently to evaluate me for a uterine prolapse.

She laughed when she saw that I was on progesterone. *"Why would you need this?"*

She seemed like she didn't believe that I had a uterine prolapse either because of my age . . . but, sure enough, when she checked me she sheepishly confirmed it. I wanted to take my progesterone pills and throw them at her arrogant face.

Instead, I left and never saw her again. I later told my functional medicine doctor that my body was falling apart.

I still bleed so heavy. If the bleeding could stop maybe at least some of my health could come back. It's terrifying, too, to think I could get pregnant in this state. I am constantly fighting a battle to increase my iron levels and I sometimes wonder if an iron infusion could help me. If I had a hysterectomy, at least I wouldn't bleed out all of the time. But if I have Lyme disease I read that surgery can worsen it and bring out more dormant bacteria. I still feel like Lyme disease is a possibility for me, but I don't know if I am going to the right doctor for it. I have read that testing is so unreliable.

To feel present again would be a blessing. I am tired of feeling like I have a hangover all the time.

We have been going fishing on cooler days, and I have been going on short walks to help clear my mind and build *strength* again. Walking is so hard for me, but on cooler days I manage.

Health care for women is *pathetic*. Treatment for POTS and chronic illness is *pathetic*. The treatment options only mask symptoms . . . there is no place to figure out the actual cause. The places that may help cost thousands of dollars. I looked into facilities in Minnesota and Texas that specialize in healing the underlying cause of POTS. *We cannot afford either of these facilities.* Tim is already drowning in finances so I don't even bring it up to him. You have to spend so much money finding and resolving issues on your own and the system is set up for us to fail.

Something needs to change.

August 3, 2020

Russell and Eliot are swimming in the little pool now. Eliot is so tan this year. Tim tans like this as well. Russell has more of a light skin tone like me. Russell was in T-ball this summer and his final game was Tuesday. My mom helped me get him to practices. I wouldn't have been able to do it without her.

Russell is very much into nature. He is a lot like me when I was younger. He has been very testy though. He challenges me a lot and wants his own way. He is still sad about the yellow house and I still find pictures that he has drawn of our yellow house with a sad face on it. Sometimes I feel like I can't handle his emotions while I am dealing with my own. It's so hard to be pulled back into the loss of our old life when I see these reminders. I try to hep him with his grief and moving on, and I need to find something to help him channel his grief and anger.

Tim and I debate on and off about taking him to a counselor. He hasn't been as happy as he used to be and it's so hard to see. It all began with the loss of our home. He has had crying outbursts where he brings up the yellow house even when it wasn't even remotely related to what upset him in that moment. This tells me that he has been internalizing it. He also sometimes complains about light and sound sensitivity. Sometimes I worry that what I have is genetic and he will get it someday. *I pray not.* The best I can do is to ensure we have all of the right causes.

I'm still homeschooling, and it's the best decision right now for our family. Eliot is still having some speech delays. It's just so hard to understand him. He doesn't seem like he even wants to try . . . he is the same way when it comes to being fully potty-trained. He wants his own way all of the time too. He is also very sweet and wants my approval. He is a mommy's boy and cuddles with me all of the time. He used to be all about Dad until I got sick. Then he was with me all of the time . . . almost as if he knew that I needed him or something. It's nice that if Russell doesn't want to play Eliot will play on his own. I feel bad often because I can't do as much one-on-one with Eliot as I did with Russell.

My health issues make everything difficult and I get as much done as I can before I'm symptomatic again, and then I have to rest. I try to get all the basics done like cooking, cleaning, and school. Eliot loves to paint during school. He gets so wrapped up in his artwork—it's fun to see. I love my boys so much. *They are my driving force for me to keep trying to heal and find answers.*

Sometimes I wonder if anyone believes me.

Does God even hear my cries anymore?

September 24, 2020

The boys are playing in the sandbox. They probably have the water hose inside of it right now, but I don't mind. I have supper in the oven and today was another hard day. I can't do a lot without symptoms . . . especially since my iron dropped again. I see a hematologist tomorrow. We are going to try an iron infusion. I have a surgery scheduled for a partial hysterectomy in November. The plan is that the surgeon will also see if there was any internal injury or missed endometriosis from my last surgery as well. My functional medicine doctor feels that since my symptoms got worse after the last surgery and there is no major improvement after completion of her protocols that it is possible I have an internal bleed or missed endometriosis causing the iron deficiency.

If the iron infusion does not improve my symptoms I will keep the surgery date. I looked at reviews for this surgeon, and my functional medicine doctor even spoke to her on the phone. She has good reviews, and some of my trusted local doctors recommended her. I *hope* that I make the right decision. My functional medicine doctor keeps telling me to think positively that this surgery will help me heal. It has to. I don't know what else could be causing my health issues. It has to be this. I *hope* it truly isn't Lyme disease. I pray that God will guide me and the doctor's hands and bring healing to me.

6

A Wave of Loneliness

October 7, 2020

It's a beautiful day today, but I have been so incredibly irritable and crazy feeling with the signs of an oncoming migraine. Lately they have been worse, though, with spinning sensations . . . *when will this go away?* My skin is still orange from the overload of iron that I received from the iron infusion. The doctor apparently gave me too much . . .

I ended up in urgent care a few days later and the nurse got spooked and made me go to the taped-off COVID ward. I told her what happened with the iron infusion. I expressed my concerns with my health conditions and acute issues putting me at risk if I did develop COVID right now . . . especially if I was placed in the COVID ward. I told her I wanted to leave and she turned around and got another person to stand with her in the doorway and they told me *I could not leave.* My symptoms were too *similar* to COVID. My symptoms have *always* been similar to COVID . . . daily . . . for the last two years.

I was so sick and nearly fainting from the overload. I wanted to walk out, but I didn't have much *strength* in me to fight and it was pretty obvious they weren't going to make this easy. I didn't want to be put in the COVID ward in my condition with all the sick people . . . especially with *high* ferritin and iron. But because I did not have Tim with me that day, I didn't have much of a choice.

I have found, throughout my illness, that it is best to always have an advocate with you . . . and in my case one that has a *"murder face"* when he looks upset. When I walked behind the taped-off area there were a lot of people crying. It was very disturbing. I wondered how many other patients were being forced back there and not getting the care they needed because of COVID. I wondered how many were afraid because they did have a diagnosis of COVID. It was uncertain times, but I certainly knew I was iron overloaded because I had the infusion two days prior.

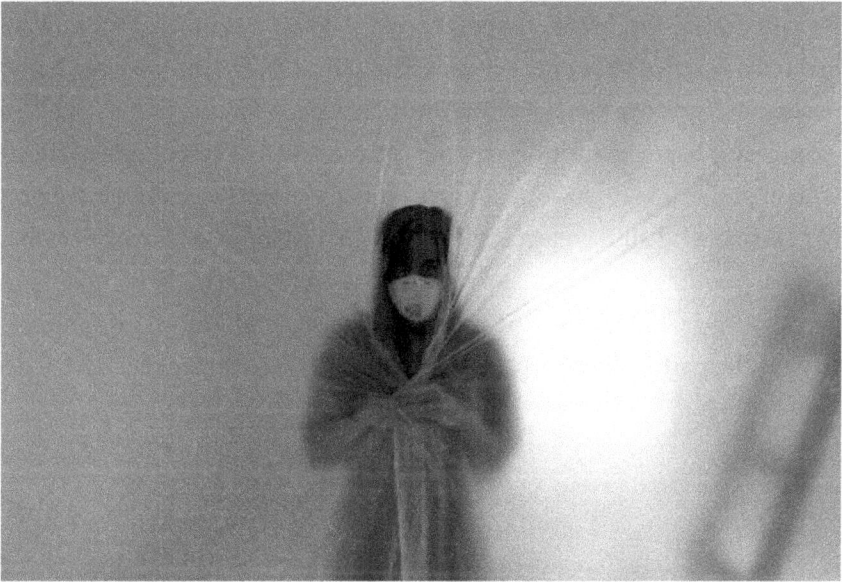

We can't let you leave . . .

When the doctor finally came to see me, she was very upset that the nurses brought me there. My labs showed a very overloaded iron level and both my kidney and liver levels were affected. She said she doesn't see this very often and is unsure why the hematologist gave me so much, but to never let this happen again . . . not that she was *blaming* me . . . she seemed more flabbergasted by the amount the doctor gave me. She was very concerned about the state of my liver and kidney levels. She was upset, too, that I was brought to the COVID unit . . . unfortunately, my quality of life on a daily basis mimics an acute COVID case. Whenever I go to the doctor, I don't even know how I am supposed to respond when they ask me if I have experienced any dizziness or breathlessness. I understand why it can be challenging to determine who has COVID and who doesn't, but I wish they would have let my labs come back before placing me in that unit.

Tim was very upset about the experience I had at the COVID unit. He wanted to go in there and yell at them. In all reality, he wouldn't have to yell, he would just have to *look* at them . . . but I talked him out of that. It really wasn't their fault, they were just following protocol, but now he had to be worried about me being exposed to COVID. And we went home upset that I was overloaded with iron, a new problem.

Since this happened, I have experienced more severe spinning sensations with migraines. I also have a lot more pressure in my head and ear ringing. My ferritin and all iron levels were so high, but at least I have been able to have a couple of periods to lower it. They will recheck my levels right before surgery to make sure it's at a low enough level. If it is, I will be safe to have the partial hysterectomy.

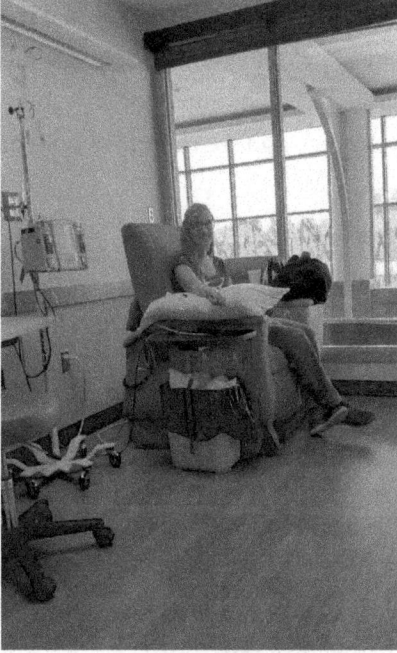

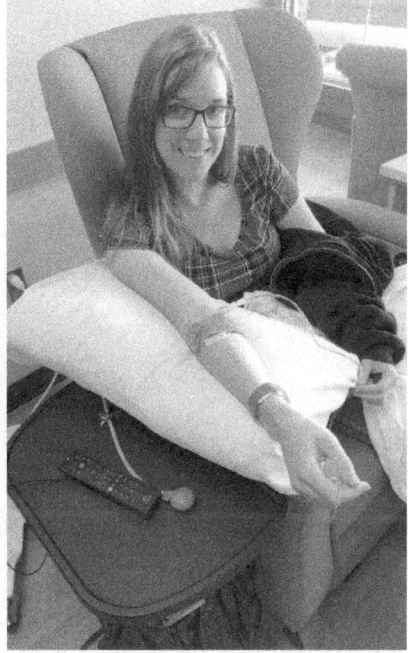

I could feel the overload happening during my iron infusion.

Previously, during the iron infusion, I was trying to use my positive mind frame instead of listening to my body. I tend to overworry now because of my many past bad experiences. I felt the overload happening. My temples started to tremor, I felt way more out of breath, and my heart was racing. I did tell them this, but they were not concerned. The last few weeks have been a pretty bad flare because of these recent complications . . . but I'm hoping that as the iron comes down it will eventually be at the level I needed. With the hysterectomy, I won't bleed it out anymore. Maybe I can finally feel an optimal ferritin level. I *hope* it can balance.

* * *

My partial hysterectomy is scheduled for November 3. I almost wish they could at least remove my right ovary because that always seems to

89

be the side where I get ruptured cysts. I am hoping that an optimal iron and ferritin level that is able to stay at a stable level will help me heal. The doctor will hopefully get a good look in my abdomen for any missed endometriosis or injury from my last surgery and we can move on from there.

I'm trying very hard to have a positive mind frame even though my POTS condition has been worse since last summer.

* * *

Russell turned six yesterday. I feel like homeschooling is going well for now, but I worry about how I will manage during my recovery period after the surgery. Russell is learning to read and is counting well and also learns a lot about Jesus.

I just want to be cured so that all of us can get out of this house more and go on adventures. That's all I want. Even before the COVID restrictions, my health has prevented me from being able to do a lot of things that I want to do. When the restrictions came into place for COVID everyone actually got to experience what chronically ill people miss out on normally . . . *fun, isn't it?*

I just don't want my body to get triggered and misfire any longer. I am intolerant to heat, cold, and exercise, which makes my triggers difficult to avoid. My sympathetic nervous system goes crazy and my autonomic nervous system goes haywire. I get lightheaded, have hearing issues like whooshing in my ears, heart race and palpitations, blood pressure shifts, breathing difficulty, pressure in my head, migraines, vision issues . . . it's very hard living this way. I have to be so careful with what I choose to do every day and I deal with these issues daily.

I am angry that my POTS isn't in remission. It's discouraging, but I keep fighting. I don't have any other choice but to get up every day. I have children. I just *hope* my hard days don't affect them negatively. I do my best, but my mental health struggles are challenging because of my physical limitations. I get overstimulated often and that is very difficult to deal with while having children in these age ranges. They are just being normal happy children, but sometimes their screams while playing or even their laughter overstimulates me and sets off my migraines. Sometimes I feel so overstimulated that even their touch makes me feel startled.

I don't want to be this way anymore. I want to be happy and free. I want the *fear,* worry, and depression gone. I want myself back. I want to be able to be around the normal noise of my children without my symptoms triggering.

I saw a therapist a while back and she told me to write notes to my loved ones in my journals if I am ever really afraid. I decided to do this again as my surgery draws closer.

October 8, 2020

Dear Russell,

I want you to know that I prayed for you every day. Every day that went by without a child in my womb I prayed harder. I love you so much. I love your smile and those dimples. I love that you have a big heart, that you care so deeply about others. I am so proud that you are my son and I pray that you have the happiest life possible. I want so much to see you grow up and be active in all that you do. It makes me sad that we can't go on the adventures we once had. I really *hope* we can soon. I want you to always remember how much I love you. That I always tried even when my body let me down. That I felt the hurt in your heart whenever you were sad. Mommy is always with you and I am trying my hardest to get better for you. I love you Russell and I am always in your heart and am always with you. Jesus loves you too.

Love,
Your Mommy

Dear Eliot,

You bring so much joy and laughter into my life. Your cuddles always warm my heart. Your sweet smile brightens all around you. I know that

God put you into my life at the right time for a big purpose. I want you to know how much I love you, always. It was very hard for me to take care of you while I was sick but you held my hand on the hardest of days and I know you knew and you always helped me feel better when you held my hand. I love you and love seeing you grow and your eyes twinkle when you smile. I love you Eliot.

Love,

Your Mommy

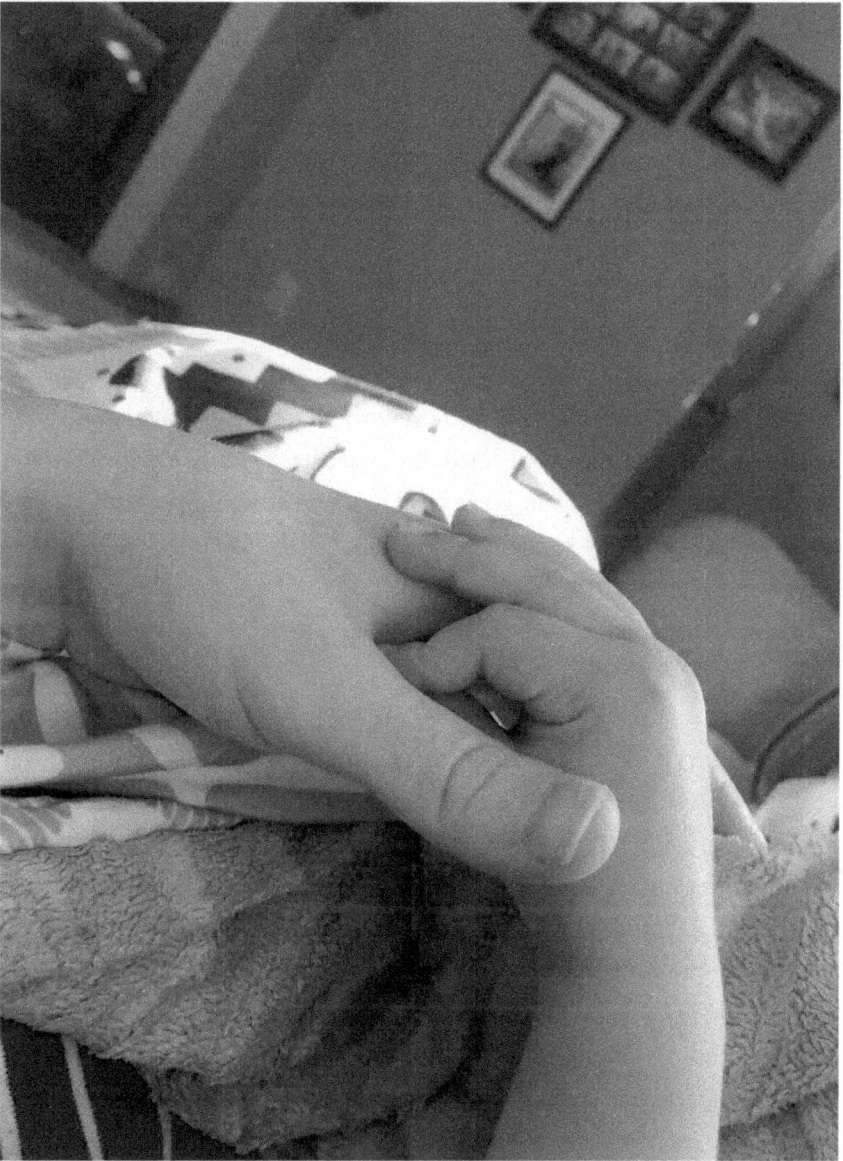

. . . you held my hand on the hardest of days.

Timothy,

You are all that I have ever wanted. You are my best friend. I am so happy that I get to be with you and grow old with you. I'm so sorry that my health

93

issues have put so much emotional strain on you. All I want is happiness and contentment again. I just want to dance with you. Laugh with you and have fun with you. Please always love our children and show them affection and attention. Always remember to talk to God. I love you. I will always love you. No matter what. *Forever* and *always*.

Love,
Your Sweetheart

Mom,

I don't even know what I would do without you. You have no idea the impact you have on me every day that you are here. You are my best friend. My life is full with you in it. Never feel that you are unimportant. You are loved and cared for by so many. I love you.

Love,
Your daughter, Whitney

December 12, 2020

The surgery did not go as planned. I lost so much blood. There was an internal injury that caused a large hematoma. I had to have three blood transfusions. Because of COVID, I was alone in the hospital. They would not let my husband come back. He did not know this when he left, otherwise he would have stayed, but our children needed him too.

I knew something was very wrong when I stood up and all I could hear was static in my ears. My head felt terrible. I didn't know if I would survive. The isolation that I felt in the hospital was like an old friend, as my entire health struggles had been isolating enough already. But it was worse to not even be able to feel the warmth of my husband or children to pull me back into reality. It was like a prison or a nightmare that I was trapped inside again as *waves* of debilitating symptoms hit me repeatedly. A similar sensation that I had felt with my health battle over the last couple of years but worse, because this time I was really alone.

I couldn't believe they wouldn't let my husband or children come in, even if they wore a mask . . . even though we had remained in isolation the week prior. We did this just to make sure my children didn't get sick with something acute and pass it to me after surgery. None of it mattered, and I remember being so *grateful* to just be alive when I left those doors . . . even in a worse condition.

It took several months to recover. I had to use a chair while showering because I could hardly stand upright. I retained so much more ferritin and iron and I was overloaded again. I was in and out of the ER many times after this. All of my symptoms were increased. I was bedbound again for a long time. I had to have a repeat CT scan because of all of the damage.

During the surgery, the doctor never went back in to see if I had missed endometriosis. If I didn't have an internal bleed before, I did after . . . we don't even know what caused the internal bleed. She told me later that she planned to medicate me with birth control if I continued experiencing endometriosis-related symptoms. I was not happy when she told me this. She *knew* my history with birth-control-related problems and was *told* by my functional medicine doctor that women with POTS often do not do well on birth control. I wanted to *fix* the problem, not put a Band-Aid on it, and she *knew* this. The bioidentical hormones were only able to help so much.

I often wonder if she didn't go back in because she knew I was bleeding internally. She said that she didn't see any bleeding when she closed me up. She sounded genuine and very sorry but I was left with more complications.

```
I didn't write a lot in my journal during this time. I was
trying to mentally erase it.
```

* * *

After these complications, my out-of-state functional medicine doctor asked me to find a local functional medicine doctor to help us. She was very upset that this happened to me and wanted someone local who knew of local specialists or surgeons if we ever needed help again.

Over time, I did improve to my baseline, but not without extreme suffering and my flares were worse. I experienced a lot of spinning sensations and increased tinnitus and muffled hearing. The pressure was so severe in my head I felt it may burst. I don't know how I got through that time. My mother, Tim's mother Terri, and my husband helped me during this time frame when I was recovering from the physical complications. When they had to return to normal life, I sat back and struggled with the daily tasks of being a mother. Most days were more of a blur where all I could do was the basic and somehow I still managed to homeschool my children. I didn't have a village for homeschooling at that time and knew of no other homeschool mothers.

I felt like I had made the worst decision ever, but in all reality I couldn't have predicted the complications that occurred. Had they not happened, I do feel I would have noticed improvement with my POTS disorder. Over time, the fainting episodes and severe heart rates did improve because my iron was no longer depleting with every menstrual cycle. But my ferritin stayed above 400 and that resulted in a disagreement between my two functional medicine doctors concerning whether the ferritin was from a form of secondary hemochromatosis from blood transfusions or from inflammation. Later we found out the cause and how to help it.

＊

It wasn't until April of 2021 when I decided I could journal again. I was trying to heal from the emotional and physical medical trauma. I was also still trying to get my quality of life back while raising my two children.

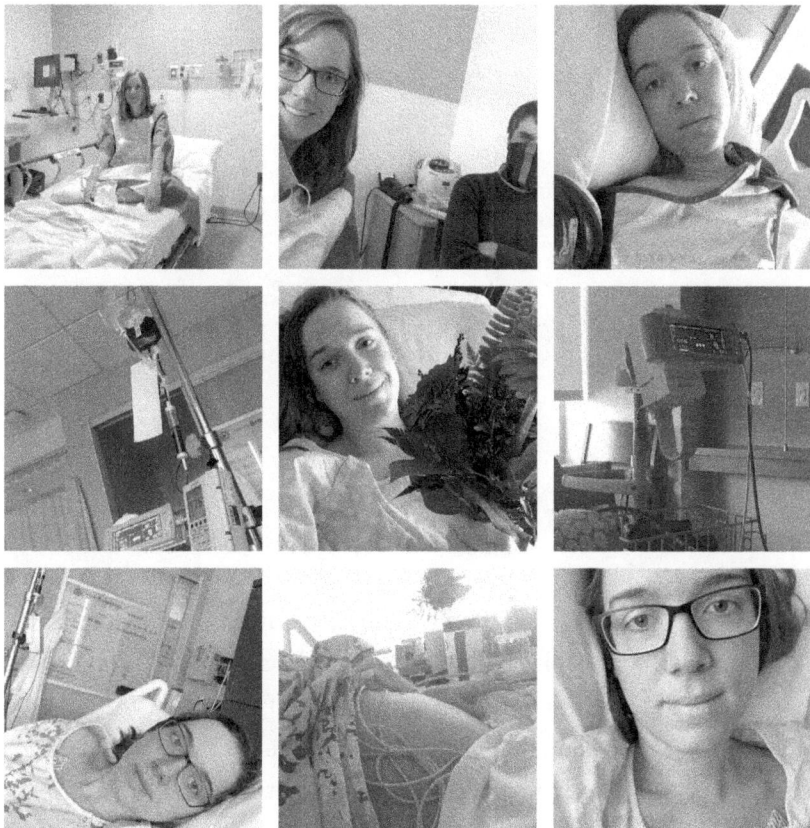

The surgery did not go as planned . . .

Where are you, God, when you said you would *carry me*? My legs feel heavy . . . am I dragging you as I beg of you to *help me*?

7

A Perfect Storm of Issues

April 16, 2021

A part of me is trying to block out the trauma I experienced from surgery. It took me two months to be able to get out of bed or off the couch more often and get out of the house again. I could only get up to do basic tasks for the kids. It's so defeating and isolating being this way. I couldn't even stand up without my head filling up with so much pressure. I was extremely foggy, weak, confused, and breathless. The sound sensitivity was very scary. I couldn't escape it. Even when I slept I would awake with heart rate issues.

It's so *awful* that people just have to live this way . . . that there is nothing they can do. *I am still hopeful that I can heal.*

I am working with a new functional medicine doctor locally who also is an MD and is a member of the American Board of Family Medicine and a Certified Practitioner of the Institute for Functional Medicine. My out-of-state functional medicine doctor suggested this. She wanted me to find someone closer to me to help us with my case.

So far, my problems are both genetic and environmental. This new functional medicine doctor feels that I have a mitochondrial disease while my out-of-state functional medicine doctor does not.

Another suggestion through my out-of-state functional medicine doctor was to go to a brain injury facility called The Functional Neurology Center. She gave me two names of specialists from that specific location. Coincidentally, one of the specialists just moved an hour from us and opened up his own center. He has seen a lot of conditions like mine. The stories he has told me have been very eye-opening. After a week of therapy with him he found right cerebral findings and other issues. He was suspicious of a brain injury. He has been very kind to me and I will always be *grateful* for his care and determination. He offered a lot of suggestions and we enjoyed the week of therapy sessions with him.

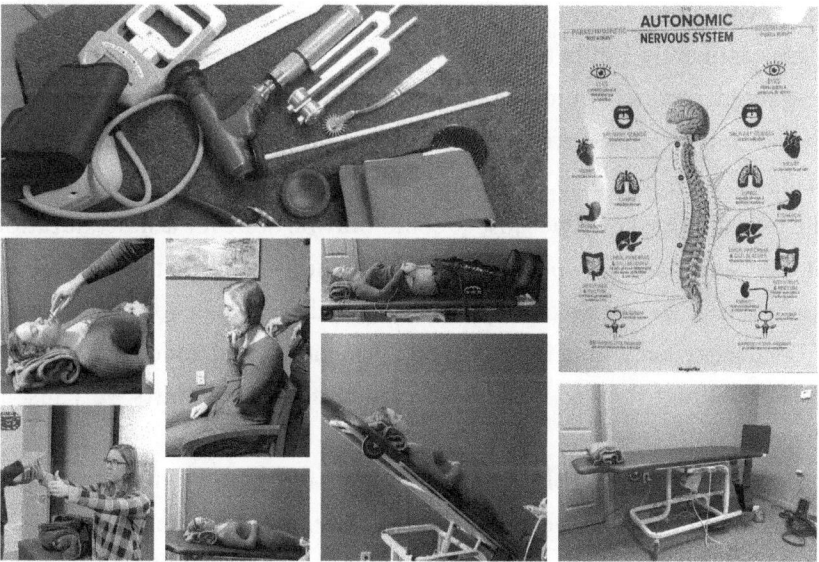

Some people come into a certain season in your life . . . and that purpose is to guide you.

My brain specialist sent me home with physical therapy ideas to help improve my symptoms, but he too is suspicious that I am dealing with Lyme or parasites of some kind. If I continue to struggle, he feels Lyme disease should be reevaluated. *My brain feels so inflamed.*

I have done parasite treatments before and passed really long-looking worms. It's absolutely disgusting and terrifying. When I showed the pictures to my out-of-state functional medicine doctor, she apologized that we had missed this and told me to contact my local gastroenterologist to see if he can figure out what type of parasite it is. I sent the images to him and he wanted me to bring the specimen in for testing so that we could treat it properly with the right antibiotic. There was a suspicion that it could be a tapeworm or ascariasis (roundworm infection).

My mind went to the time my mother told me that her mom had once passed a tapeworm the size of her leg. I was disgusted with the idea that I may have parasites in me like this and wondered how in the world I would have ever gotten them in the first place.

Unfortunately, I didn't have the specimen anymore because at the time I doubted anyone would test it for me anyway. I got a sample cup from the lab and began to retry the treatment in hopes that I would be able to bring a sample to the lab. Getting the sample took several months of trying the parasite treatment because it could only be done for a short duration of days and during a specific time of the month. I didn't always pass a specimen. It was an absolutely degrading feeling to have to check and see if I had passed anything . . . over and over again. I had done stool samples in the past that showed no signs of parasites and those tests were just as disgusting.

I was finally able to collect a sample after a few months of the treatment. I took it in to the lab and they called me later and told me they disposed of the specimen because it was supposed to be a worm, not stool. *Are you kidding me!?!* I told them it was not stool and had they taken it out they would have seen how it uncoiled in length from my wrist to my elbow. I was very upset and defeated and gave up at that point. Everyone was so unreliable.

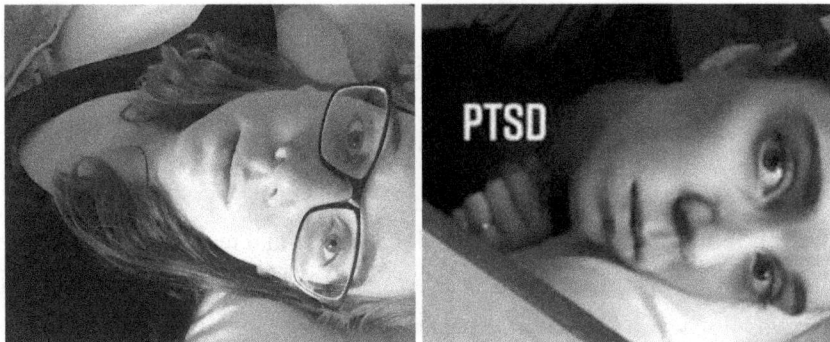

I didn't want to share this part of my life but I felt it was necessary. What I experienced was absolutely terrifying. I took the specimen to the lab as directed and they called me later saying they threw it away because they mistook it for stool. They never tested it . . . After that, I lost all faith in the medical system.

* * *

I have had so many issues with labs . . . it's upsetting. It takes so much out of me to go to the lab anyway, and then they just mishandle my labs or screw something up. I didn't try to get a sample again after that.

There many people who claim that *all diseases* come from parasites. Parasite cleanses are constantly being advertised as the *cure-all* solution. I feel that there a lot of factors that can cause disease, not parasites alone. You could have mold, systemic candida (overgrowth of yeast), heavy metals, hormonal imbalances, Lyme, or other environmental toxicities that build up in your system. If parasites are the only problem and a parasite cleanse heals you I would count yourself lucky.

I feel that it is important to find out your specific underlying cause so that you don't cause damage to your body by constantly treating something that may not be causing a problem.

Do I believe that parasites are a part of the problem for myself? *Yes*. But not the only factor.

Later, when I met my new local functional medicine doctor, she said that everyone has parasites, some are harmless and a normal part of the gut flora. If the body is overrun by a certain kind they can be very damaging.

* * *

I had the appointment with my new local functional medicine doctor. She agrees that my issues are from a *perfect storm*. What I liked the most about her was how soft-spoken and patient she was. She also responds very quickly to my questions and ensures me that I can email her questions through the portal when I need to. Her demeanor fits more with me as she is very calm during our appointments and I feel less stress when we discuss my concerns.

The detox issues that I have, along with environmental toxicity, caused gut issues, hormone issues, adrenal issues, and nutrient deficiencies. My immune system couldn't keep up with the overload.

Since the hysterectomy, my food sensitivities have been a lot worse. I used to eat things and get rashes or heart palpitations. Now sometimes I feel like my throat is going to close up. I don't understand it. I did the full gut protocol with the out-of-state functional medicine doctor, so why is it worse and not resolved by now?

My local functional medicine doctor put me on another regimen right now for mitochondrial health and certain food restrictions. If nothing improves we will test for SIBO, mold, or Lyme. I always suggested SIBO and Lyme disease to my out-of-state functional medicine doctor, but she felt what we were doing was good enough to get rid of it . . .

* * *

I have been eating very healthy. I never cheat. I don't eat gluten, dairy, processed foods, refined sugars, and certain oils. I also juice and eat healthy fats.

Unfortunately, I am still getting ovarian cysts. I had a four-inch cyst burst about a month ago. I was seen by a gynecologist on a Friday and ultrasound imaging was ordered and completed. I saw the results that night. Unfortunately, since it was a Friday I didn't hear back from the doctor, but in the scan it said a cyst looked like it was rupturing. A hemorrhagic cyst.

The following morning, I woke up vomiting and it continued all day. I had severe breathlessness, leg pain, and couldn't stand without heart race. It was awful. No one else in my family was sick. Since I have POTS, I knew I was getting dehydrated. My husband took me in to the ER because I was not able to hold anything down. I didn't want to go to the ER, but it was a Saturday and my doctors at Mayo always said it was common for POTS patients to need fluid, especially with an acute factor worsening their symptoms. I felt very brushed off at the ER. The entire staff acted like this was just a stomach bug and anxiety. I explained to them about the cyst and how with my POTS I need fluids if I get really dehydrated. They kept saying they couldn't give them to me and they could only give me a medication for nausea.

I left the ER and a few hours later I was nearly fainting so we went back in. I was in very bad shape.

The doctor on call came in and scoffed, "Back again to try to get fluids, I see?"

Like I wanted to even be there . . . He still would not give me fluids. He said something about a fluid shortage, but when I was sent home I was given a sheet on anxiety and somatoform disorder. I remember looking down at the sheet and feeling like there was a pit in my stomach. I read the letter out loud to my husband. He was upset, too, and told me I needed to contact the hospital and have them remove anxiety off of my chart. I found out later that the POTS diagnosis wasn't even in my chart. Even *after* my hysterectomy complications.

The next day was just as terrible, but I had to lie down in bed all day because if I tried to stand up my heart rate was close to 200bpm and I was nearly passing out.

The following Monday, my gynecologist called me about the hemorrhagic cyst. I told her about my symptoms and asked if they were related. She said absolutely, and with the severity it could have indicated more serious things going on like an ovarian torsion or infection. *Funny* . . . when I told the ER about the cyst they said it was a small cyst that wouldn't cause those symptoms and it was most likely a stomach bug that I was dealing with. They sure have no idea what they are talking about. I did a simple online search and could tell you what was happening was related to the ruptured cyst. *It's almost like Google is more reliable than doctors.*

As the nurses whispered in the hallway and gave me the sheet on anxiety and somatoform disorder, I told myself that was the *last time* I would go to the ER. I would rather *die* than be treated that terribly *ever* again . . .

I don't understand why my face gives people the impression that I am making stuff up. I don't understand why so many have gaslit me and blamed my conditions on anxiety. Even when I have a history of POTS, aura migraines, and hemorrhagic cysts. I don't understand. There are few solutions to problems like mine, only birth control has been offered to reduce these cysts, which has caused me numerous problems in the past. I still remember bleeding every day for over a month when I tried the IUD. Then the mood disorders, acne, and cysts that grew even when I was on birth control. Every birth control I have ever tried, especially since having children, resulted in some negative side effect and the risk of blood clots is not reassuring.

My experience has shown that we have a very broken medical system full of people with *no empathy*. There have been a handful of good doctors, but the rest of them don't give a shit about you. They are just there for the money. They blame everything on anxiety. Always do. Frankly, I don't think the majority of them know what the hell they are doing.

I called the clinic and asked for a complaint letter to get anxiety taken off of my chart and POTS, ovarian cysts, and aura migraines on it. That way if I ever go to the ER I stop running into these problems. I got the letter, but I was so emotionally defeated that I never completed it. I still haven't. My husband kept asking me if I got it done. I told him, "No, but I will." In all reality, I just don't even want to deal with them anymore. I just won't go to the ER again. If I could only find a reliable primary doctor this would not keep happening.

A PERFECT STORM OF ISSUES

*So many times I feel so near death
and no one can help me.*

II

Part Two

Blanketed by POTS...
"I am meant to heal, rebuild, and restore. My body is working
for me, not against me. Healing is possible."

8

Setting Healthy Goals

August 1, 2021

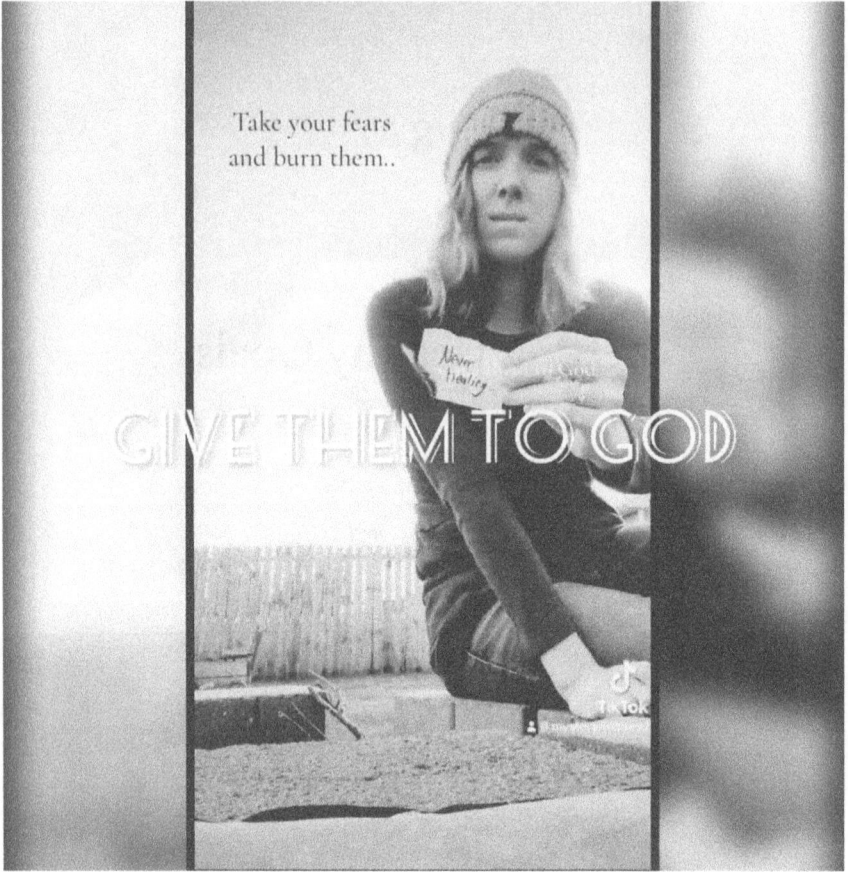

Take your fears and burn them . . . give them to God.

I need to heal. I want to heal. I hope to heal soon. May God bring complete healing to me in these pages. I am grateful that I took my kids to the park today. I am grateful that I saw family and was able to be there with my sister when she needed me.

So much of what this illness has taken from me is *time*. The hardest part has been having to miss out on so much and not being able to be there for others. The grief over the loss of myself is great, but the heartbreak associated with the loss of time is overwhelming.

This new journal is so beautiful. I look forward to filling its pages and *hope* there are more positives in this chapter of my life.

This fall Tim and I will be celebrating our tenth anniversary. I am so *grateful* for each and every day with him. Even on the bad days. He may not have always been able to understand what was going on with my health regression in the beginning, but he always *tried*. He was *always* there for me for every appointment and every medical test and he *still* is. We have both had to learn and grow together because of this experience.

I really wanted to have a big party this year to celebrate ten years of marriage. Tim wanted to renew our vows with the priest. I wanted to, too, but I was worried that I would have an episode during the ceremony and lose control of my body in front of others. I wouldn't have any way to hide it standing in front of others. It's so hard not knowing if I can tolerate something or not.

We would have had a big wedding party at the local gardens. We wanted to have all of our close friends and family with us. We wanted to dance and eat delicious food . . . hopefully we can do that someday. Sometimes, when I feel sad, I look at all of the memories of Tim and I together, especially when we went to D.C. for our friends' wedding. We danced that night and had so much fun.

We have been wanting to take dance lessons for years now . . . but my limitations prevent me from doing that.

I have learned that we are all fighting hidden battles. Some things you have no control over. Breathe slowly and deeply. Let it go; it doesn't matter. We are meant to be with others. Not alone and isolated. Practice forgiveness and understanding.

August 16, 2021

My goals for this year . . . first and most important is to heal my soul and spirit from the trauma I have experienced. I need to find an inner peace from my external suffering. Next is continue to heal physically. That would be wonderful if both healed in the same time frame. I need to find a way to escape what I am going through physically.

Meditation is helpful. Journaling is helpful. Photography. Projects.

Positive distractions. My health coach, through my local functional medicine doctor, has been very helpful. She gives me a lot of suggestions to help me with my emotional struggles. I speak with her about once a month and am very *grateful* for her help and advice.

I have discovered something new this summer. I feel relief from my pain and symptoms when I swim. I was surprised to find that I was able to tolerate the heat as long as I could get into the water. My heart rate calmed down and I felt less air hunger, pressure, buzzing, and dizziness as soon as I got into the water. The only challenge is the sensitivity I have to the chlorine, but I can be outside in the heat as long as I am in the water. The *waves* crashed around me while I swam with my family. I heard their laughter and real laughs escaped my lips too . . . it was the happiest I have felt in a long time. It was the most real laugh I have had in a long time. This is a huge discovery for me and I am so *grateful*.

* * *

Whenever I begin to feel closer to God, the dark shadow of my past haunts me in my dreams. His dark presence hovers over me. I know that it is a spiritual attack. I talked about the issues concerning my night terrors and health struggles with my former priest when he counseled me recently. My spirit has been weakened from all of the physical and emotional trauma I have experienced.

So much medical gaslighting. I will win with the help of God.

* * *

Mom and I have been going on short walks. She has been telling me that she is having issues on and off with double vision. *Is it the Bartonella* from the cat bite? My mind races. She has been experiencing some symptoms similar to mine. *God* . . . is this some kind of *genetic* disease?

What is happening? She is worried on and off about her vision. She went to the eye doctor, but they don't see a lot wrong. I still can't go to her

112

apartment very often. Something environmentally triggers my heart race and allergy-type symptoms. I feel so bad, but she has to come visit me most of the time because of this. This illness impacts so much of my life. *Could it be mold?* I just don't want my mom to become sick like me.

* * *

November 9, 2021

I am meant to heal, rebuild, and restore. My body is working for me, not against me. *Healing is possible.* This too shall pass. My pain is my *purpose.* More than trillion cells are intently listening to how I speak to them. I am built with the infrastructure to heal. My only limits are the ones I set for myself. Don't give up. You will heal. I promise.

9

I Should Have Been My Own Doctor

November 18, 2021

What is it like to be chronically ill? It kind of feels like you're drowning. It feels like waves rushing in, crashing into you. Like a current you will never escape.

Today I am struggling. I try to be uplifting, but I struggle to see an end to this suffering. My moods today were all over the place, indicating an impending migraine. Which I did experience. It always begins the same way: depersonalization, fogginess, extreme rage, extreme light and sound sensitivity, and then, it hits. My hearing is affected. I feel slurred. I get very sad. *Am I okay?*

I believe that in my lifetime I will heal, but the days of my children being small are ever fleeting. My dreams in life were so *simple.* I wanted to be a mom and live in the country. I wanted love, laughter, and to never be lonely again. Such simple things.

* * *

The mold test came back positive. I was diagnosed with mold illness, CIRS, SIBO, and SIFO (small intestinal fungal overgrowth) through my local functional medicine doctor. I don't understand why things were not done

114

well enough before to get these things out of my body. My out-of-state functional medicine doctor was always so convinced that if I had these things the glutathione and diet would resolve them. I feel like I could have been better a lot sooner had these things been treated properly.

I am told that I have to take certain type of binders (medications to lower certain levels) to get this type of mold out of my body. Previously, I was on no binders at all for possible mold. *Would I have even needed the hysterectomy if I had been diagnosed properly?* I no longer faint all of the time because of heavy bleeding . . . heart rates above 150 out of nowhere are very rare now. But I still have such pressure in my head since the surgery. My blood is very thick and the ear ringing and vestibular migraines have been terrible ever since I was overloaded from the blood transfusions and iron infusion.

The mold illness has stolen my dreams from me. I am so very tired. I still have *hope.* I still wonder if I have Lyme disease. *At this point, I may as well have diagnosed myself with all of my conditions.* I feel like I have been my own doctor this whole time.

My local functional medicine doctor said that, even if I do have Lyme, what we are doing is focused on strengthening the immune system and that will help eradicate it. So we are focusing on the other factors now. Not a lot is covered by insurance for the tests and supplements. This is all *so* expensive. The Lyme test that I want to do through IGeneX is almost $2,500. The one that my local functional medicine doctor offers through Vibrant is $900. We can't afford the best tests and with the other costs right now we can't even afford the Vibrant one. I am trying to *trust* my doctor. I *hope* she is right that targeting the immune system will be enough.

I worry about my mom more now. Is she living in mold? Is this why I can't breathe well at her place? Is this why my heart rate acts up in a MCAS (mast cell activation syndrome) attack? Is this what is progressively affecting her vision? I feel so stuck, like I might know what is going on with her but I can do nothing to help her. *Or is it the Bartonella still living in her body?*

Her health has been regressing ever since the cat bite, but she moved into that apartment at around the same time. If things continue to get worse for her, I will have to do something to help. When I mention the possibility of her apartment having mold I know it overwhelms her, especially with my recent diagnosis and how my doctor has said it has affected me. And she has mercury fillings breaking off into her mouth when she eats. I've mentioned to my sister that she may need them removed, but my mom is low income. My sister's dentist seems unconcerned about the fillings. But they are breaking into her mouth. *In pieces.*

Someone I knew locally had the highest level of mercury build up in her body that her doctor had ever seen. She almost died from it and was bedbound for several years before getting a diagnosis. She had to get her silver fillings all removed and then have the mercury chelated from her body. She has been completely healed for several years and feels better in her 60s than she did in her 30s. *And my mom's fillings are breaking off into pieces into her mouth . . .* This can't be safe.

I know it is overwhelming and scary. It is for me, too, knowing these things and not being able to do anything about it. I tread very carefully when bringing up my concerns with my mom because it overwhelms her. Who wouldn't be overwhelmed? Especially if you cannot afford the care to help these conditions. Healing from these things should be an opportunity for all, not just for those who can afford the care . . .

God, why is this happening to my mom?

* * *

The physical parts of this illness are hard enough, but the mental, spiritual, and emotional parts of grieving the loss of my self are the hardest. Now I have to worry about my mom on top of it because I don't want her losing her health like I did. I am constantly battling myself to have positive thoughts. It is the most challenging thing when I continue to experience the trauma that put me here. I experience such extreme suffering every day. And I don't want my mom to.

The world I enjoyed so much is now too loud, overstimulating, the lights are too bright, and the smells and other environmental factors trigger me. I just wish so badly that Jesus could come down and save me from this nightmare. Like he saved Mary . . . and the blind . . . and the paralyzed. But it is not so simple, and he is not here to save me like he did them. Sometimes I wonder if he doesn't want to. I have to do the hard work. The meditation, the exercise, positive thoughts, food . . . I have to do this.

When I completed the SIBO protocol, I had to add in one food at a time and wait for a five-day period before adding another. I had to keep a food journal and write down any new symptoms after each food. It felt so impossible to do this since I was still experiencing symptoms even when eating the safe foods. Sometimes the environment would even trigger my symptoms. Food and just breathing certain air became such a challenge, but I never lost any weight while doing these diets. I kept my calorie intake the same and I ate plenty of the healthy foods.

I spoke with a woman online who suffered with Lyme disease. She told me she had ulcers all over her gumline, and her Lyme doctor told her that was where the Lyme was harboring. This is very scary as I have had repeat issues with ulcers and mouth sores since the early stages of the onset of my illness. I still wonder if I have Lyme.

I just want peace and happiness, and for my children to have a new image of their mother. I love them so much and they deserve so much more. They deserve adventure. Today is hard. Tomorrow may be different. The sun is welcoming. I *hope* soon my new life as a healed mother will begin. You can heal. This too shall pass. Don't give up.

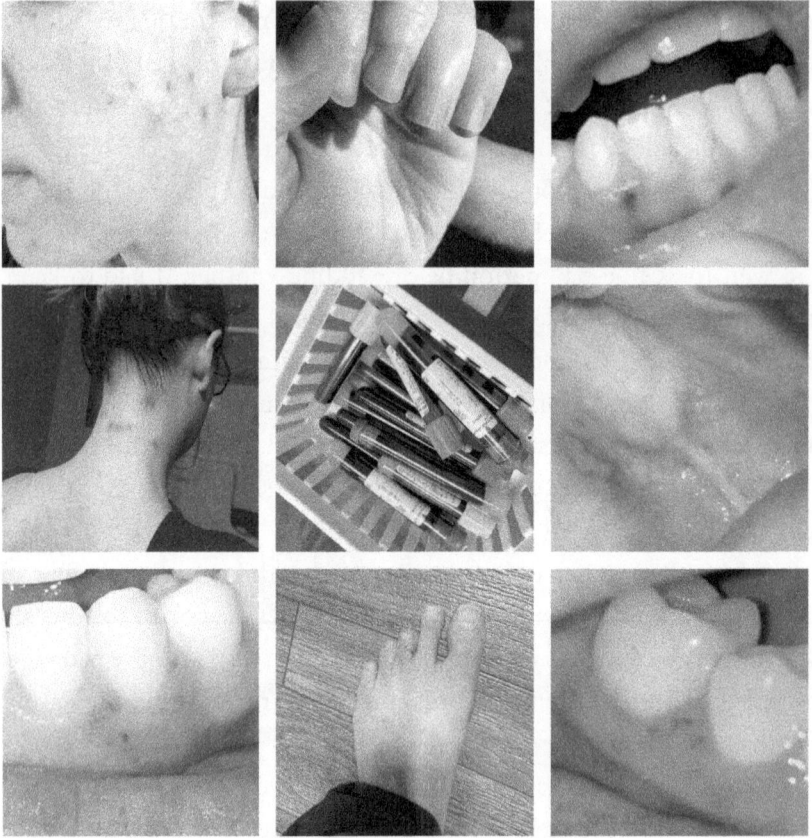

The world I enjoyed so much is now too loud, too bright, and too overstimulating. I watch as the blood pools in my feet as my heart races . . . I cannot breathe.

December 7, 2021

Today was cold with slow snow showers. We went outside and I did some things in the snow with the kids. We did a little sledding. My mom still helps me a lot. She comes over and folds my laundry and helps with chores without even asking me. Because of her, there is usually always a snowman every year. She brightens up my life and doesn't even realize it. On my darkest days, her presence has kept me going. *I don't know what I would do without her.* Sometimes she has mild symptoms that are similar to mine. I always wonder if something we have is *genetic* or if maybe she has had a mold exposure. My son, too, has some similarities. Part of me fighting so hard for my answers is so that if something starts happening to them we will have the answers and they won't have to go through what I did.

*** *** ***

We did a little sledding today, and my mom and I built a snow mountain with Russell. It was very hard for me physically, but I did it. I felt nauseated a lot today but kept my spirits up by wrapping Christmas presents. I often wonder if the nausea is from the fatty liver. That has been this way since my surgery complications. I love Christmas. My *hope* is that by next Christmas my health has improved.

If I wanted to, I could make Christmas a dark time because that's when my health regressed a few years ago. But I *choose* not to. I *choose* to see the beauty in every day and a *promise* for better days to come.

*** *** ***

Today I put my health issues in a box and burned them in our fire pit outside. I am giving these worries to God: mold illness, aluminum toxicity, iron deficiency, high ferritin, SIBO, leaky gut, PCOS, MTHFR, COMT, oxidative stress damage, free radical damage, cell damage, mitochondrial damage, POTS, dysautonomia, hypothyroidism concerns, aura migraines, vestibular migraines, high inflammation, hormone imbalance, and nervous system dysregulation. I did the same thing with my worries of missed diagnosis: Lyme disease/tick-borne illness, colon cancer, MCAS.

I hear . . . *"Don't worry, my dear one. I am here with you. I will not abandon*
you.
Never . . . will . . . I."

119

10

The Dark Shadow of My Dreams

December 12^{th, 2021}

These dreams never felt like dreams.
They felt real.

Recently, the dark shadow has returned in my dreams at night. This always seems to happen when I draw *closer* to God. And it disappears when I feel *further* away from God. I experienced this dream often before my children were born and a few times after. The dream is always the *same*, but the only thing that changes is the location that I am presently in. I am always in my room. I see myself lying in bed as if having an out-of-body experience. First, it was in my room at my home growing up. Then, it was the room when we lived in the trailer. Later, my room in the country. And now, in our present home.

THE DARK SHADOW OF MY DREAMS

He is in my doorway . . .

I see myself lying in my bed, asleep. The dark figure stands still . . . *he stares at me*. Then, as if skipping a scene in a movie . . . I see him right next to my sleeping form. He is hovering over me. *Just a black shadow . . . a figure with no face.* I can feel myself writhing around in bed, struggling to escape from him. But the harder I try . . . the more *I cannot move.* I can hear and feel myself *screaming,* but no sound escapes my lips . . . because I am trapped inside of my dream. I realize that the person who is writhing around and screaming is actually myself outside of my body. I watch as *the shadow figure comes closer and closer* to my sleeping form. I can see my husband lying next to me . . . I *scream* at him to *wake me up,* but he cannot hear me. I try to shake him, but when I move my arms are so heavy. *I cannot wake him.* No one can hear my screams and my body is frozen in time. As the figure draws *closer* I feel myself gasping for breath . . . I *cannot* evade him. I have *no control. I cannot escape . . .*

When I finally pulled myself from this dream I would be gasping for air and extreme terror would wash over me, keeping me awake. If I awoke groggy, I would be ripped back into the nightmare and the dark figure would hover over me, getting closer and closer to my face again.

He never had a face . . . just a *shadow* . . . I could not see his face . . . but he could see mine.

If able to stay awake, I would always say the Lord's Prayer and beg God to protect me. It wouldn't be until much later, during the darkest times of my life, when this figure would return.

I often wonder if it is from some repressed trauma from my childhood . . . I researched sleep paralysis and spiritual attack . . . I wondered if it *was* some form of spiritual attack.

The counseling sessions with my priest began about a year after my physical illness started. I brought up the dream because it bothered me so much. He confirmed that it *could* be a spiritual attack. He asked about my history, and I told him that I may have experienced sexual abuse as a small child, but I did not remember it. My mother experienced similar dreams years ago. She was abused by her cousin . . . who took his own life on her wedding day. My priest was always very curious about this. He told me that sometimes something as extreme as him ending his life on her wedding day can evoke a generational curse. He gave me a prayer to say if the dream ever happened again . . .

"In the Holy name of Jesus, I ask for freedom from any curse or bond put upon my mother and her family by *****. Jesus, free me from this bond. Amen."

Afterward, he blessed our home and we prayed over my health struggles.

Oddly, when the figure would *not* return in my dreams it correlated with the darkest moments of my daily life. But the times that I felt I was becoming *closer* to God was when he would return.

Whatever it was . . . I did not like it. It was not welcome and never is.

December 15, 2021

This is the me that nobody sees.
The tightness in my chest makes it so hard to breathe.
The burning of my flesh that I cannot escape.
Was it something I ate?
Something absorbed into my skin?
Perhaps . . . whatever air that I breathed in?
Or mold on a surface?
An air freshener?
Dust?
God. This is endless . . .

The invisible nightmare is worse.
My heart races, it skips a beat.
I lose control of myself.
The room spins.
I feel like falling over . . .
Like I'm constantly drunk . . . but not the fun part.

Close to a panic attack, but it never was one.
Am I losing my mind?

The extension of my gut and the ripping inside, as if something is tearing me apart.

The internal tremors as my body shakes . . .
The overstimulation is hard to take.
The nightmare that I wake up to every day.
But don't forget to be grateful.
And have positive thoughts . . .
Because if you do not THEN ALL PROGRESS IS LOST.
The blinding migraines.
The ringing in my ears, as if my head is hooked up to an electrical current.
The blinding lights.
The constant "I can't breathe," "my heart is acting up," or worse "Mommy can't,
she is sick again . . . "

And the PTSD from feeling near death over and over again.
And the anger inside—that I try to let go—toward all who didn't help me and left
me blanketed with a diagnosis that's near impossible to heal from.
Why didn't anyone help me?
Why didn't they listen?
And the thoughts of how so many others are going through this . . .

The sad reality that I face because, after research, I suspected the biggest reasons
for my illness the first summer I became sick.
Now three years later finally diagnosed with them.

The blanket was draped over me and I am worse off now than I would have been
then.
Now the reactions are starting to show on my skin.
Making me suspicious of mast cell activation. But it's all from chronic
inflammation.

So now what I will do is put them all in a box.
All of my worries.
My frustrations.
All of my fears.

WAVES

The past hurts and the people that I must forgive.

I put these all in a box and give them to God.
Because at this point only he can carry me through these trials.
. . . and give me strength, for all of mine is lost.

I will continue to enjoy the small joys of each day, the small accomplishments.
I will not lose hope.
Because all hope is never lost.

Blanketed by POTS.

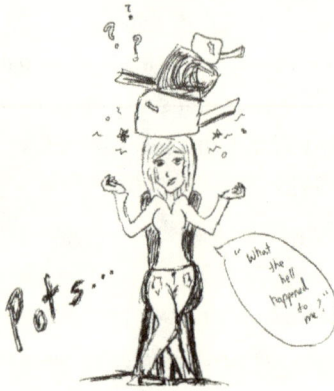

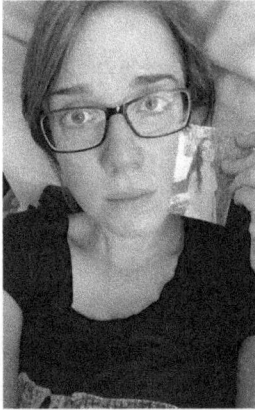

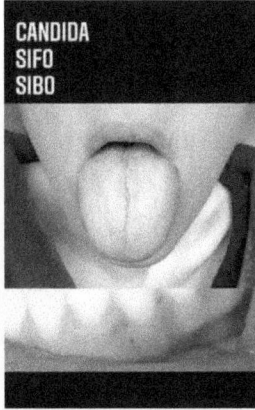

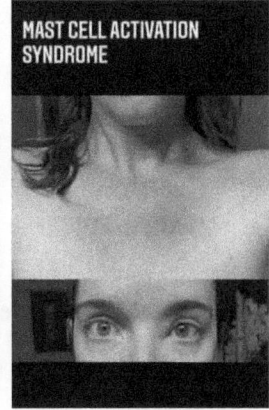

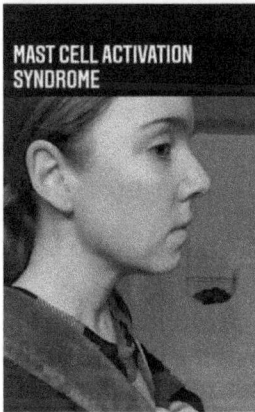

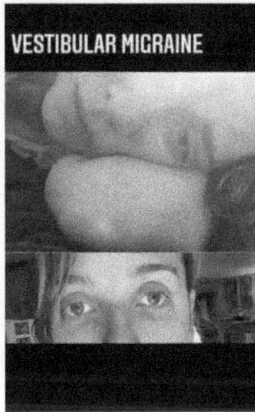

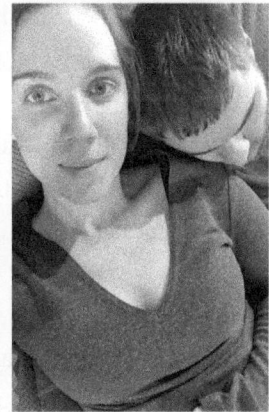

Things that were said to me by doctors, mostly when I was alone: "Your blood pressure is like this because you are at the doctor's office." (Later it was the same at home.) "These blood sugar levels are only concerning if you are having symptoms." (I told them I was and they sent me home anyway.) "Sometimes these things just happen and there is nothing we can do to help your condition." "Well . . . you look healthy." "Why are you even here?" "You will grow out of this . . . you are a tall girl." "You are too young to be sick. Your labs are normal . . . oh, and I like your glasses." "You are young, healthy, and vibrant. All of your labs are normal." "You look so normal." "You need a psychiatric specialist." "Mayo will find nothing." "You are a strong, healthy girl." "Have you ever considered this could all be in your head?" The doctors treat me differently when my husband is with me. I don't like going alone.

I am *grateful* for:

- my husband
- how well my children played today
- the nice weather
- my neighbor's kindness
- my mom
- our ability to start replacing things
- deep breathing
- a warm home
- the ability to afford healthy food
- God and his love

After writing all that I did today, I had a good cry and meditated in the sauna. I listened to *The Chosen* soundtrack. I feel more restored and as if another light has lit within me, giving me the drive to fight another day.

January 8, 2022

You can develop myocarditis from a virus, a parasite, mold, inflammation issues, fungus/candida, and sometimes vaccines. I have mold, fungus/candida, inflammation, high ferritin, fatty liver, and am fighting a virus on top of it all. Lord God, please help me get through this flare.

I am starting to get concerned that this is more than just a usual flare. I try not to, but when I regress like this I worry that it will be my new baseline. When I bend I feel more breathless than normal. I am so weak, and eating or drinking fluids is not improving my symptoms. I don't want to worry Tim, because I know I have been evaluated for myocarditis in the past and it was negative. I *hope* this is all related to detox and is an immune flare from a recent trigger. I have been on a mold protocol for a while now and am doing infrared sauna treatments.

We got lucky and found a really nice one for an affordable cost online. It was brand new when they put it in a hotel gym, but the entire room was closed because of COVID, so it just sat unused for two years and they decided to sell it. There was something minor wrong with it, but Tim can fix anything, so it wasn't a problem.

It's so hard to know if what I am experiencing is ever serious or not. My symptoms daily are hard enough. I don't like getting reevaluated when things get worse than my baseline, but I don't know what to do. Something happens to me that I don't understand when I get hit with an illness accompanied by a fever. I feel like I develop recurring fevers for 1–2 months after an acute illness. I always *pray* this is not my new baseline.

11

Hope and Perseverance

January 17, 2022

I am still here. I am still fighting. I go between beginning to heal, wishing for death, and then when I feel close to death I beg for God to save me . . . even if I have to be sick forever . . . just so my children do not lose their mother.

W e built a snowman today. The weather was very nice and it was the most amount of physical exertion I have been able to do in the last month. A vestibular migraine occurred on Christmas Day, and two days later I was hit with a virus that has since set my POTS symptoms into overdrive. Definitely a *"bucket overflower"* with the amount my immune system is already dealing with since I have been doing the protocol for mold. More than likely MCAS (mast cell activation syndrome) and my newest diagnosis of CIRS (chronic inflammatory response syndrome) are partly to blame, along with the acute virus.

I'm also working on something new. It's called brain rewiring from limbic system impairment. Our limbic system helps regulate specific behaviors we use daily. I am doing some minor things right now on my own. The challenge is to have fewer worrying thoughts and lower responses to my symptoms. Repetitive constant thoughts have to be rerouted.

I have been practicing visualizations, with the main focus on walking with God and God healing me. I imagine the simple things that I will do when I am healed. I use positive memories too. If things go according to plan, I will start a six-month program to help retrain these systems and connect to how I was before all of the trauma.

The diagnoses of CIRS, mold, and MCAS gives closure but also causes my mind to race. The impossible feeling of ever being able to avoid these mycotoxins, replace things that were in our exposed home, and the restrictive food is *overwhelming*. How can someone replace things in their home when they are spending so much money already because of poor health? God . . . the food. I know that I am stuck in a pattern of negative thinking. My mind is hard to slow and turn off. I need to heal my mind, and, possibly, the body will follow.

I am *grateful* for:

- the ability to build a snowman
- being alive
- being there for my children
- a warm home
- healthy food
- clean water

I will heal. My body is listening. Let's tell it what we want and what it must do. Choose your thoughts carefully.

January 24, 2024
HOPE
"We boast in the hope of the glory of God. Not only so, but we also glory in our sufferings, because we know that suffering produces perseverance; perseverance, character; and character, hope. And hope does not put us to shame, because God's love has been poured out into our hearts through the Holy Spirit, who has been given to us." Romans 5:2–5 NIV

* * *

What suffering have you experienced that has produced *perseverance, character,* and *hope?*

The daily suffering and fears with chronic illness. Feeling out of control.

My health coach has told me that one of my strongest character traits is *perseverance.* This Bible reading connected with me so much. I am still *persevering* daily and *hope* for a positive change soon. In the past, my journal entries were so simple. The little things in life felt much bigger.

I was always in more of a calm state. On my own, I am working on ways to heal my limbic system/neuroplasticity and dysregulated nervous system through meditation, grounding, and DNRS (Dynamic Neural Retraining System). Following this trauma, there are PTSD symptoms that need to heal. I am not perfect, and these thoughts are hard to control. *Will I ever get better? This is hopeless. Why do I feel this way? Why did this happen to me?* These thoughts trap me in a constant victim state that I am trying to break free from. *Healing trauma is so hard, though, when you are still experiencing it.* There are constant thoughts of uncertainty as to whether or not we are on the right path . . . because so many things were missed before.

I still wonder about Lyme, Bartonella, and Babesia. I remember researching so much the first year on Bartonella . . . I thought my head might explode. It could have been transmitted by either a tick or a cat bite. I have had plenty of cat bites in my life and odd stretch marks that came out of nowhere after a bite years ago. But the testing has been negative . . . I'm trying to put *faith* in this new doctor and *trust* that we have the answers. I often wonder if what I am doing is enough. I battle a lot of thoughts.

The mind is very hard to control. I use prayer often and try to leave all of my worries to God. But sometimes *I wonder if it's his voice telling me that I don't have all of the answers and not my own.* I try to channel my negative thoughts and change them to positive ones and I have been talking less about my daily symptoms to Tim.

I feel closer to God lately, but sometimes this darkness still hangs over me. I try to stay in the light.

* * *

Russell and Eliot are both looking forward to the new *Sonic* movie. We are happy to take them to the theater to see it. COVID cases are still high, but will they ever not be? We wouldn't be overly concerned if I wasn't having these health issues . . . high ferritin, high oxidative stress, and mold issues affecting my immune system. The thing about COVID is that nothing has really changed for us. My health issues started before COVID, so even then I was taking more care to try and avoid illness because we didn't know what was wrong with me.

Tim had COVID last March. Thankfully, it didn't affect him much, but he did have loss of smell for a while. I'm surprised I never got terribly ill. I was with him every day. I saw some family members last month and whatever that was definitely tanked my immune system for a while. I was negative for COVID and strep. I had the worst POTS symptoms, and my GI issues have increased since then. My abdominal pain is a lot worse too.

The mold protocol diet/sauna/binders/antifungals were increasing symptoms prior to the acute illness. I originally felt this was because of *die-off* . . . but then when the symptoms are prolonged, a *Herxheimer* reaction from die-off seems unlikely. When targeting mold, candida, and fungi, a Jarisch-Herxheimer reaction is an adverse response to the toxins released by bacteria and fungi when they are killed by antibiotics and antifungal medications. Symptoms of candida/mold die-off can be frightening because they come on suddenly and make you feel very bad, very fast.

Later, when trying to improve my GI issues and issues with acute viral overload, my primary doctor and I decided I would try ivermectin because it can help with other viral infections and parasites, both of which are suspected in my situation. I didn't have any negative side effects from the ivermectin, but no major improvements either.

I am very careful with the things I choose to put into my body, and I did have somewhat of an internal battle about whether or not I should even try the ivermectin. The last medication I was on was an antibiotic called neomycin for methane dominant SIBO. I had to stop that after only two days because I was developing terrible tinnitus. I couldn't even listen to my music on my headphones anymore because the ringing in my ears was so loud. That really worried me.

I went on the antioxidants CoQ10 and NAC, and over time the ringing did improve. I was worried it would be permanent, and the medication (neomycin) has been put on my allergy list.

Many people in my chronic illness group are developing long-haul COVID, which is basically POTS/dysautonomia. Some claim it happened after COVID, while others say it happened after the new vaccine. Whatever this *syndrome* is, it is affecting people very *similarly* to how I have been affected since 2018. From all the testing I have done, I really believe it's a combination of mitochondrial damage, cell damage, inflammation, and high oxidative stress levels. These are the things that show up in my testing as a result of my specific underlying factors. It makes me wonder how many long-haulers also have mold, Lyme disease, or heavy metals hurting their cells and immune system. *The perfect storm.*

I feel like figuring this out wouldn't be terribly hard. A program should be put in place to help patients find the underlying conditions and treat them. Then these long-hauler syndromes could reverse. Our medical system is failing us. Finding answers should be better organized and covered under insurance. There is a time and place for medication, but not everyone wants to just suppress their symptoms. Some want to discover the cause and heal. The body *can* heal. It seems no one wants to do the hard work, and insurance companies deny everything, so we are left chronically ill and suffering.

February 13, 2022
  I am *grateful*:

- that I made it to my nephew's party
- that I was able to go to the farm
- that my children are healthy

- for my husband's dedication
- for my mother's help
- that Terri listens to me
- that I was able to visit with friends
- for nice walks
- that I may be getting help with lowering ferritin
- for the option for ozone therapy
- for happy past memories
- for smiles and laughter
- for Annabelle's company

12

Angry and Depleted

I am still here since my regression from the acute illness. It must not have caused myocarditis. My symptoms have improved some. Most people would think I may have had COVID, but all the tests were negative and, in all reality, with an already compromised immune system/high ferritin, any virus would cause cytokines to spike . . .

I think that is what happened.

I have been trying to do the sauna more often again now that my lungs aren't suffering as much and the tightness in my chest has improved. Tomorrow I have my first ozone therapy session to help improve the fungal infection and mold overgrowth. I'm very *grateful* to have this option since I have mold, SIFO, and systemic candida. We need to wipe it out.

I see a hematologist, as well, in March since I tested positive for one hemochromatosis gene. My local functional medicine doctor suggested this because she and my out-of-state functional medicine doctor functional medicine can't seem to agree on whether my high ferritin is coming from *acute* inflammation or from the retaining of iron from the blood transfusions. I feel like the highest likelihood is because of the blood transfusions. I know I had an injury during surgery, but my blood has been so thick since the infusions and my out-of-state doctor is telling me that even with the one gene I could still retain iron from blood transfusions. She wants me to do therapeutic phlebotomies to lower the amount of ferritin in my body and thin my blood. My ferritin is close to 500 and before all of these complications with iron overload it was at 7.

I don't know how I feel about seeing another hematologist. Honestly, it has surprised me how little they seem to care about ferritin levels. I won't be surprised if they don't have a solid answer for me either. My out-of-state doctor has a hematologist on their end who has confirmed that the issue in my case is from the blood transfusions and Secondary hemochromatosis. I can't get orders for a therapeutic phlebotomy from out of state easily. It may not be covered by insurance. My local functional medicine doctor has to be on the same page . . . so I have to go through this process.

It's difficult when doctors don't agree. I never meant for it to be this complicated. I always just meant to find someone local to help us. If this is indeed the problem then I will have to do phlebotomies (blood draws) to lower it. I will not donate my blood, though. I am still concerned that I may have Lyme, and I don't want to give this disease to anyone else. I will find a way to make sure they throw the blood away afterward.

If the levels are from inflammation alone, that is still a problem since high ferritin and inflammation can lead to high cytokine issues. It's complicated, but I understand it. I am just so ready for this to be done. I don't want to struggle anymore doing simple tasks. I want to move on from this.

I am trying to be patient and *trust* the process and God's timing, but I am feeling a little angry and depleted. I fall back so often with my thoughts. Every day starts out with debilitating symptoms. If I get any reprieve in the evening, a new day just starts everything all over again.

I can't even imagine waking up feeling refreshed and standing up feeling normal. I don't remember what it feels like to have energy or not feel overstimulated all day. I can't remember what it feels like to breathe normally most of the time. I live life feeling as if I am choking, dying, or having strokes all the time.

* * *

I feel so trapped in this body. I want to do so many things . . . My symptoms make it impossible to do anything out of the house while supervising my children. It can be isolating. My son Eliot doesn't even know that I am sick. Russell remembers how I was before all of this.

The other day when Tim and I were talking about my chronic health issues, Eliot stopped me, confused. "Wait, you are sick? What?"

Well, at least I know I'm doing a good job of not stressing them out over it every day.

Russell calls it my "*chronicle*" illness . . . as if I am from some type of a famous fiction novel series. I can't help but chuckle every time I hear him say this.

I am so very *grateful* for my children, but it can also be so hard breaking up fights all day long and taking care of them and entertaining them all day every day. But the thought of being here alone is terrible too. I at least have distractions all day. This is the best option right now for our circumstances. I don't know what the future will look like, but we make our decisions year by year. I love that I can homeschool. I just wish I felt better while doing it.

* * *

I have attempted more walks with my mom. She tells me often that her vision is getting worse. This worries me so much. I feel powerless in how I can help her.

She comes over almost daily and it's very challenging for me to have internal worries of something like the cat bite or mold causing her issues. I want to fix it for her, but I can't even seem to fix myself . . .

* * *

I get so defeated with the environmental and food reactions. My out-of-state functional medicine doctor says she feels my reactions are worse because of the high ferritin. It creates so many more inflammatory issues. I feel she is right because I've been increasingly more sensitive since my surgery. I just don't know what to do because my local functional medicine doctor agrees that the ferritin is causing issues, but she thinks it's from an inflammatory factor and should go down on its own as we lower my mold levels . . . but it's been months and it hasn't lowered at all.

There is so much stress, too, with this mold illness. It has been recommended that we replace most porous items. Do you know how impossible that is? My doctor said she cannot tell us to replace everything at once, but it might help to try replacing some things. The Shoemaker Policy for mold says to replace *everything*. How can people afford to replace all of their things while extremely ill and suffering? If you do buy new, you have no idea what warehouse a brand-new couch was in before making it to the store. There has to be a level of mycotoxins on most things.

Is the problem really even mold, or is it your immune system going crazy from something else, like Lyme? I've even read about people doing mold avoidance. They leave their home and everything in it and they travel in an RV or sleep in the back of a truck to *heal*. But how could I ever uproot my family again when my older son is still having grief over the loss of our last home? And then my doctor told me that even if I do buy new I have to worry about VOCs (volatile organic compounds) in the products, because when you have CIRS your immune system will react to those things as well. So that's great. I was looking at new organic beds. We can't afford them. So what we have done is gotten rid of some things and used ozone on a lot of the others. I had to go through a lengthy process of stripping all of our clothing too. This is exhausting. Sometimes I feel like I am stuck in something that is killing me slowly. And ozone can kill you, too, so be careful with that.

This entire experience is so heartbreaking. I look at things now in a much different way. I cannot even be normal anymore because I have all of these things I have to avoid while I am healing. I can't even be around certain fragrances anymore, or certain toxins like cigarette smoke. My heart will race, I get itchy, and I feel like I'm going to have a brain aneurysm.

As far as we know, there are no other mold issues where we are living now . . . but it's always in the back of my head. If this is *really* why I am so sick, it has destroyed so much of my life. I just want my life back.

I have read, too, that some people with mold illness will leave their home and everything in it. Everything. And they are still sick. Some people remediate their house, but they do not replace any furniture and somehow they are still able to get it out of their body and heal. That makes me wonder if, for some, it isn't even mold keeping them sick but Lyme.

I'm so frustrated with how long this process takes. The suffering is extreme. I want to take my kids to the zoo on my own again. I want to take them shopping and go out to eat and drive with no symptoms. I had it so good before. My life was so perfect and I didn't even realize it. I still had things to complain about. Sometimes it feels as if God no longer hears me. If God can take all of this away, why hasn't he? *What am I supposed to learn from this experience? Who am I supposed to help?*

My dreams of what I wanted to experience with my children are fleeting before my eyes. They are not going to be this little forever and have a *fraction* of the mom that I was *meant* to be. *Trusting in God's timing is hard when the time they are with me is so short.* It would be so wonderful to be able to do the things I used to be able to do with Russell before becoming sick.

Please, God, let me heal by spring. Please.

* * *

I really *hope* there is something to this ferritin like my out-of-state functional medicine doctor says. I have never experienced a normal ferritin level. It was either extremely low or extremely high. She says that secondary hemochromatosis from infusions can cause CIRS, and when the liver has to deal with all of that excess iron it makes the body in a state where CIRS and MCAS increase because the liver cannot expel the excess iron. Since the liver can't expel all of the toxins, my body is more sensitive to the food and environmental triggers. She feels that lowering my ferritin through phlebotomies will help all of this, and killing the candida should put me into remission. POTS will reverse. God, I *hope* so. This makes sense to me . . . especially because I didn't have some of these issues until after the transfusion complications.

Sometimes I really wonder why I had to have such a *failure* of a surgery. If it would have gone perfectly, I do not feel I would be dealing with these increased symptoms or fatty liver again. I'm sure a lot of people would think that I made a terrible decision. But when I was fainting with most periods, it made it very difficult to keep trying with the oral iron. I tried very hard for a very long time to heal naturally. I really did. And I thought I picked a safe surgeon.

My local functional medicine doctor—who is working with the out-of-state functional medicine doctor—doesn't seem so sure about the theory of the secondary hemochromatosis and blood transfusions causing the retaining of ferritin. She thinks a secondary form is unlikely because that usually occurs right after an infusion. I feel that this theory is a likely possibility, but we will see what the hematologist says.

I get nervous about how my body will react to the phlebotomies, even if it *will* help long term. With POTS you already have low blood volume in your head. But my blood is so thick . . . maybe this would bring relief.

Honestly, I wish I didn't have to think about these things anymore. I want to think about nothing but nonsense and plan fun gatherings with friends. I don't want to suffer anymore and try to be my own doctor all of the time. I'm tired of researching and contemplating what the best decision is. I just want relief.

* * *

Yesterday I spoke with an excision specialist for missed endometriosis. I don't have any plans for surgery, but if I ever need a surgeon in the future I am making sure I research one thoroughly enough to feel confident that the surgeon won't hurt me, while also respecting my boundaries for therapies.

He stopped me mid-conversation and asked if either myself or my husband were in the medical field. Both Tim and I laughed and said *no*, but he told us we both sound like we could be doctors. We have had to become *"doctors"* throughout this process . . . we had to *learn* and *research*

139

in order to get *answers* because no one else could. This is not the first time I have been told that I sound like a doctor. Some of you may laugh when you read this . . . but I am serious when I say I had to become my own doctor throughout most of this process. I didn't ask for this. This was the hand I was dealt.

I told him that I was diagnosed with CIRS and MCAS. He was very interested in my case. Some women with CIRS have MCAS because of the histamine response to certain hormonal fluctuations. He said it's very concerning since he has seen cases rising drastically in the last ten years. I was relieved to know that he was aware of this condition.

I found this surgeon online through a group for missed endometriosis and scar tissue correction. If I ever need someone who actually does the job right, he is my first pick. I still experience a lot of pain.

At the end of our conversation, he told me that endometriosis was missed in 90% of cases where the woman had a previous exploratory surgery before finding him . . . 90%. That's huge. And so very sad.

February 20, 2022

I am *grateful* for:

- more answers
- more understanding
- my children's joy in the simple things
- being able to call Terri
- a surgeon who actually cares
- my mother being so close
- Tim's laughter and smile and how his eyes light up
- a warm home
- no mold in my home
- my mom quitting smoking
- my dog's comfort

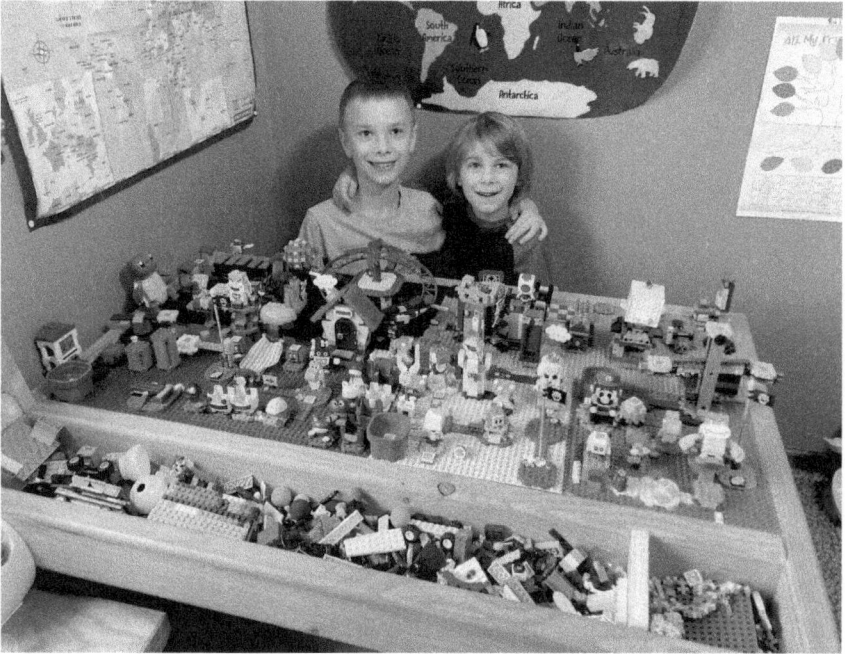

The boys are building a Mario Lego set tonight. It will be fun to set up a permanent table and add on to the Mario World. Tim is a talented woodworker. It's so nice that we are able to build happy memories for them from the comfort of our home.

13

I Just Want to Scream

February 22, 2022

I woke up this morning to Russell crying.

"Mom, you are not blessed. Why can't God fix you so that you can be better?" He had a deep sadness in his eyes and confusion written all over his face.

He cried, "I want my *real* mommy back, the one *before* you were sick. Why did we move into the yellow house if it had mold?"

He thinks that is the only reason that I am sick. He wants me to be better, and he expressed a lot of sadness.

He finished by saying, "I love you more than anyone, and I want you to be a real mom before you go to heaven."

I don't know what caused these feelings today. He must be internalizing things he has overheard. My heart breaks for him.

I *tried* so hard for so long to keep the reality of my health issues from my children. I tried to make it look like everything was okay. I still do, for the most part, but this has been going on for so long now. Sometimes we have no choice but to take the boys with us to the doctor's office . . . and Russell is smart. He listens to everything the doctor says and wants to learn more.

I feel that most of my health issues *should be* kept from my children at this age . . . but I also feel that creating a false sense of reality can be damaging.

142

If things do crumble it makes it very hard to climb out from the rubble.

I feel that I have failed in protecting him from these big emotions that he is feeling. I tried very hard to keep him in the dark concerning my health. It makes me want to heal even more. I am trying so hard. I grieve often over the loss of myself and I know that he does too.

February 23, 2022

I have been learning that the limbic system can become impaired by severe infection, toxicity, inflammation, trauma, or stress. When this happens, the limbic system can maladapt, producing an exaggerated stress response that results in the inappropriate activation of the immune, endocrine, and autonomic nervous system functions.

The limbic system controls emotion, motivation, memory, and behavioral regulation. The key components are the amygdala, thalamus, hippocampus, and hypothalamus. This system is a complex network of brain structures and plays an important role in regulating various aspects of human behavior and emotion. If the limbic system is impaired from chronic infection or toxicity, it can cause chronic health conditions. I *hope* my doctor has found all of the underlying infections so that it will be easier to heal this system.

Positive thoughts to focus on after telling your limbic system to stop:

- Read a novel or poem
- Listen to happy music
- Dance
- Go through happy family photos
- Make a poster with places you have visited
- Make a wish list
- Watch videos with exotic destinations
- Watch family videos
- Watch funny pets
- Write affirmations

- Read a motivational quote
- Paint or draw
- Do yoga or stretches
- Jump
- Call a friend
- Cook
- Have a cup of tea
- Watch a movie
- Take a bath
- Take a walk
- Write a gratitude journal
- Hug yourself
- Tell yourself a compliment while looking in the mirror
- Do breath work
- Epsom salt foot soak with face mask
- Play a game with your kids

Exercise and analyze your thoughts:

- Set an alarm for every 50–60 minutes. "Are my thoughts and actions supportive?" "What am I thinking?" "What am I focusing on?" "How am I acting?"
- Then set a timer for two minutes and listen to your thoughts.
- After that, set another timer for two minutes and write all of your thoughts down.

"I love you, God. I need you. Allow your Holy Spirit to guide my mind. My thoughts. My actions. Be with me always. And forever. Do not let me fear or crumble. Do not allow the darkness to win. Carry me, Lord—my Savior—as we walk this path together."

Gratitude:

- I am alive
- My children are healthy
- I have a warm home
- Fresh organic food
- Option for ozone therapy
- My feelings are heard
- God, always
- My husband's embrace
- My mother's love
- That I am going to heal

Actions and behaviors around health:
What do you think you have to do to heal?

- No sugar
- No grains
- Lower histamine
- Low oxalate
- Low salicylate
- Avoid certain environments
- Supplements
- Bright light avoidance
- Pressure change avoidance
- Organic food only
- Replace all furniture

Why do I believe this?

- Because of past reactions
- Research and groups
- Protocols
- Doctor recommendations

Why do I feel that I have to do this?

- To heal
- To not experience symptoms

Does this belief get me to where I want to be?

- It has not

Many people heal from chronic symptoms without avoiding all of these things.

February 24, 2022

Hello. It's me again . . . I've been so foggy and sleepy off and off. I know I write this a lot. Hopefully soon there will be a shift. Recently I have been practicing more positive thoughts and limbic system exercises. Part of my exercises through my health coach is journaling things that I am *grateful* for and thinking often of old positive memories. I decided to go back and dig into my past journals to read about the happy times in my life. I went to open the fireproof safe where I have kept the last 15 years of my journals . . . and *all of them were covered in mold.* One of the journals has a leather cover and, because of the lack of fresh air in the firesafe box, it had started to mold.

I don't understand how the thing that has possibly destroyed my entire life is now destroying the last 15 years of my happy memories. I am just at a loss. I won't throw them away. I will have to ozone them and put them somewhere where I'm not constantly breathing the mold in. But I can't even go back right now and read my past happy memories. *How is it possible that so much can be destroyed by one thing?*

To shift my sadness . . . I will talk about something else. The weather yesterday was beautiful. I felt alive again, even though the heat still makes my heart race and jump around. WHAT ARE THE POSITIVES? *Focus on the positives . . .*

Russell tried Tae Kwon Do with the homeschooling group for the first

146

time on Monday and he *loved it.* He ran around the room excitedly when we got home. "This was the *best* day of my life."

I am so *grateful* for Amanda. She drives my son to every practice. She has been so kind to me. I never could have expected someone like her to come into my life and be so understanding and kind. She brightens up my life in so many ways without even realizing it.

When I was still healthy, I had set up a Tae Kwon Do session for Russell, but I had to cancel it when my health issues began. I never thought I would be able to take him. Because of her kindness he can finally participate.

I have noticed a shift in his anger and sadness too . . . his Tae Kwon Do master is helping him in more ways than he understands . . . Russell needed this and I am so *grateful.*

March 25, 2022

I am really not doing very well with this pretending like I'm healthy thing. How do you do this when you feel so sick? Every part of my body is so affected by this. My eyes. My hearing. My gut. Nervous system. Heart. Detox pathways. Hormones. But I am trying to rewire my brain.

Will this ever end? STOP.

* * *

I have had a really hard morning. It started last evening with bad stomach pains. It progressed today with really awful breathlessness. I have felt extremely dizzy and am having difficulty breathing. Just awful. I am not sure why I have the increased breathlessness lately. I still have high ferritin, despite the ozone therapy and mold protocol that I have been doing. The pain seems to be coming from my stomach and liver. The pressure is really awful today. I don't like to think too much about the cause anymore, but when my symptoms are this severe and long-lasting, I worry that something more acute is wrong with me. It's so hard to tell. I'm trying to keep myself from worrying over it.

It's very windy today. I am still unsure if the ferritin issues are coming from inflammation, but I have a lot of pain in the liver and lower/upper abdomen. I just wish we could understand and fix the inflammation if that is what is causing it. Every time I see my local functional medicine doctor, she has me stick out my tongue and says the line is a sign of inflammation, but she doesn't know where it's located. I hear a lot from her about how she can *see* signs of inflammation.

Lately I just feel very lost. I have not had improvement with the breathing issues, swollen lymph nodes, and sore throats. Ever since my surgery I have had so many sore throats, and before then I had so many mouth ulcers and cystic acne all over my neck. I'm always fighting something. The mold made sense, but why am I not having improvement? I am doing the protocol. I am not cheating on food. I haven't for over a year now . . .

I'm so tired of going back to the unknowns when I don't have improvement with protocols. The reality is so difficult to tolerate. I'm not sure why everything has worsened so much since October/December. The only new therapies have been from the mold protocol. I just don't understand. I know you can have *herxheimer* reactions, but eventually there should be *improvement*. I feel like everyone blames everything on detox or *herxing*. I just want to scream.

14

Trying to Find the Root Cause

April 30, 2022

My husband has been struggling because of my chronic health issues. The finances drown him. He feels alone and isolated with this burden. When I try to talk to him about things he shuts down. Sometimes *I feel like I'm the burden*. He tells me that I am not . . . but it's hard to not feel like one. I know he doesn't mean to shut down when I try to talk with him about my feelings or conditions. It's just so much to take in. He is trying to provide for us and he is there for me for every appointment. I don't blame him for having trouble handling all of it at an emotional level.

I have struggled with feelings of being a burden since the *beginning*. At my lowest times, I battled thoughts like it would be better if I was just dead. When those feelings are really bad, whispers sneak in like, *A funeral would be cheaper*. The whispers can become so loud . . .

Tim doesn't have a lot of people to talk to, either, about what we are going through. It's really difficult to tell people what is wrong with me. Sometimes I feel like some of these conditions are too unbelievable and they embarrass Tim. No one really knows what is wrong with me. We mostly just tell those who ask that I have POTS, but most people don't even know what that means. Tim and I have gone through many ups and downs and have had to learn so much together to understand all of it.

Because of the stress, Tim struggles with chronic acid reflux (GERD). He originally tried the medical route to solve it, but just ended up in a worse condition and was diagnosed with SIBO (small intestinal bacterial overgrowth) and gut dysbiosis. He has struggled with stomach issues for many years, and I have often wondered if gut dysbiosis was connected to his excess worry. Even before my health issues began, he struggled. His issues worsened because of my regressing health and the finances on top of that.

We have not asked for any help concerning my health issues. We sold our home so that we could afford my care. We were hoping that would be enough to get my health better because we could then afford outside treatments.

I understand that it must be hard to see your wife sick. I can't imagine seeing Tim's health regressing like mine has and not being able to fix it.

The feelings of isolation are difficult. I can't talk to my husband about certain things because I would just make his own conditions worse. He is the only provider in the family and I have to run everything by him before moving forward with my care.

It's so unfair how expensive it is to get better. It is such a *burden*. The medical system is set up for the chronically ill to fail. There are no programs to help us get better because of the lack of understanding in these types of diagnoses. There is *only* symptom management.

* * *

I just found out yesterday that the mold level in my body is now very low. So the protocol is *working* . . . but I am still sick. My local functional medicine doctor feels that because we have not seen extensive improvement that this was *not* the main underlying cause. She said it was something that built up and caused damage and issues but, unfortunately, there is usually *more than one cause.*

We have to do more extensive testing. I am considering a comprehensive test for Lyme, but it's so expensive. My doctor is assuring me that we are targeting my immune system, which is the best thing you can do anyway for chronic Lyme. First, we are moving forward with a chelated heavy metal panel, a comprehensive stool test, and an immune system panel to check immune function, cytokine levels, and oxidative stress levels. She feels these blood tests will be more helpful right now.

My mind once again has been in overdrive. If we don't have the main root cause, then could it be candida? Perhaps I have a different heavy metal level that was missed before? Is it a parasite or Lyme disease? Or could it be something structural like a CFS leak? A CFS leak was evaluated long ago, but I was never evaluated properly, according to my doctor. I was also never evaluated for a cranial leak, which has been a suspicion as well. Recently, we did a sample of the fluid from my nose and it was negative for CFS fluid. CT myelograms sound very invasive, and when my previous lumbar tap and MRI scans showed no signs . . . it seems unnecessary to move forward with such invasive testing.

It just seems so endless. I don't want to do this anymore. I don't think anyone realizes how defeating this feels. It's so embarrassing to tell people that something is wrong and not get better from treatment. I don't want to do tests anymore. I don't want to fight anymore. I just want to *live* instead of survive. I go as long as I can on one path. But I know there is something wrong with me. If I could just lie down and not have to get out of bed another day, I could just accept my position in this life. But I am a mother and my children need me. I cannot give up.

I deal with brain injury symptoms daily. It's as if my brain is still very inflamed from something. What is it from? Was it only mold? When I really think about it, some symptoms are mildly better. But not enough to feel that was the main root cause.

Somehow I manage to not completely go crazy or become trapped in a deep dark hole from dealing with these chronic symptoms and possibilities. I am still here for others. That is why I fight. I don't fight for myself alone, but for answers for those struggling with similar issues. *There has to be a reason for all of my suffering.* I fight for my children. I fight for my husband

. . . he works so hard for us. I just *hope* a shift comes soon. My husband doesn't deserve this and neither do my children.

I am sorry, Tim, that I get mad at you. I know you are going through so many things too. I know that it is hard.

FEARS

1. That my children will never have the mother that I once was
2. That I will never be able to experience memories with my children without being sick
3. That every day is going to be a struggle
4. That every day will be spent surviving, not living
5. That I will die and my husband will completely lose himself, and my children will no longer experience the adventure and joy that I bring to them
6. That my children will become sick like me
7. That my brain and nervous system is forever damaged
8. That I will never heal
9. That the darkness will take over me
10. That I will lose my mind
11. My vision forever being this way
12. That no one truly believes me
13. That I will forever be trapped in this nightmare
14. That I will poison my body further if I do more invasive testing through CT, MRI, spinal tap, CT myelogram, or surgery
15. That food will always be the enemy
16. That I did this to myself by accepting certain tests, procedures, and surgeries in the past
17. That God does not hear me
18. Death of loved ones
19. That I am too damaged to be fixed
20. That the metals, mold, fungus, or Lyme is trapped inside of my brain and has caused irreversible damage. *My doctors tell me it can cross the*

blood-brain barrier . . .

21. That I will never be able to properly breathe again, exercise, or enjoy the heat
22. That I am just a burden
23. Not good enough as a wife, mother, sister, aunt, friend, or daughter
24. That my symptoms will always keep me from enjoying life
25. That I do not deserve to be healed
26. That I have been abandoned by God
27. That my illness will continue to affect everyone's health and mental state
28. That my family's emotional state is my fault
29. That I will die this way
30. That no one can help me
31. That we are missing something
32. That I will become worse
33. That I will never be able to repair my limbic system

I give these fears to God because they are too much for me to bear any longer.

May 1, 2022

What would I do if I were well?

1. Drive and spend the day going to different places and eating wherever I want
2. Go on walks in the heat
3. Time with my friends while feeling normal
4. Shower and get ready without symptoms
5. Stand up
6. Drop off and pick up my son from school
7. Go to a movie
8. Go grocery shopping
9. Go kayaking
10. Go visit my family in Rapid City (I miss them so much)

11. Dance lessons with my husband
12. Breathe normal
13. Be there for others
14. Help others
15. Be free

Hear me, my God . . .

I pray for change, and drastically, so that life can return to a comfortable peace. I can take my son to school and experience life without overstimulation and illness. God, please let us be close. Please heal my brain and nervous system. Please return my body to what it once was. Restore me. Redeem me. Please, God. You can do all things. Christ, my Savior. Amen.

May 26, 2022

I am in a flare that is making my entire body and immune system tremor and scream. I just want to *run away from my body.* From *everything.* But I cannot. This seems so endless. *I feel so alone in all of it . . . I am trapped here and there is no way out.*

15

Suffering Wears Me Down

I have been praying for relief, but it has not happened, so I have resorted to praying for death even though I don't want to die. And when I feel close to death, I beg for God to *save me* to keep me alive for my children and husband even if I have to *suffer forever.* How messed up of a concept . . . but the suffering is wearing down on my *mind and soul.* Each time I regress with illness the feelings become stronger. I feel like I am drowning in the *waves.*

There is nowhere for me to run. I cannot escape my body. The only thing I can escape is my mind when I meditate with prayer or music. I just *hope* that God forgives me for every negative thought I have had and for the challenges that I have faced within my soul because of all of this. I always *hope* my family knows how hard I tried.

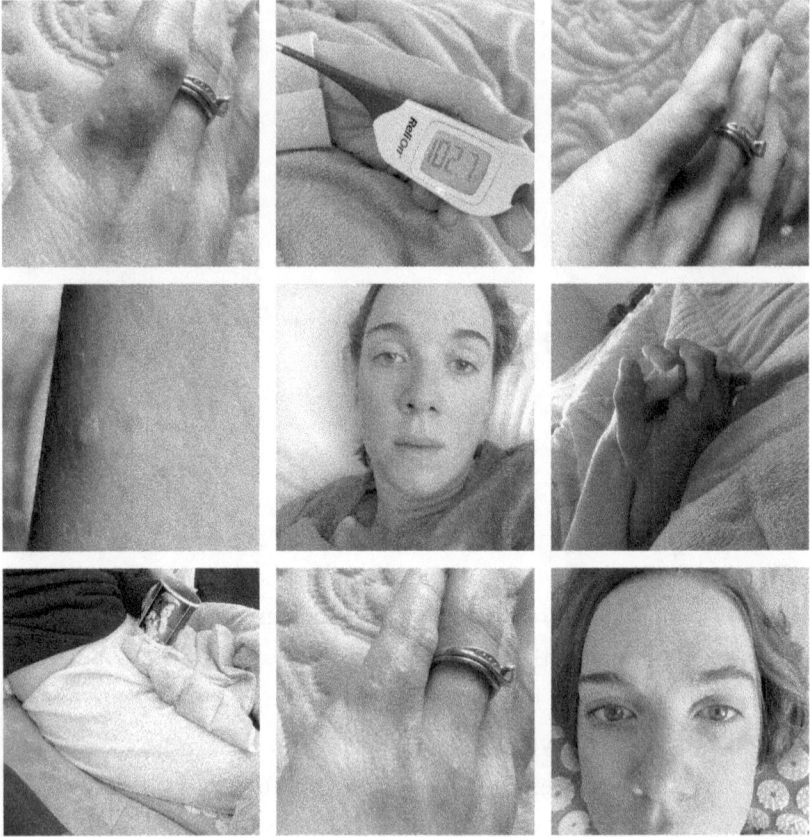

My condition regressed after this day . . . I began vomiting after almost every meal . . . and asked myself repeatedly, am I okay?

What I find *especially* challenging about medical trauma and chronic illness is that it is very hard to *heal* from this form of trauma. In order to heal from *trauma* you have to remove yourself from the source. How can you do that when the source of your trauma is your own body? You cannot escape your body, making the cycle ongoing. You can try to channel it the best that you can during flares, but the flares tend to enhance the medical trauma, leaving you in a worse condition than you were in before.

* * *

These letters were written to my family when I was going through an extreme illness that resulted in a very bad regression in my chronic illness. I thought I was going to die.

Dear *Russell,*

If I go to heaven God will fix me there. I know it is not what we wanted. If I had the *strength* I would stay with you here every day, even if it meant I would be sick. Sometimes we don't have a choice and it isn't always fair. But life isn't meant to be forever. It's just a stepping stone to a better future for all of us in heaven. We may often question what the point is and why some have to suffer. The point is to be kind to others. Bring joy to others. Have strong *faith.* Always question things. Don't follow along with everyone just because. Talk to God often. Let him be your guide. Life will always change and people will come and go. Some will never truly leave because they leave behind a piece of themselves in your heart. That is where I will be, in yours. I won't ever truly be gone and I will always be waiting for you. Life will have its challenges . . . its spiritual ones . . . temptations and suffering. With God you can overcome them all. I love you more than ever. You will always be under my wing and I will be in your heart.

Mommy loves you.

You are never alone.

Lean on *Jesus.*

Dear *Eliot,*

To the one who brightens up our day. You wake up in the morning always looking for Mommy, a panic appears on your face and tears stream down your cheeks when you think you can't find me. I want you to know that nothing could keep me from always being by your side. When I go to heaven someday, I will still be with you. You may not always feel it, but you can listen for it in the quiet or feel it on a soft breeze. A gentle brush against your cheek. I will always be with you, even when you cannot see me. It may feel unfair and empty at times, but don't let it ruin your joy when I do go to heaven. Life is a stepping stone for all of us to a permanent paradise where we will be together and there will be no suffering. No *fear* of not being able to find Mommy . . . In the meantime, remember how much I love you and how I am watching you grow every day. How I am still here because a part of me is in you. The point of life is as I told Russell . . . and the end is meant for us to reunite in heaven with Jesus. Life will always have its challenges, but don't let it turn your heart black. Always look toward the light and know you are not alone.

Mommy loves you.

Dear *Timothy*,

This is the second time I have written to you because of thoughts that I may die. And you look at me with *fear* in your eyes when I tell you I am unwell. A deep concern of what you would do without me here. I understand it too well. Do you remember the quote I picked for my dad's funeral? *Don't grieve for me for now I'm free.* That would be the same pick for me. I have been fighting this battle, and my body and soul are weary. I am not giving up, but I want you to know that if God's only way of relieving my suffering is by bringing me to heaven, I need to be okay with that. Do I ever want to be away from you and the kids? *No.* You are what I live for. What I fight for. And I will fight as long as I can. But one of the biggest burdens for me when I feel so close to death is if my husband and kids will be okay. I need to feel like you would be. If God's plan is for me to continue living in this condition then I guess I will just have to keep fighting. But if God takes me please don't lose your joy. Don't lose your light. Because then it will be lost in our boys too. Cling to God and know that I am at peace. Don't be angry with God . . . we are not in heaven, and on Earth there is going to be suffering. Suffering is not done out of spite by God. Hold on to the kids . . . adventure with them. Don't fall into a darkness. Don't get stuck. Know that we will all be together someday. Surround yourself with people who will light up your life. And know how *sorry* I am that this experience has caused you great suffering as well. Don't sit at home with the kids. Keep involving yourselves in church. Find joy. Always

SUFFERING WEARS ME DOWN

remember and hold on to the good memories and share them with our children. Tell them our stories. A lot of joy left my dad when my mom got sick and had to go to the hospital. I could see the change in his smile. The way the light just left his eyes and he often looked hard at the world. Don't let that happen to you. Find happiness and love and joy. I love you so much, Tim, and I'm so sorry if I did not heal.

Love, *your Sweetheart.*

I love you. I will always love you. No matter what. Forever and Always.

June 21, 2022

I feel lately like my body is not even trying to heal anymore. The last two days I have had diarrhea and low back pain that radiates up my spine and sits at the base of my skull. I can hardly turn my neck. I have severe pain in my abdomen near the gallbladder and intestines. Everything I eat comes back up yellow or dark. It's difficult to do anything. I have been having a fever and chills, too, with sweats. I often feel like I have mild fevers, but this is different. The fevers have been 104 degrees . . . and *no one in my family is sick.* My stool test recently came back showing gut dysbiosis and an infection of some kind. I don't feel that is causing this specifically, but I just don't know anymore. For the last three years I always feel like I am fighting an infection with low grade fevers. I don't understand why . . .

I just keep thinking back throughout my life and what went wrong. What triggered this? I don't know why I am having all of these increased symptoms acutely. It seems to reoccur every few weeks. But this is the worst one. For so long these relapses and extreme flares have been blamed on *herxing* the mold. But the levels are so low now. It's almost as if my body is trying to get rid of some other infection that we don't know about.

If I hear the words *detox reaction* or *herxing* one more time I feel like I am going to explode.

I just don't know anymore if there is any *hope* in my body healing. I have had so much toxicity build up, causing damage to my cells and mitochondria, and my oxidative stress levels are so high. All of the tests recently came back showing this. My local functional medicine doctor

159

doesn't seem to be able to tell me why my oxidative stress is high, and she says it will age me very quickly. I already feel like an eighty-year-old inside. It's very scary to hear that the damage done to my body is *going to age me drastically*. Sometimes the words said to me by my doctors are very traumatizing and make it harder for me to have a positive outlook. I am not worried about the wrinkles on my skin but by the internal damage and regression in my ability to function normally.

The mitochondrial damage, oxidative stress, cell damage, nervous system dysregulation, limbic system impairment, and acute inflammation—that only God knows the location of—is overwhelming. I feel like the damage is from my brain and nervous system and that is the reason my gut is so bad. Not because of the food. My immune system has to be in overdrive from all of these toxins and infections throughout my body, and that's what makes me so sensitive to everything. The pain is increasing so much . . . the POTS. It all feels so impossible. I don't know what to do moving forward. I'm considering the Lyme test, but it's another expense that I have to burden my husband with.

All of the work that I have done . . . the protocols, all of the things I have tried for my gut . . . they just seem so pointless and futile. But then I remind myself I *did* reverse intestinal metaplasia. I did that. Through food. But there still seems to be some underlying factor that keeps reinflaming my gut and causing these acute fever-like regressions.

My local functional medicine doctor says a lot of these issues that I am still experiencing could be coming from all of the trauma I have experienced from the chronic health issues. In my day-to-day, I utilize the exercises. I try very hard to be *positive*. I complain very little to others. I don't tell everyone around me what I tell my journal. *I use my journal to cope with my pain.* I don't feel like I have an outlet to be truly honest about my suffering. I am often met with disappointment, or I stress out the people I love. Even with my doctors, they seem to want me to always be untruthfully positive. I understand it, to a point, but I feel like I have no one to grieve with on the hard days. I just lie alone and suffer.

I put a smile on for the outside world and I do everything I can for others.

But inside, my body is screaming.

* * *

My out-of-state functional medicine doctor has been completely opposite, she doesn't feel that the limbic system is the main factor, and she is still suspecting the ferritin is an issue. She still suspects a possible infection or bleed of some kind.

I wish that every single doctor and naturopath that I have would just come together in one room. Set aside their differences and look over all of my labs and scans *together*. They could *learn* from each other and find a better way to *help me* and others like me . . . I never expected there to be so many different opinions concerning what to do with my care. It makes it very difficult for me to feel confident in the path that I *choose*. I didn't ask for this. I am trying to do what everyone says will help me.

* * *

I was looking at the bacteria levels that are elevated in my stool test. Some can cause IBS. My local functional medicine doctor says that this bacteria can also trigger autoimmune diseases. When I showed the test to my acupuncturist, he said it's a very tricky one to eradicate and it can hurt the kidneys. My doctor agreed. I have to go on antibiotics for it . . .

Is there any hope at all?

The tests seem never-ending, because now my two functional medicine doctors and my primary doctor are all recommending doing a HIDA (hepatobiliary iminodiacetic acid) scan because of these increased issues.

Why?

I just want to be a mom. A wife. But I lie here in bed just trying to survive. And wondering what the point is over and over again. *Why?* To see how strong my *faith* is? I don't even know anymore.

I found out recently that I have an eye disease called Keratoconus. I have to have a surgery on my eyes called corneal cross-linking.

I am scared, and the doctor who diagnosed it asked, "Have been evaluated properly for a CFS leak?"

Because of these findings, it was suggested to do a spinal tap to check the pressure. I didn't want to do this, but the findings could show if I had a CFS leak. It was terrible, but I did it. My pressure results were *normal*. Go figure. Another invasive test that probably just hurts me worse . . .

No one else in my family has this eye condition, and I am not an eye rubber. After the normal pressure result, I talked to both of my functional medicine doctors and my brain health specialist. They all feel the condition is a result of the inflammation from the toxicities I have had. The mold, heavy metals, and perhaps Lyme. It brings me back to the times when the pressure was so bad behind my eyes that I had to have Tim put my head in a vice-like grip between his hands as I cried . . . *Tim, something is very wrong* . . . It was the only way I got relief. Funny how I suffered so much and needed help and now have permanent eye damage because no one *listened*.

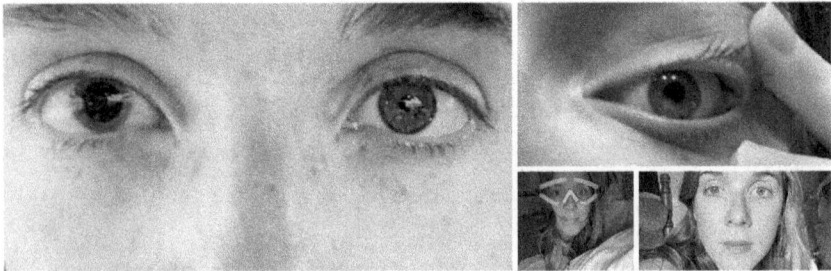

"Have you ever been evaluated for a CFS leak?" the doctor asked.

The surgery was pretty terrible. It burned when he scraped away at my eye, and then I had to lie there for over an hour with a bright light beaming into my eyeball. Afterward, my vision was as if someone had smudged fingerprints all over a window, and the lights were so bright I had to wear two pairs of blackout shades for several months. The first day at home, my eye burned most of the day. I still made it to Russell's swimming lesson practice, though, to take pictures with my one eye a day after. I had to have two surgeries at separate times. The second time I actually broke down and started to cry to Tim . . . I told him I didn't want to do this again and I didn't want to be here . . . I didn't feel like the numbing drops worked very well at all during the second surgery. It hurt terribly when he scraped at my eye, and I felt like I was having a panic attack during the procedure. I will admit it this time . . . that was a *panic attack*. I hid it well, though. The doctors didn't even notice. I have been through so much trauma that my nervous system suffers from it. After this experience, I noticed I would start to shake more when I became stressed . . . I still battle this.

* * *

I found out recently that, because I had the corneal cross-linking surgery, my insurance will not cover the specialized contacts for keratoconus. The surgery was recommended by the specialist to prevent me from hopefully ever needing a full cornea transplant in the future, so of course I had the surgery. *But,* the contacts are only covered under insurance if you have *not* had the corneal cross-linking surgery. The contacts are $2000 per eye. Lately, I have been trying to manage as best I can with the contacts I already have. I have to move them often because my eye is coned now, and they will spin on me and become blurry. Glasses no longer work for me because of this eye disease. I feel sick when I wear them because everything looks like a fun house. I often wonder what kind of backward world we are living in . . .

16

My Mom's Health Issues

July 19, 2022

My mom came over today, like she has been doing every day for the last year. My mother is my best friend and has been here more days than I can count.

When I was younger, if someone would have told me that my mother and I would see each other every day I would have laughed in their face and not believed them. I am so *grateful* that I was able to try and understand the struggles that my mother had and forgave the time I lost with her. If I had not, we wouldn't be together today. My first lesson concerning *patience with prayer* was in regards to my mother's situation. As a child, I cried out over and over again for God to heal my mother. I experienced discouragement and anger toward God when it didn't happen. I begged for God to heal her and allow her to be with me. Now, years later, my prayers are answered at a time when I need her most. It's sometimes difficult to understand God's timing or unanswered prayers, but throughout my life I have *seen* answers, even if they didn't come in the way that I expected.

My mother struggled with many health issues when I was a child. I was mostly raised by my dad and grandmother. There were a lot of things I didn't understand concerning my mom as I was growing up. She did not have POTS or *chronic* migraines, but she did experience ovarian cyst growth, endometriosis, gut problems, fibromyalgia, diverticulitis, and aura migraines. She had surgery to remove her uterus and ovaries in her 30s, and no hormone therapy after that because she was a smoker.

Her biggest battle was with the anxiety and depression spells . . . Her depression was somewhat caused by the abuse that happened to her growing up, but I sometimes wonder how much of it was being caused by her other imbalances. She had mental health diagnoses of bipolar disorder, anxiety, and depression. Oddly, she has not had to take a single medication for bipolar disorder in the last twenty years. There were many failed attempts at medicating her for these mental health struggles. My mother told me that the first time she started self-harming was when she was twenty years old, right after she was in the psychiatric hospital and placed on a medication called Haldol. It only made her worse.

In her words: "I don't keep track of how long I was put on any of those medications because they all made me feel like shit."

Even before I became sick, I tried to understand her situation and become closer to her . . . but when I actually started to experience some of the symptoms she had as a mother, it made me able to understand her even more. She didn't have the support that I do. She may not have been fainting, but there were things she was battling every day. I sometimes wonder why.

* * *

We ate almond flour bread together and then went outside. Mom put birdseed in the yellow birdhouse. It was a pretty normal day.

But then she sat down and she seemed off. "Something is wrong, Whitney. My lips are tingling and I can't breathe very well."

I sat down with her. I looked at her mouth and it was swelling, then her face, eyes, and legs began to swell after that. She was red all over on her legs, right where she would have wiped the birdseed dust off. *But she has been exposed to this many times before . . . was it the almond flour?* Her heart rate was high and she was breathing funny. This was some kind of a severe allergic reaction. *Mast cell activation?* I've been worrying that her health

165

was going to continue to regress . . .

Her symptoms are so similar to mine. They are getting worse. I gave her an antihistamine and we jumped in the car and drove to town.

By the time we got there it had calmed down. She saw her primary care provider and she was prescribed an EpiPen . . . but this has never happened before. *What caused it?*

August 3, 2022

I am proud that I can admit my fears. I am proud that my biggest strength is perseverance.

I am *grateful* for:

- being able to go on a short walk today
- my husband
- my children
- my mother
- beautiful weather
- friends
- Terri

I will overcome.

17

Visualization Helps

August 4, 2022

What I Visualize Often

This was inspired by a meditation. I revised the visualization to my own liking and experience. *I hope it can help you, like it has helped me.*

- *I am with God. The sand in between my toes is warm. I am not alone because God is with me. I am so close to the water that some of the waves touch my feet. The rushing sound of the waves calms me. The sun warms my skin and the fresh air sends energy through me. There is a thick rope around my waist connected to an anchor that trails behind me. The anchor weighs heavy with my accumulated fears, worries, and thoughts about the past and future. They hinder me. They have held me back and kept me from healing and having inner peace . . . from joy and freedom. With each step the rope gnaws into my skin. God points to something glimmering in the sand ahead of me. I walk toward it as I drag the heaviness with me. When I come closer, I realize it is a blade from ancient times . . . there is an energy link between myself and the blade. I look down at the blade and realize suddenly that my name appears on the handle. A part of me is curious, but God reassures me that this blade was here for a reason . . . life has given me the chance or choice to deliberately cut the rope and let it all go to God. I cut the rope and let go of all the worries and unwanted feelings I have been dragging with me. I feel a sense of relief as God picks up the pieces. I fall to the ground, overwhelmed with the weightlessness of my body. God picks me up, and there is only one set of footprints in the sand. I no longer have to carry all of my burdens on my own . . . because God is carrying me . . .*

A*ll that is left to heal is oxidative stress and limbic system impairment. A bad bug will be squished in my gut with this antibiotic. I will persevere. I will win because God is with me.* I tell myself this over and over again. (Words from my health coach and local functional medicine doctor.)

August 5, 2022
My diagnosis then:

1. Mold
2. Mast cell activation syndrome
3. Heavy metals
4. Parasites
5. CIRS/POTS
6. Candida/yeast
7. Gut dysbiosis
8. Intestinal metaplasia
9. Vestibular and aura migraine

My diagnosis now:

1. POTS from oxidative stress damage and mitochondrial damage
2. Gut dysbiosis
3. Vestibular migraine
4. High ferritin

How to heal them:

1. Limbic system rewiring
2. Kill off bacteria with antibiotics
3. Antioxidants and glutathione support
4. Food: onion, garlic, eggs

Mind:

1. 4-7-8 breathing
2. Tapping
3. Gratitude list
4. Rerouting negative thoughts
5. Visualization and prayer
6. List what you are proud of

Supplement:

1. Antioxidants
2. 5-HTP
3. MitoCORE and PQQ

I am proud of myself for going to the park with my children today and watching Russell at swimming lessons, even though I can hardly see from the cross-linking surgery. I felt terrible, but I still took pictures of my son swimming, and I was there. My world is mostly blacked out right now as I cannot see out of the one eye properly until it heals. The lights are so much brighter I can hardly look outside. But I made it.

I am *grateful* for:

- weather
- forgiveness
- Mom
- Terri

- Tim
- my children
- a cozy home

August 7, 2022

I am proud of myself for pushing through another day of crippling symptoms and vestibular migraines. The constant pressure in my head and spinning was awesome . . . not.

I am *grateful* for:

- my family

"Tim and I are going to a Halloween party tonight! I'm so excited! He is going as Two-Face and I am going as Catwoman. It's going to be so much fun. I can't wait to try the sweets and dance all night with him." (Visualization homework)

August 8, 2022

I am proud of myself for taking care of my sick children without feeling overwhelming anxiety.

I am *grateful* for:

- God

August 9, 2022

I am proud of myself for being more active today.

I am *grateful* for:

- contacts
- my husband
- Russell

"Tim and I are going out dancing tonight! We both are so excited and have so much energy." (Visualization homework)

August 12, 2022

I am proud of myself for going to Dollar General on my own today and making chocolate bars with Russell. I didn't eat any, but at least I got to experience his joy.

I am *grateful* for:

- bravery
- a cozy home when it rains

August 14, 2022

I am proud of myself for getting through these last few high-flare days.

I am *grateful* for:

- the beautiful weather
- financial stability
- my kids' joy
- my husband's diagnosis that will soon bring him relief

Healing is possible. Never give up. You are loved. You are wanted. You are needed. God loves you.

18

Mold Ruins Another Experience

I have been trying to get Russell involved in a homeschooling group. We had him all signed up, and Tim and I attended the meeting. The classes are held in an old brick building at a church. We walked down the steps and it hit me like a thick fog. Mold. Tim and I saw it all over the walls. I couldn't believe it. We had already paid for the school year. *What are we going to do?* My chest started to tighten the longer I was in there, and I could feel my heart rate pick up off and on. I felt itchy and hot.

While we were in the church basement, my husband kept looking at me worriedly. We both quietly went back up the stairs. I sat on the steps, feeling very embarrassed, and didn't know what I was supposed to say. I knew Amanda would be there any minute and the plan was for her to take Russell on days when I was not well enough. *What am I supposed to tell her?*

Mold has destroyed so much of my life, and my health coach and doctor both told me a big part of healing is avoidance of these types of environments. I still had this feeling like *maybe I am overreacting.* Tim reassured me that I was not. He said his eyes burned just from being down there for a short time. *I can't expose myself or my child to this . . . especially when I am still healing.*

Knowing what I know now about mold exposure means that I would

172

not ever feel comfortable with my son going to school in that type of environment. It cost us so much time, money, and energy to lower the mold levels in my body. The ozone therapy was so expensive. The months I have spent using the sauna and all of the expensive diets and supplements . . . and we still don't know if my immune system is dealing with Lyme disease. I can't erase all of the dedication I have put in with the food and limbic system rewiring. *We can't do this.* If we do find Lyme, it will only weaken my immune system more, making the Lyme harder to eradicate.

This is one of the hardest aspects of this illness. I hadn't even thought to check the environment first. It's so upsetting that I have to live this way while everyone else just walks happily into that church basement. *But they don't know how bad it can be.* Later we have to explain our personal situation to the director, which I never intended to do . . . I keep my health issues very private from people who don't know me well. The only person I have been comfortable in sharing with, outside of trusted family and long-term friends, has been my fellow homeschooling mom, Amanda. She has been so wonderful and has pulled me out of many dark times without even knowing it.

We were able to get our money back, but it's so disappointing that I will be spending another year homeschooling Russell alone. Both Tim and I agree . . . we won't allow him to be exposed to that level of black mold. There were spots of it on the walls. It was visible, so who knows the level of contamination beneath the surface.

I grew up in a house that had a moldy basement like this. It wasn't a big deal for us growing up. We didn't know it could hurt us. But now I do know, and I won't do that to my son. I have heard that the homeschool group has grown so much since COVID. They expanded into two other locations and this location was the only one they could find. We had to put a hold on the homeschool group right now. I want to be a part of Russell's schooling.

It took me over a year to feel comfortable enough to allow Amanda to drive my son to Tae Kwon Do. The director of the group suggested finding another placement for him at a different location. I don't know anyone well enough and want to be there as much as I can.

The embarrassment of running into another problem like this at a different location was too overwhelming for me. We decided we would wait and hopefully next year will be better.

* * *

Later, I was invited to a family picnic through the homeschooling group. I really struggled in the heat with my pain that day. A kind woman came up to me and expressed how the pastor, too, had a difficult time with the mold in the building. I do not know the level of his symptoms. She brought up the limbic system. *So she knows . . .* I listened to her and understood what she was saying. There is a time and place for limbic system balancing, but, in my opinion, putting yourself in a moldy environment on purpose is dangerous. I didn't share with her the other health issues that I have faced. I didn't talk about the heavy metals, genetic detox concerns, or the possibility that I still am struggling with Lyme, candida, and the excess acute inflammation from the high ferritin levels. I didn't want to talk about the details because it can cause me too much stress in certain environments.

It's nice when people care and understand and I don't really have to explain myself. But we were at the picnic to try to get to know people for next year, perhaps. I didn't want my health issues overshadowing everyone's joy.

There are events I would like to attend . . . but I still need a driver for most things. I don't want to burden anyone by asking if they can pick us up for field trips. A lot of them would be too difficult for me to attend right now anyway, unfortunately, and I have such *trust* issues with people I don't know well enough to take my kids.

* * *

The following week, I had to talk about our experience at my next doctor's appointment. We told her what we ran into at the church, and I was trying to make sure I wasn't overreacting. She told me *absolutely not*. She said there is a *difference* between that situation and proper limbic system retraining. She would not suggest that I expose myself or my child to that level of mold repeatedly and was surprised that a school setting would allow children to be in there. I'm honestly surprised that the church hasn't done anything to remediate the problem.

Tim and I did express our concerns with the director about the potential dangers for the children going to that location. We felt obligated to say something after our own experience . . .

It's upsetting that *mold* had to ruin another experience for my child and me.

September 28, 2022

I could not get ahold of my mom this morning. I got in my car and drove to her apartment. *Her car is here . . .* She has not been feeling good for a long time now. Her vision has been getting worse . . . she has been having heart rates issues similar to my own . . . *what is happening to her?* Her bike was still there too. I knocked on her door . . . no answer. *Oh no . . . if I go inside will I find her dead on the floor?* I turned the handle slowly, preparing myself. I left the kids in the truck just in case something bad happened. My mother is like a second mom to my boys, and I didn't want them to see her if I found her on the floor. When I walked into her apartment she was nowhere to be found. Her phone was there though. *What if she went on a walk and passed out or had a heart attack?* I turned around quickly, intending to drive all over town until I found her.

Her neighbor opened the door across the hall right as I was about to leave the building. I asked her if she knew where my mom was.

Her face kind of turned pale and she said, "Oh no . . . you don't know."

My heart started to race.

She continued and said, "She was taken by ambulance to the hospital this morning . . . I am so sorry."

I went outside, trying to hold it together. I took deep breaths before I got in the pickup so I didn't lose it in front of my kids . . . My hands were shaking. I called Tim. I lost it then. I told him what happened and that I was going to go to the hospital but didn't want to bring the kids with me in case something bad happened to my mom. All of the memories of our life together flashed before me and the times between her and my children . . . *she is like a second mother to them*. Then my phone rang. I pulled myself together before answering, thinking it was going to be the hospital with terrible news . . .

"Whitney . . . ," my mom whispered in a small voice.

She told me she was okay but she had to call me on her neighbor's phone from the hospital. She had an episode that morning. They didn't find anything wrong with her in the CT or EKG, and her labs didn't show any obvious signs of the cause. *Thank God* . . . I don't know what is happening to my mom, *but I am going to find out.*

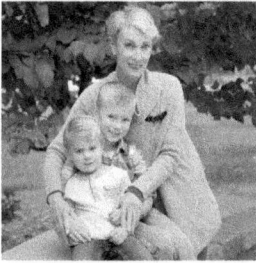

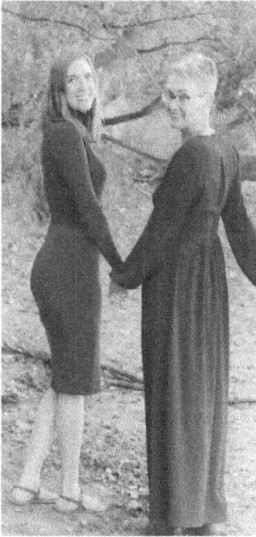

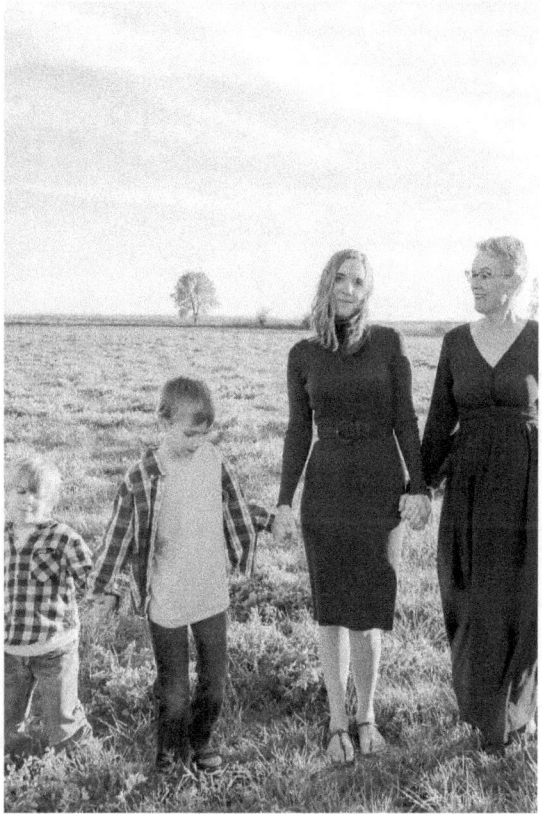

. . . she is a second mother to my sons . . .

19

Why Won't Jesus Heal Me?

October 27, 2022

I have decided recently to try my out-of-state functional medicine doctor's therapy recommendations for lowering the ferritin by doing monthly phlebotomies. I will also be doing her candida protocol once my testing comes back. She says I have insulin resistance and estrogen dominance too. I am going to retry her bio-identical hormones and see how I feel. I have never had a lot of results with progesterone since my hysterectomy. Because we never know when I am ovulating, it's more difficult to balance.

Organic Poultry	Organic Meat	Organic Seeds & Nuts	Organic Fish & Sea Food "wild catch"	Organic Plant Source Protein
• Eggs • Goose • Pheasant • Quail • Chicken • Turkey • Duck	• Pork • Beef • Organ meat • Venison • Beef • Goat	• Walnuts • Flax seed • Sunflower seeds • Pine nuts • Pumpkin seeds • Chestnuts • Almonds • Macadamia • Brazil nuts • Sesame seeds	• Wild Salmon • Shellfish • Anchovies • White fish	• Peas (green or yellow) • Sprouts • Beans (once a week) • Tofu • Chia seed • Lentils

Organic Fruits	Organic Vegetables	Organic Fresh Herbs & Spices	Organic Oils & Fats	Organic Grains & Pasta noodles
• Avocado • Limes • Peaches • Strawberry • Blueberry • Kiwi • Goji Berry • Blackberry • Apricots • Grapefruit • Currant • Cranberry • Plums • Raspberry • Pomegranate • Mulberry • Green apple • Cranberries • Lemon • Kumquat	• Beets • Cucumber • Broccoli • Asparagus • Radish • Olives • Celery • Zucchini • Sauerkraut • Okra • Lettuce • Kimchi • Green peppers • Chives • Collards • Onions • Peppers • Kale • Green onions • Fennel • Garlic • Eggplant • Cauliflower • Cabbage • Seaweed • Tomatoes • Turnip • Spinach • Snow peas • Rutabaga	• Basil • Thyme • Parsley • Ginger • Garlic • Bay leaf • Cayenne • Mint • Nutmeg • Dill • Cumin • Cloves • Cinnamon • Cilantro • Oregano • Paprika • Sea salt • Vanilla • Turmeric • Red chili flakes • Sage • Rosemary • Ground pepper • Sage	• Extra virgin olive oil • Sunflower oil • Walnut oil • Coconut oil • Avocado oil • Flaxseed oil	• Buckwheat • Wild rice • Red rice • Millet • Quinoa • Amaranth • Whole Oat Flakes • Black rice • Rice noodle • Oat bran • Brown rice

Candida Grocery List (p. 172 & 173)

Dairy Alternatives	Sweeteners	Snacks & Others	Foods to try as Gut Improves	Foods to Avoid
• Unsweetened Coconut milk • Oat milk • Hemp milk • Unsweetened almond milk • Other unsweetened nut milks • Flax milk	• Xylitol • Stevia	• Buckwheat • Seaweed crackers • Nut butters • Hummus • Japanese rice crackers • Apple cider vinegar	• Squash • Potato • Sweet potato • Pineapple • Bananas • Carrots • Sourdough	• Chocolate • Beans • Yeast • Cream • Processed food • Cheese • Milk • Sugar • Barley • Spelt • Mushroom • Soy • Alcohol • Peanuts • Rye • Mustard • Ketchup • Caffeine • Vinegar • Mayonnaise • Wheat • Peanuts • Cashews • Salad dressing • Legumes • Honey • Syrup

I can only eat the food items in these categories for the first six weeks: Organic Meat, Organic Vegetables, Organic Poultry, Organic Fish & Seafood "wild catch," Organic Plant Source Protein, Organic Seeds & Nuts, Organic Oils & Fats, Organic Fresh Herbs & Spices, and Dairy Alternatives. After the six weeks is complete, I can add the food in from these categories: Organic Fruits, Organic Grains & Pasta Noodles, Sweeteners, and Snacks & Others. After three months I can add the category: Foods to Try as Gut Improves. After four months is complete, I can occasionally add foods from the Foods to Avoid category.

* * *

My ultrasounds only show fatty liver, nothing else remarkable to explain my pain. My out-of-state functional medicine doctor feels this is partly because of the long-gone ferritin retaining from my surgery complications and blood transfusions. She said when excess iron sits in the organs like that it causes a lot of organ inflammation. My recent inflammation testing and cytokine panels from my local functional medicine doctor were also unremarkable. So this is what pushed my decision to try the phlebotomies, because there are no other levels of inflammation seen in other testing. My out-of-state functional medicine doctor also feels the candida is inflaming my gut and there is still a suspicion of missed endometriosis or a small internal bleed or some sort from surgery. I wonder this often, too, but my debilitating abdominal pain issues began this summer . . . after the fever episode. Prior to that I had a lot of other symptoms . . . but not this vomiting and increased pain and fog. I would think if this new pain were related to surgery complications it would have happened sooner.

It's difficult to make decisions. The plan, to begin with, was finding a local functional medicine doctor to help my out-of-state functional medicine doctor. I didn't expect that they would disagree on a lot of things. Many times, when I see my local functional medicine doctor she points out signs of inflammation. As I mentioned previously, the line she sees when I stick out my tongue is a sign of inflammation, but she doesn't know where it's coming from. When I was diagnosed with CIRS and oxidative stress, again, I was told these were signs of inflammation somewhere. Then, with the ferritin levels, that was always a *sign of inflammation.* At my last visit with her, she seemed very set on the idea that it is my limbic system mainly keeping me sick. She asked me where I keep getting all of these ideas that I am struggling with inflammation when my recent interleukin 6, C-reactive protein, and cytokine levels were normal.

I didn't really have it in my heart to say, "*From you. From everyone* who has repeatedly told me I have signs of chronic inflammation."

But I did feel that way . . . and I am sorry I felt that way . . . but over the course of the last year, inflammation was blamed on so many of my conditions by so many specialists.

As if she read my mind, she said, "I know I need to be more careful with how I speak to patients dealing with complex symptoms like yourself. I am still learning that."

It made me happy to hear her say that. *Yes . . . that would probably help many . . .* but it's okay . . . and I am not angry at her.

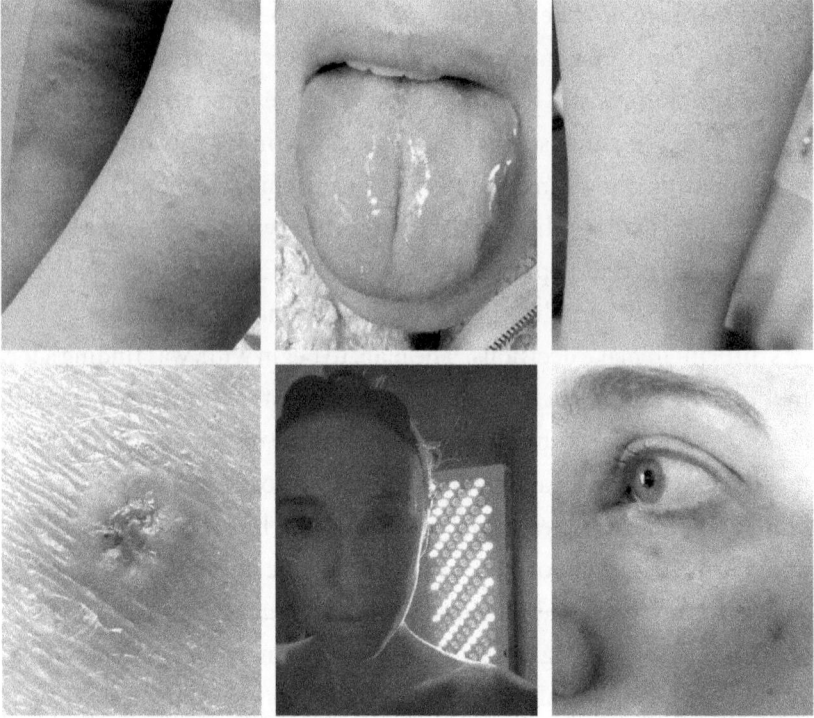

"Where do I keep getting all of these ideas that I am struggling with inflammation . . . ?"

If my out-of-state functional medicine doctor is correct on the ferritin being from the retained iron and hemochromatosis, I could have resolved that so long ago by donating blood. Perhaps by now I wouldn't be dealing with the fatty liver and extreme GI issues. My local functional medicine doctor can't answer *why* I still have high oxidative stress levels. She said she has not found the cause to that yet. I don't feel that is from the limbic system alone. The tests show that my cells are hurting. The limbic system cannot possibly be the cause of this . . .

The hematologist was really no help either. He said it *could* be from inflammation or it *could* be from the blood transfusions. He said the form of hemochromatosis that I have *can* sometimes result in retained ferritin from blood transfusions, but *not* always. So I had to make my *own* decision on what to do moving forward based on all of these facts put together, plus my lab results showing low inflammation markers.

* * *

I am *not* upset with my local functional medicine doctor. I am *not* upset with either of them at all. I am *not* upset that my out-of-state functional medicine doctor was part of the reason I made the decision to have a hysterectomy. I am *not* upset that she may have missed the mold and SIBO. I am *not* upset that my local functional medicine doctor may have missed the solution to the high ferritin.

This has been an exhausting debate. I am just so tired. I am too tired to be upset. I am doing everything that my doctors are asking me to do. Even the nervous system things. My day-to-day is spent grounding, visualizing, breathing, tapping, and redirecting my thoughts. I mostly write about my struggles here, because journaling the pretend visualizations were making me feel sadder. I believe that my limbic system is impaired, I can feel it from certain stresses that never used to faze me . . . but it's from all of the trauma and continued findings with other medical conditions. It's because of things that went untreated, like the retained ferritin straining my central nervous system even more. I have a hard time believing that *everything* is from the limbic system alone when I still feel very sick. How do you heal the limbic system when you are still experiencing the trauma that put you there?

* * *

I have been doing acupuncture for several months now for suspected gastroparesis. Because I had not seen my acupuncturist for several months, I could tell when he saw me again that he was very saddened by the weight I had lost due to the vomiting spells and the issues with pain when I eat. He is determined to help me. He feels that I have Lyme and has been talking about a live blood analysis evaluation. He doesn't have the equipment yet, but he wants to do that for me sometime since the other testing is too expensive for us right now. I know he just wants to help.

My sore throats have been crippling. The headaches, migraines, sinus headaches, dizziness, heart race, night sweats, stomach pain, liver and abdominal pain, and brain fog are so challenging from day to day. Acupuncture has been helping with the pain flares, so maybe I do have a mild case of gastroparesis. We plan on doing the therapy for several months because it can help the nerves work better on their own again . . . but the underlying cause is still there and it's like an endless battle.

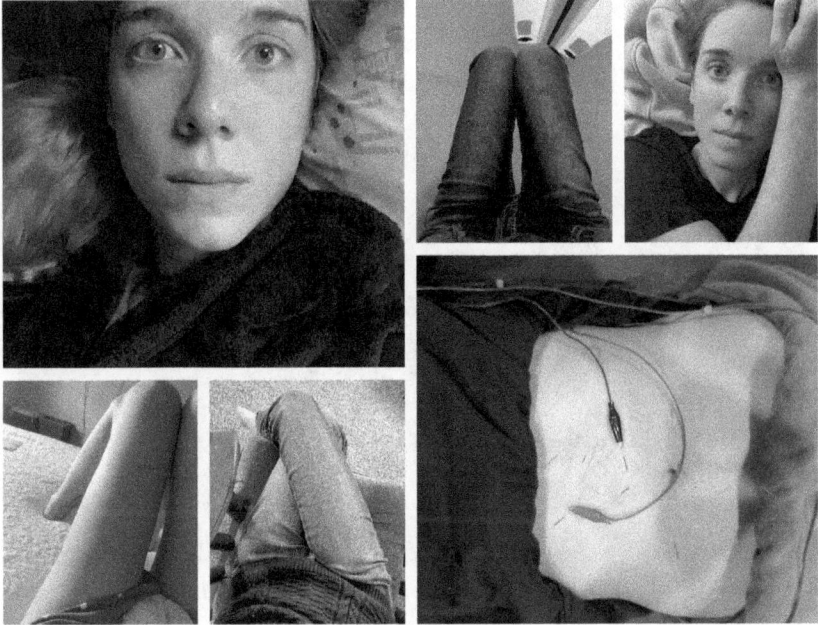

The pain was so intense. I would often vomit from the extreme pain and nausea after eating. I lost around 55 lbs in a short time frame. I was a skeleton of my old self and cried when I looked in the mirror. As I looked in the mirror, a memory flashed in front of me . . . a previous doctor sits at his desk, barely acknowledging me, and says, "Your stomach issues could be mentally induced." Because he ignored my pain, I am now in this condition . . . years later. I want to scream, but no sounds come out of me anymore. I want to cry, but the tears have all dried up . . .

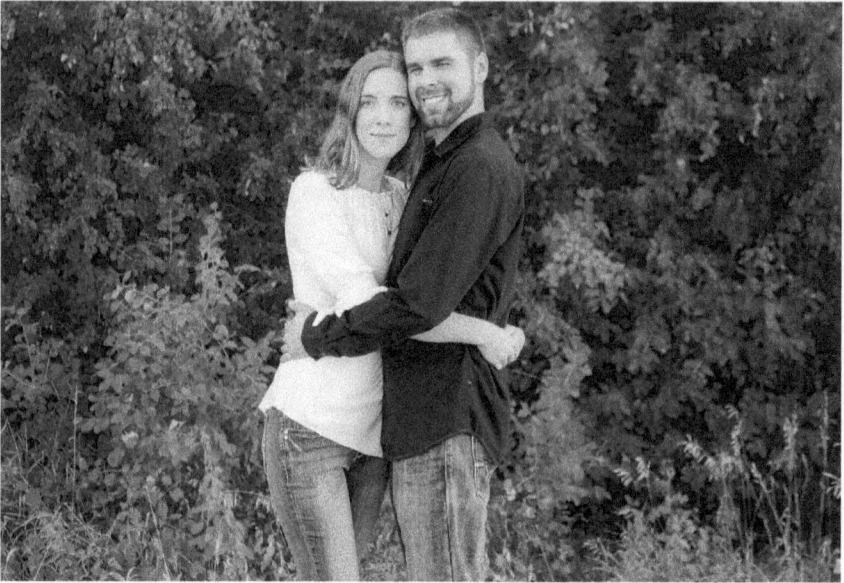

As the weight fell off of me, it fell off of my husband as well. The extreme stress eats away at him.

October 28, 2022

I have done the first blood donation for the high ferritin and secondary hemochromatosis condition. I did not want to do a standard blood donation because I don't want *anyone* getting my blood. We had to fill out a medical form to get it done at the hospital. That way they discard the blood afterward. I wanted to make sure that no one could get Lyme disease from me because I really feel that Lyme disease is a possibility. *I don't want anyone going through what I have gone through by getting my contaminated blood.*

* * *

When I experienced the high fevers in June, they really affected my spinal area and brain stem. I had so much pain in that area I could hardly turn my neck. I feel like it just inflamed the autonomic nervous system *again* and right now I feel like I'm back to square one.

186

I have trouble grasping the reality of my situation. The duration of my illness is disheartening, and I can't help but wonder . . . if I hadn't had those surgeries, would I be where I am at today? Sure, I don't faint anymore or deal with as troubling of heart rates because I don't bleed heavily anymore . . . but I feel like the medical system failed me. If I had found these underlying causes and corrected the infections, then the issues may have resolved without needing surgery. And then I feel like a failure because I try all these protocols just to get hit with something acute and end up at square one again. The odd thing, too, is that sometimes these acute flares are only happening to me. No one else in the family will be sick . . . it's almost as if I am regressing every month. I don't know what happens to me, but if I experience anything with a fever I feel like death is knocking at my door.

My local functional medicine doctor told me I need to stop fearing these acute flares. The thing is, I don't *fear* the acute illness. What worries me is when I begin to *feel* how it is affecting me after it's done. After the fever is over, what I experience is not normal. A year ago, if I got a cold, sure I would not be feeling the best, but it was nothing like what I experience now. The way I regress is *not* normal. I believe her when she says my immune testing came out okay . . . I do. But something is happening to me during these flares, and whatever it is does not show on labs. I was *never* afraid of illness until *after* I started to regress in this way.

* * *

It's embarrassing going to these doctor visits with little to no improvement, despite all of my hard work and dedication. I do not cheat. I take every supplement they recommend. It costs us so much money, and we can't do anything else in life right now besides pay for my protocols and therapies. And then I just keep *failing.*

When my out-of-state functional medicine doctor suggests there may still be something wrong that needs to be explored through another surgery, the thought of going under the knife is unsettling. I remember before my second surgery, when I was still convinced I had Lyme, I read somewhere that surgery can bring out dormant bacteria. I was worried about that with my last surgery, but I was told my results were negative per CDC testing and I believed that.

I knew the Lyme disease tests were terribly inaccurate, but I didn't have the resources at the time to help me. I remember years ago, when I was healthy, I was shopping at a book store and came across a very interesting book calling Lyme *"the great imitator"* of disease. I didn't have any debilitating issues then and had not been looking for a book like this, but it caught my eye. That was one of the reasons I even decided to look into Lyme disease during the first year that I was suffering. No one told me in the beginning about ILADS (*International Lyme and Associated Diseases Society*) or about the importance of Lyme-literate doctors. Sometimes I still wonder if my functional medicine doctors don't know *enough* about Lyme disease and maybe I need to go elsewhere. But starting all over again is so painful and expensive. I feel like Tim would just lose it emotionally if we had to start somewhere new.

* * *

I see everyone around me functioning at a normal level and I look at my children with the thoughts of *they are my main driving force and the reason that I am still here today*. I cannot leave them, even if I am suffering. I have no other choices but to keep trying or accept the condition I am in and try and find ways to manage it better. I have thought on and off about getting a wheelchair or certain mobility aids that can help me take my kids to more places. I think of Tim and how hard this is for him. All of this is just so hard to grasp.

I am told over and over again that my biggest *strength* is *perseverance* and I feel that dwindling some days.

Some days I just want to say, *"Damn it all . . . "* and eat an entire pizza.

I have worked on my diet for all these years, to show only mild results. I have just done so much and I am at a level of exhaustion that I cannot explain. I have been trying to escape my reality in any way possible, but it is so hard when I am still experiencing trauma daily.

But here I am. I am still *persevering* as I stand in front of a red light daily . . . pouring myself out to God in my deepest prayers and meditations . . . trying supplement after supplement, and bleeding myself dry with phlebotomies and lab draws. I try to *trust* in God's timing, but then remember that it isn't his fault that I am in this condition. Disease is in this world. God didn't make me sick. The world did. The doctors who gaslit me did. It wasn't God.

What the hell happened to my life? I feel destroyed. But I still grasp on to this small fiber of *hope*. Throughout the day, I trick myself into thinking that things are okay and will get better. But sometimes I have trouble believing it.

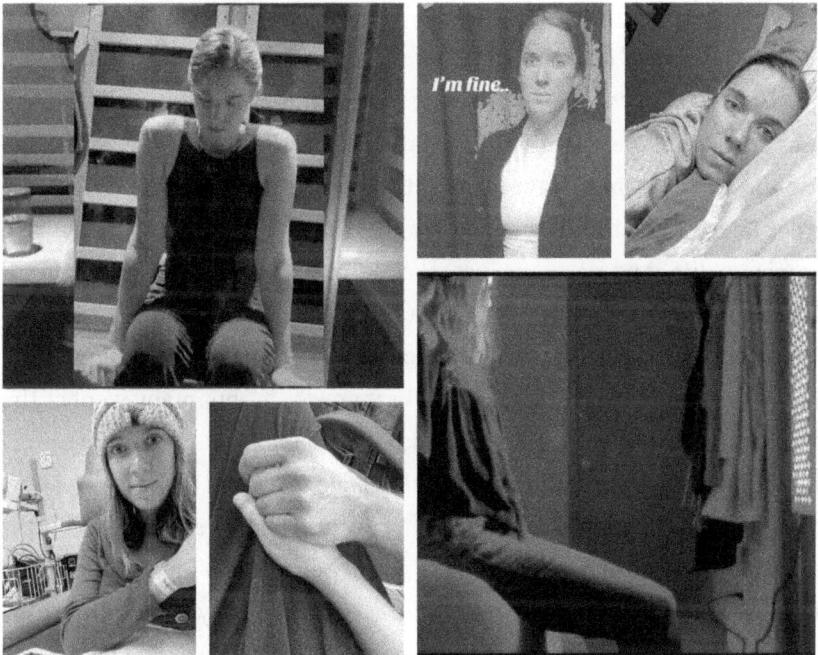

I pour myself into the sauna, red light, and phlebotomies. I try to trick my mind into feeling like I am better, just to stay stuck at the same spot . . . it is an endless battle and I am tired.

I decided not to do the 5-HTP. It's a supplement for depression. Sometimes I have thought I was depressed, but when I really think about it I am just deeply saddened and hurt by everything that has happened to me. I *want* to do the things I love. I *desire* to be well again. I have been *promised* over and over again by doctors that I will be healed. They convinced me that if I just did this protocol—or that one—I would be *healed*. I can *heal*. Sometimes I wonder if anyone used me by taking advantage of my suffering. But I really don't think this has been the case. I was told that I would heal over and over again. So I cling on to that for my future.

I can't do the things that I want because of the body I am in. *I feel trapped here.* If I were *depressed,* wouldn't all that longing and want go away? Isn't the feeling of sadness over the loss of one's health normal? Does everything have to be a mental health diagnosis? Can't a person just feel *sadness* and *loss,* or *nervousness* about what has happened to their body? Loss of oneself, loss of hopes and dreams . . . wouldn't that normally cause sadness? *Is it so hard to understand that sometimes what people really need is a hug and not a pill? Is the human condition really that hard to grasp?*

Then I switch perspectives to what I am *grateful* for. I have so much to be *grateful* for . . . but I have learned that the one thing you *need* to have in order to enjoy the things that you are *grateful* for is *your health.* It can be so simple . . . *life.* And everyone just takes advantage of health. They find silly things to *complain* about or *stress* over out of *boredom* . . . not realizing how *good* they have it. And then there are all of these *claims* that if you *view* your health as that important then you make it an *idol* . . . but many wept as they went to *Jesus* for *healing* . . . and you know what he did? *He healed them.* He didn't say *you are acting like your health is more important than worshiping me, go away!* No. He knew they were suffering and he healed them. *Why can't he heal me?* Because it is not like it used to be . . . I can't just walk out the door and run into Jesus like Mary did. He called her by *name* and she was *redeemed.* The woman *touched* his *cloak* and she was healed. The world is full of disease, and I don't blame God. I used to. It got me nowhere. It just filled me with anger and hopelessness. I think it's okay to ask God to heal you. Even if it doesn't seem like he is listening. Maybe I need to scream it again like I did when I longed for a child . . . but I feel like this time is different.

Maybe I am not meant to heal . . .

* * *

All of the darkness has come up since my illness. I just want healing from all of it. During my day-to-day, I focus my attention away from my circumstances. I play with my children. I take them to the park when I can. I throw birthday parties for them and attend Russell's Tae Kwon Do lessons. But it's a daily battle . . .

I am easily frustrated with certain complaints of others and have a hard time relating to anyone anymore unless they are close family or friends . . . It's not that I don't believe they are truly struggling, but because I have no control over my struggles and they do, I find most complaints so *fixable*. So many create struggles out of boredom . . . Sometimes I fall into jealousy. *It would be so nice to have such easy problems.* Everyone has problems . . . not just me . . . *but life can be so easy when you have your health.* It's so much harder when you have no control of your body. I have never made a big deal about small things, but I notice that so many do. It's like they are bored. *I wish I could be bored.*

* * *

Sometimes I really struggle with circumstances. Why did this have to happen to me when I am raising small children . . . *Why?* They don't deserve this. It is so difficult to raise young children with all of these barriers to get around. They get this *unhealed broken version of me.* I worry about how my outbursts will affect them in their life later. I try so hard to hide and keep them from worrying over my conditions. I don't want them to *fear* life or illness or mold.

Sometimes it's hard for me to see people being able to function normally in life that are much older than myself. Of course, everyone has specific things they deal with, but no one that I know of has the debilitating conditions or POTS, MCAS, chronic migraines, and reactions to everything in life, with no control of their body. The people that I am around can still run after their children, run errands, and go grocery shopping, even if they are much older than me . . .

Russell turns eight this year, and it is yet another reminder that I have spent half of his life sick, and he is growing up. I struggle to complete any task and am missing out on precious moments while they are young. *I will never get this back.* I don't have many years of his childhood left. I do the best I can at making memories at home. My condition is so unpredictable, though, that it is difficult to plan things, and a lot of times I can't be a part of activities because of symptoms flaring.

I try very hard to make every birthday special, even if we have to have them at home. I decorate for every holiday and come up with fun activities on the days where I feel well enough. I try so hard and everything that I do for them is a struggle, but I do it for them because I love them so much. It just makes me so angry that I have to struggle like this with every task. I get so angry at my body and struggle with feeling envious when I see other people able to do normal tasks with little effort. I know you aren't supposed to feel envious and compare but it's hard not to . . . especially in my condition. I always try to remind myself that others can have it worse and to be *grateful.* I fail a lot in this battle.

The constant feeling like I am near death and the flares that make me feel like it's the end for me are difficult to experience over and over again. Feeling like I am in a drunken state every day is not ideal. The symptoms this last year where I feel tremors in my head, pressure, and as if I have a chronic sinus infection are so disheartening. Those symptoms got so much better after lowering the ferritin.

I had to treat the gut infection with an antibiotic. I don't know if it really resolved . . . I feel worse, but that stool kit was over $500 and I would hate to have to do it again. Maybe it just made the fungus worse, but I was told this gut bacteria can trigger autoimmune conditions and can hurt the kidneys, so what was I supposed to do? Just keep trying to treat it with garlic oil?

I did the best I could with the help that I had.

20

A Shadow of the Person I Once Was

November 28, 2022

Most of my days have been spent in crippling pain and a thick fog. I feel out-of-body with how extreme this fog gets. I don't know what has happened to cause this regression, but it is persistent and these GI issues are becoming worse. Ever since last June when I had the fever and GI issues, I have been vomiting on and off with the crippling pain. I'm losing so much weight. I am down to 110 pounds and I used to be 157 pounds.

The pain starts in the upper left abdomen, it moves down to the mid- and lower back, then radiates up to the liver area and goes down the right mid- and lower back. It happens a lot when I eat. It almost feels like something is stuck. I had a CT scan done, per my out-of-state functional medicine doctor's request, *because* of these issues. The only thing they see is fatty liver and some signs of possible scar tissue. No kidney stones. No signs of a blockage. There were some mild signs of inflammation in the gallbladder, but it resolved more recently when I had an ultrasound done. Great . . . *more radiation* showing *nothing* that can be treated for this pain. I don't understand what I did wrong or what triggered this. I've been doing acupuncture for potential gastroparesis for a few months now. That seems to help the flares.

I feel out-of-body a lot during these abdominal flares. *Am I okay?* I get very foggy and they are usually surrounded by back-to-back headaches and migraines. The area between my liver and right side is again flaring, and I just don't know how I'm going to continue to live my life in this state of distress. How can I take care of my children when I'm in this amount of pain?

My out-of-state functional medicine doctor is still attributing it to the ferritin that was retained for so long. I am still doing the phlebotomies, but it takes months to get the levels lower. I have had improvement in vestibular migraines and ear ringing since donating my blood. But these stomach issues seem to be coming from something else. My out-of-state functional medicine doctor says that I am in a state of acute metabolic acidosis and a respiratory alkalosis state. She says this is all from systemic candida gone too long, the ferritin and parasite/potential Lyme disease, or a derivative of Lyme disease. I'm assuming co-infections . . .

My out-of-state functional medicine doctor tells me that the secondary hemochromatosis is either from the hemochromatosis gene or an acute internal bleed, and this is causing my liver to continuously be in a state of acute inflammation. The liver struggles with the high ferritin, and the candida, Lyme, and parasites are the cause. I completed three weeks of the diet and supplement plan for candida and parasites. Sometimes I wonder if this is die off or herxing, but these increased issues began in June. How long can die off go on? I go back and forth between *I am going to beat this and heal* and *Will I ever get better?*

My options right now are trying this protocol for candida and suspected Lyme/parasite or going forward with the exploratory surgery if I don't have improvement with the protocol. I have a surgeon that is a specialist in missed endometriosis and scar tissue that I feel is trustworthy, but I don't know if this will even help me. What if it's another situation like last time? But I'm vomiting all the time and in extreme pain now and I can't understand how this is okay to just be left to live this way. It seems like no one can really help me and no one can give me an answer or not as to if the surgery will even help. I even sent off all of my recent scans to this surgeon, but he says, unfortunately, for the conditions we think I have there is no other way but to go inside and look. I can't understand how a person can have symptoms like this with nothing obvious showing up on imaging.

It always feels like there is a blockage, but there are no signs and there are no signs of compression issues either. The reason I went back to try something different with my out-of-state doctor was because I was not improving with my local functional medicine doctor's mold protocol. The last thing I did with her was the ozone and antibiotic for the gut infection. Sometimes I wonder if something I did with her has triggered these increased vomiting and GI issues. Like it woke up another dormant bacteria that needed to be treated, but it is now just running rampant because we can't find it. For the longest time, I blamed my symptoms on *herxing*, but I feel that at *some point* there should be *improvement* if it's die off. There has not been. It's very difficult to go out in this state. I never know when I am going to get a vomit attack and it puts me on edge while doing anything.

I don't agree at all anymore that these issues are coming from limbic system impairment alone. I wasn't having these issues before June. I am vomiting after almost every meal, having extreme pain, brain fog with the pain, and my liver is fatty with signs on and off of my gallbladder having inflammation.

If anything, my limbic system is just going to be harder to fix because of this additional trauma. My recent labs and scans show that these things are happening. For the longest time, during my scans I was told everything was normal, until the last one when the person told me that I still have a cervix. I said it was removed. Confused, she said there definitely is one. I emailed the surgeon out of Minnesota and he said that leftover cervix could definitely be bleeding, causing acute inflammation and the retaining ferritin.

I called the doctor who performed my last surgery and was told there was absolutely no way that was a cervix, since it was removed. Upon further looking, in the newest CT scan, she said what they are likely seeing is the surgical cuff, but because of the complication of the hysterectomy and the development of the hematoma, when the hematoma began to dissolve it appears that it grew into the surgical cuff, creating connected scar tissue and the appearance of a cervix. *Lovely* . . . for months this finding was *missed* in all of my other scans as I was repeatedly told they were *normal*. I even read the reports myself to make sure.

If this scar tissue *is* bleeding, it *could* be a cause of acute inflammation and high ferritin. If it bleeds on and off, my body absorbs that blood and that causes the ferritin retention and irritation of the liver. I sent over the images to the surgeon in Minnesota and he said that could be the source, or at least part, of the problem. But he wasn't sure . . . It was missed in every other prior scan because they thought it was a normal cervix. My medical notes list partial hysterectomy. I feel they should have known this.

So here we are. Two years after my hysterectomy. At this point, I won't be able to avoid surgery unless a miracle happens. I can't keep vomiting like this. I didn't do well with surgery the last two times, and I don't ever want another blood donation ever again. I have learned how contaminated they can be with Lyme and other infections. They are not cleared of these things. I feel like I am dying for at least two months after surgery. I can't breathe and have stroke-like feelings and pressure in my head. I have constant feelings of panic because of the extreme symptoms. I have been told this may be because of the oxidative stress levels that I already have and the anesthesia. Last time I felt it was because of the internal bleeding and blood transfusions.

But if I actually had a surgery that *fixed* a problem and didn't cause more, maybe I would do okay. I'm praying that God would give me a clear sign on what direction I should take. If this is a part of what I need to help me heal I need a sign. But if it is not, I need God to tell me in some way. *But I don't hear anything.* I don't know what direction to take because everything seems so unclear. If the vomiting continues I will have the surgery. If it does not, I will do the different testing for Lyme disease. Even if my functional medicine doctors don't feel the testing will be very beneficial . . . that is the path I will take if my vomiting stops.

I don't ever want another person's blood put into my body again and have the risk of infection or extreme iron overload again.

The surgeon said I can go in and donate a unit of my own blood and save it for the surgery. So we have to figure that process out. I *hope* I won't need it. My migraines have been much less since my ferritin has come down. I also recently went on a medication called LDN and that seems to help some too. My primary care doctor actually suggested it, and my functional medicine doctors approved it.

* * *

Thanksgiving this year was very clouded. It was really difficult for me to focus, and the food part is challenging. I'm very clouded now. I hardly feel here when my GI issues and vomiting become extreme. Twice this month I had a temporary lift of the fog. I could even breathe better. People seriously have no idea how lucky they have it. I would be so *grateful* to feel that way again. I hardly remember how that felt, which is so sad. I am nearing four years of this absolute nightmare. And five months of the chronic vomiting episodes.

I struggle so much to be a mother to my children. I feel so overstimulated so often and struggle with the most troubling of symptoms. I can hardly relax, and a lot of normal play startles me. Like getting squirted with a water gun. I can't laugh like a normal person would and I instead react negatively or get triggered. I often react in an overstimulated manner to these normal things that children do.

I have guilt that I never do enough with them. I imagine all of the things I would do if I weren't trapped in this body. It's like when you are sick and you feel bad if they have too much screen time, except it's every day. I think about how little they were when I became sick and how big they are now. I can't do anything to stop it but to keep trying to get better. I *hope* they know this was not how I intended to be as a mother. It is how I have become because of my circumstances . . .

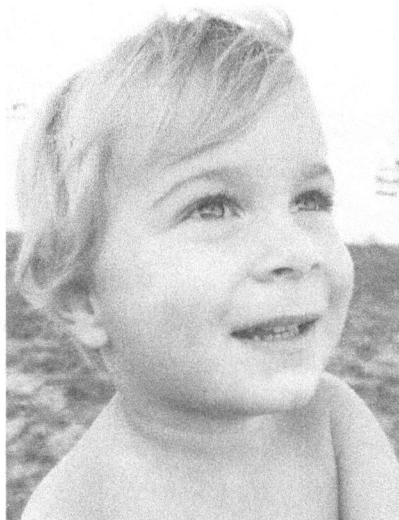

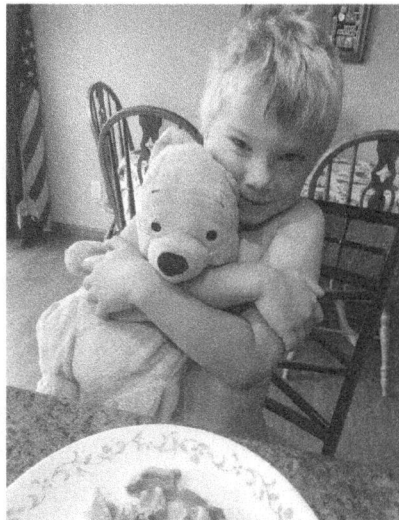

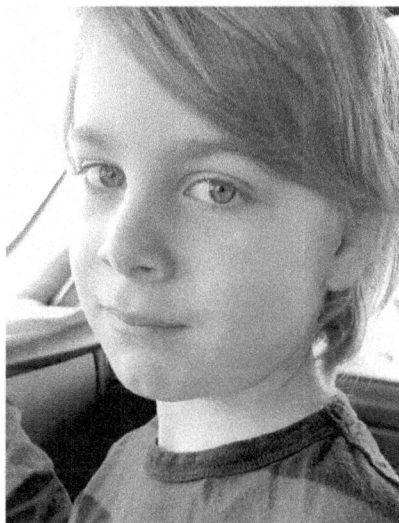

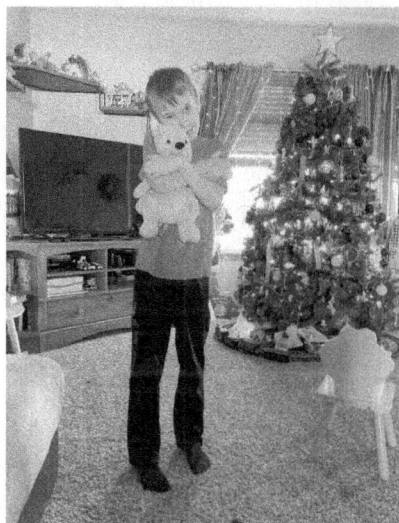

I watch as my children grow up so fast, and I struggle to even feel present . . .

Sometimes I think I can be *grateful* that this happened to me because it brought me so much closer to God, but other times I just don't understand what I did to deserve this. I don't know how I can keep living this way, and I don't know what the best decisions are. It's very possible there is nothing surgery will help me with, and I am just putting myself at risk for more scar tissue. How am I supposed to make this decision without any certainty that this is the cause to my issues and will help me, not harm me?

I am a shadow of the person I once was. A shadow of the mother that I once was. I am in this state and am here simply because I am needed. I pray for a miracle to direct me in my choices.

The most reassuring thing I hear is my out-of-state doctor's words that my blood levels look exactly like her other patients with systemic candida, Lyme, and parasites, and they are all recovered from POTS now. Completely healed. She told me about a patient that was on a PICC line antibiotic for Lyme. She was a model, but all her hair was falling out and she was bedbound. They did the candida protocol together and she finally *healed*. The other factors were keeping her sick and the antibiotics were just making her worse. I don't want that to happen to me with antibiotics, so we are continuing to treat it by getting rid of the candida and doing the therapies for possible Lyme through herbals. Sometimes I wonder if that is part of why my health has regressed so much. Maybe we are targeting Lyme right now without fully knowing it, and it's causing these *herxing* episodes. *Jarisch-Herxheimer reaction (JHR)* is a clinical phenomenon that occurs in patients infected by spirochetes who undergo antibiotic treatment. The reaction occurs within 24 hours of antibiotic treatment of spirochete infections, including syphilis, leptospirosis, Lyme disease, and relapsing fever. As the spirochetes die they emit a toxin, often causing worsening of symptoms.

I do not think my out-of-state doctor is lying to me. I feel she is doing the best she can and she wants me to heal. She says that I will be healed too. I believe her and have *hope*. But when I feel this bad it makes that *hope* less strong. I am a different person too. Perhaps what is keeping me sick is not the candida, but the Lyme.

Please God, let me heal in six months or I may be lost forever.

Summary from the loss of Entries

From December to April, I proceeded to do the candida, parasite, and herbal Lyme protocol through my out-of-state functional medicine doctor. I continued to do monthly phlebotomies for the retained ferritin and began to experience fewer debilitating migraines and stroke-like symptoms. The tremors got better in my head and I had less ear ringing and brain pressure. My blood became thinner and flowed better.

I continued to deal with vomiting episodes, debilitating pain, and brain fog during flares. Before doing an invasive surgery, we decided to do a colonoscopy and hida scan to see if there was anything causing the vomiting. Both tests were normal. Later, I did a gastric emptying study, which was also normal.

My exploratory surgery was to take place just a few weeks after the test was done for gastroparesis. Because of the negative result for gastroparesis, my acupuncturist felt that what we had been doing had been helping the nerves and he tried one other therapy as a last resort, hoping to avoiding surgery. The therapy completely stopped my vomiting episodes. It was like a miracle. Prior to this, I had lost about 55 pounds from the vomiting episodes and felt very hopeless.

I could eat again with less pain. I had less pain flares. I couldn't go forward with the surgery because we were very suspicious that, because his protocols helped my issues, it was unlikely to be related to the scar tissue seen in my scans. The phlebotomies were working to lower my ferritin levels. There were no signs of internal bleeding in the scans, so I did not feel comfortable at that time getting cut open.

Instead, I contacted my local functional medicine doctor to do Lyme testing through Vibrant Wellness 2.0. My out-of-state functional medicine doctor only did testing through Labcorp, which I had been told was very unreliable. I continued my entries in the spring of 2023 when I was completing the gastric emptying study.

21

Lost and Unsure

April 4, 2023

I am at the hospital doing a gastric emptying study. Ever since I experienced the fever illness last summer, I have had severe pain or vomiting after eating. I have lost a lot of weight and the pain still comes and goes. Fog, breathlessness, heart race, extreme bloating, and pain accompany the episodes. I get a feeling of fullness, nausea, heartburn, and sometimes anxiousness after eating. I didn't recover from these issues after my out-of-state functional medicine doctor's protocol for candida, parasites, and possible Lyme. It makes me feel like a *failure* really. I did have improvements with food reactions and I hardly ever have heart palpitations after eating grains anymore.

The nurse doing my hida scan is not here yet to get me. She was *supposed* to get me by now. It is almost forty minutes late for the first picture. I *hope* that doesn't matter.

I am still doing phlebotomies for the ferritin, and I have had improvement with vestibular migraines, pressure in head, and tinnitus since lowering it. I still have surgery scheduled for next month and am trying to make the right decision concerning that. My out-of-state functional medicine doctor wants me to do a genetic testing for a condition called porphyria. *It could make sense,* but it seems very random that she would be suggesting this now. I'm still hoping for something that can be fixed. I have to do a 24-hour urine test the next time I am in a flare to rule out porphyria.

My body has been so frustrating. Today I was lucky enough to get hit with an extreme migraine behind my right eye, but I still made it to the hospital to eat radioactive eggs and do a photo shoot. I feel breathless off and on. I still have mild food reactions occasionally, but I have noticed that has improved greatly. I don't get near as many heart palpitations after eating, either. I don't lie in bed for hours every night with heart palpitations. Those symptoms have improved a lot. It's the other ones that are hard to deal with.

The symptoms I have experienced:
Dizziness, lightheadedness, vertigo, heart race , spinning sensations,
derealization, abdominal pain, brain fog, pressure in head, tremors, severe
fatigue, breathlessness, oxygen drops, air hunger, blurry vision, double vision,
aura migraine, stroke-like symptoms, heart skipping beats, night sweats, sore
throats, vomiting, rash, heart race after eating, chills, blisters on skin, sores, and
cystic acne.

* * *

It's frustrating how I keep going back to feeling like we don't even know what is wrong with me. We don't have all of the answers. The last possibility, besides working on the limbic system, is testing for Lyme disease and co-infections.

Never give up. Keep advocating for yourself.

* * *

The boys and I recently got hit with influenza A. I had a fever of around 104 for a few days and was in a state of delirium. I was in a very bad state for about three weeks after that. The boys came out of it okay, but they both had fevers of 105. Sometimes my son concerns me as he complains more and more of light sensitivity, smell sensitivity, and headaches. He also has some attention issues and OCD-type tendencies. Tim and I noticed more recently, too, that he seems to have developed a tic and stammers/stutters on his words a lot.

I am still experiencing symptoms from the flu, while the boys are running around happily again. I am very *thankful* for their health and ability to recover, but I am still stuck and that makes it hard to take care of them as a mother.

It's been a month since our acute illness onset. When I was first sick, standing was extremely difficult. I could not breathe well at all. It was like the symptoms I get from overdoing it would happen just from standing. Extreme air hunger, chest tightness, dizziness, pressure in head, brain fog, heart palpitations, and the GI and back pain is worse again.

Whatever is wrong underlying, whether it's the oxidative stress or an infection of some kind, flares terribly now with acute illness. It's so hard. *Hope* is still present but harder to grasp lately.

No one can give me a solid answer on if I have an internal bleed either. All they can say is they *think* that I have scar tissue connecting to things. This *could* be responsible for the retained ferritin and pain. But why did the pain start so much later? It wasn't debilitating like this until last summer. I have always had some pain, but not like this. Unless the inflammation, over time, just caused it to worsen.

* * *

The last time I saw my acupuncturist he said, "Please don't let them cut you open."

He feels there is a different cause and still highly suspects Lyme disease. He feels that *maybe* doing certain exercises could help break up the scar tissue. We are waiting for my gastric emptying test to come back before knowing what to do therapy-wise.

I often feel myself spinning with uncertainty. I just don't know what to do anymore. I don't know what path to take. I stay on one path as long as I can, but when I have little relief in one area and none in others it makes it hard to have *faith* that I am doing the correct thing. Giving my *fear* to God is hard when I don't hear him.

It's just not fair how some people find their underlying causes so easily. They go through the protocols and heal. I've done this so many times and I'm not healed, and we keep finding more underlying factors. It's scary, too, to go through this . . . to see these things showing up on labs that have been hurting my body . . . it's difficult to hear. It's so scary to hear how this has hurt my cells and I just have to sit there and accept it. It's like a never-ending cycle, and then I feel like I'm failing at healing my limbic system.

I am *lost* and *unsure*.

* * *

One of my friends on *Facebook* has developed POTS . . .

It seems that so many young women are developing this syndrome. I met her years ago when I was well. We both were part of a homeschooling group together. I remember she had stomach issues, similar to mine at the time, and gluten intolerance. Now, recently, she has developed POTS. Both of her children are experiencing POTS symptoms too . . . both girls are around my boys' ages. I saw on her *Facebook* page that the doctors wondered if it was possibly from having COVID.

POTS has been becoming more known since COVID. The syndrome is exactly what I have experienced for the last several years. What is going on with our mitochondria and cells to cause these issues? Why is POTS increasing? What is wrong with our food or environment, causing so many people to have GI issues and increased GI cancer rates? I wish they would do more research, but I have a feeling they will not. It will just keep getting worse and continue to be pushed under the rug.

February 20, 2023

My gastroparesis study was negative. I am very happy to say that I don't have that. When I saw my acupuncturist and told him the results, it pushed him to reevaluate my situation moving forward. He treated a specific area that is often affected by Lyme disease, where the large and small intestine meet. I have not vomited since . . .

The severe pain and issues after eating have improved too. I was shocked when I felt the release of pain and even more shocked as my vomiting episodes continued to stay away.

Today I have been having some returning pain in the liver area and air hunger. I don't know what to do moving forward concerning this pain. *I don't feel confident that surgery will fix this.* I always prayed that if something fixed the vomiting then I would not do the surgery. *I felt that this was an obvious enough sign from God to hold off for now.*

No one can assure me there is even anything that needs fixing surgically.

I still feel like I have some tick-borne disease or co-infection problem. But I don't know what to do just yet. I am so tired. Physically and emotionally. The tests are so expensive.

I had a flare of heart palpitations one night. The sudden feeling of having sinus-related headaches and mouth sores returned. Sometimes it feels like I have repeating fevers. It's weird, because I have noticed these flares seem to revolve around certain times of the month. I used to base everything around my hormone fluctuations, but since I no longer have a period, I can't do that any longer.

I feel so defeated because I am still dealing with the same old problems. They just return over and over again to torture me. I feel like a failure and I'm hopeless that we will ever reach an underlying cause and find true healing and relief of these symptoms. I don't want to do this any longer. I just want to live again. Normal.

* * *

I am unable to do the complete brain rewiring on my own as an over-whelmed, chronically ill mother and wife. I've tried so many times to achieve that to heal my symptoms, but then I just get sicker over and over again. It's traumatic and my brain can't forget when it keeps happening.

The doctors give me *hope* and confidence, but then they make me question everything when we start to dig into other illnesses. *I don't trust anything anymore.* I don't want to be cut open. I just want to lie under a red light for hours until it fixes me. I don't want to get up and struggle every day with my symptoms. But then I have to be a mom. *My kids need me.* My husband needs me. Others need me. Everyone wants me to get better.

No one wants me to have surgery. *"I really am scared of you having this surgery." "I don't want you to go through this again." "Please don't let them cut you open." "What if they find nothing?" "What if it makes you worse?" "Are you sure this is what is wrong?" "I don't see any reason why you should undergo surgery." "This may not even be the problem." "Are you sure this surgeon is safe?" "What if you lose blood and need a blood transfusion again?" "What if you die?" "What if you have another internal bleed?" "What if your fainting episodes come back?" "What if you have Lyme?"* Everyone in my family has discouraged it.

The only person who tried to speak positive words to me was my out-of-state functional medicine doctor who had many patients, like me, that had missed endometriosis or internal bleeds. If I had any chance of going into this surgery with a *positive* outlook at all, it was taken from me because of all of the words around me that kept killing me inside. Even words from strangers that had no idea what I was gong through affected me. I was already living in trauma and PTSD from the last surgery. I was so conflicted on what to do because of my pain, vomiting, and the claim of troublesome scar tissue they could see inside of me.

I want everyone to know that I understood their concerns because of what happened the last time. But if they *felt* the pain that I am in they would understand the conflict that I felt. I understood their concerns, because what if they did find nothing to fix and it *did* cause more problems . . . I had all the same concerns that they had.

I don't even know how I am alive still. It's just reality.

I am trying to escape my reality and find a piece of myself that I lost to chronic illness. Tim has been encouraging me to illustrate and write a

Boomer book. *Boomer* was a cartoon that I created in high school. He has been tucked away in storage these last few years. I don't know if I know how to write children's books. I have been playing around on the computer doing little books out of my photography just to get a grasp on how it all works. If I do write *Boomer* books, I will use our own memories to create the stories.

I just wish I could be healed before doing this, but maybe this is something that I need right now while my mind is so overwhelmed with my condition and the unknowns.

Maybe this is what I need to escape my reality and remember who I was before all of this.

22

Friends Become Distant

February 4, 2023

I have been painting with Kara off and on this winter. I don't think she realizes how much she means to me and just how much these small things help me. I don't feel very good during our time together, but it can take my mind off my pain when I am painting with her. I am so *grateful* to have Kara as a friend. I wish I could do more with her. She tries so hard to understand what is wrong with me and is not mean or judgmental.

I am sure she questions some of my diagnoses, but I understand how hard it is to understand. I am just so *grateful* for her.

Kara was there for me, too, a few months ago when I tried hyperbaric oxygen therapy (HBOT) during the summer. I tried this a few months after I had the flare in June. Kara took me to every session and stayed with me that entire week. She understood when I had trouble breathing at the musty hotel and helped me cook food and stick to my diet while I was away from home.

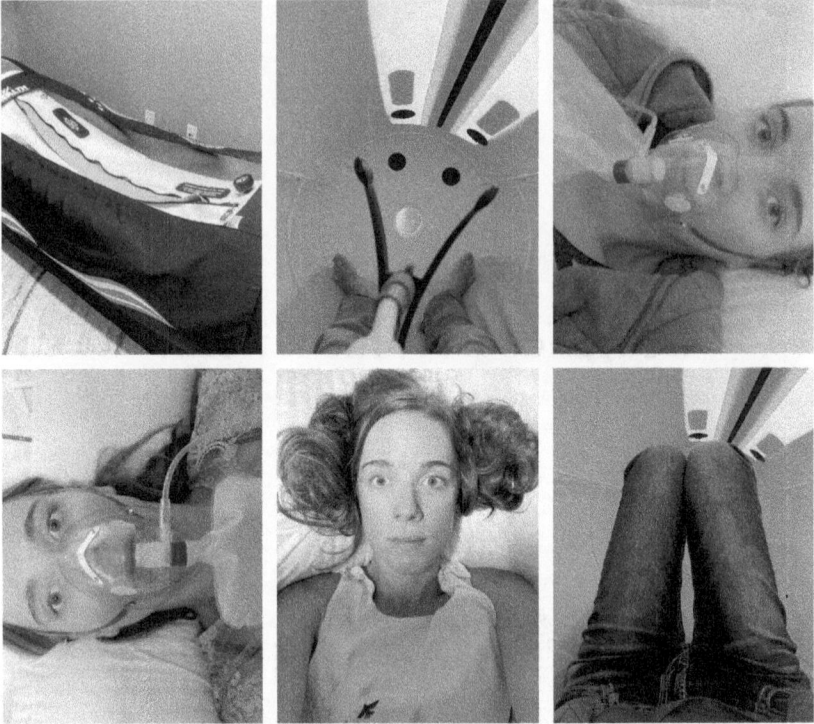

I tried so many things to improve my pain and chronic GI symptoms, but until my acupuncturist helped me, I just kept vomiting . . .

I know they don't mean to, but I have had a lot of friends become very distant from me throughout my illness. *I don't blame them.* I am *not upset* with them. But I *miss* how it *was* when we were together when I was *not* this way. I feel that most do not know how to act around me anymore because they may not understand or believe my health conditions. POTS alone is hard to understand.

I feel they were the most distant during the first year, when all I had to tell them was that the doctors felt I had a panic disorder. I couldn't even explain to them why this was happening and I felt very embarrassed, because I knew there wasn't anything externally causing it. I was happy as a stay-at-home mother, I was happy with my husband, I was finally getting my freedom back to do more things.

Later, some of my friends did try to help me brainstorm and I was always very *grateful* because a lot of times I worried about what they *thought* of me. I felt their distance meant they didn't want anything to do with me anymore. I understood, though, it being difficult to believe all of these conditions that were being thrown at me.

I was also embarrassed that I could not control my body at times. I always hid the symptoms when they were around. I always looked normal. I would often feel afraid that I may have an episode when we got together. *What would they think of me?* I know the fact that I looked so *normal* and hid my symptoms often *confused* a lot of them. *You look so normal. You look so healthy. You don't look sick at all. You must be feeling better.* I am not sure how I could have navigated this better, because I didn't know what my episodes were at the time, and it was very embarrassing for me to experience them around others.

I am not upset with any of my friends or family. I was always so appreciative when any of my friends called me just to chat or check in. It meant so much to me to know that I still had people who wanted to be in my life, regardless of my health decline. In the early stages, I struggled mostly with feelings of isolation and loneliness and concern that no one would want me in their life any longer. I am understanding that this is a common feeling for chronically ill people.

It's partly my fault because I don't share a lot with them. I don't want to overburden them and I worry they might not *believe* me, but there have been friends who still do keep in touch and help me, and I appreciate that so much.

The suggestions I have for people who have chronically ill loved ones is, they don't expect a lot. Sure, it's nice for them if their friends do a little research on their condition so they can understand it better. But the most that the chronically ill need is just someone to sit with them sometimes. Or paint with them. If they can't do a lot physically, it's the small acts of kindness that help.

I was very vulnerable during the HBOT sessions because it was the first time that we had asked for help from others. It was the first time that we really tried to explain to people what was wrong with me. I was worried that people wouldn't believe us or understand . . . it was hard enough for most of my friends already.

We were ashamed to ask for help, but my husband and I both agreed that we needed help to try these therapies. We did a GoFundMe for the HBOT, and we were able get enough money to do ten sessions. I completed eight. I was unable to complete all of them because of a flare. I purchased a red light with the remainder of the money because of the research on how it helps with the possible Lyme and with the mitochondrial healing.

My brain health specialist is still convinced that I have Lyme, so I felt the red light, for now, was the best option. He also says *I am one of the most complicated immune cases he has seen* . . . yay me.

* * *

I have recently decided to start illustrations for my *Boomer* books. Because of our painting sessions, Kara has rekindled my artistic side. Tim is very encouraging as well and encourages me to create a series. I don't know how I can ever thank Kara, and I *hope* that when I am healed we can do so much more together.

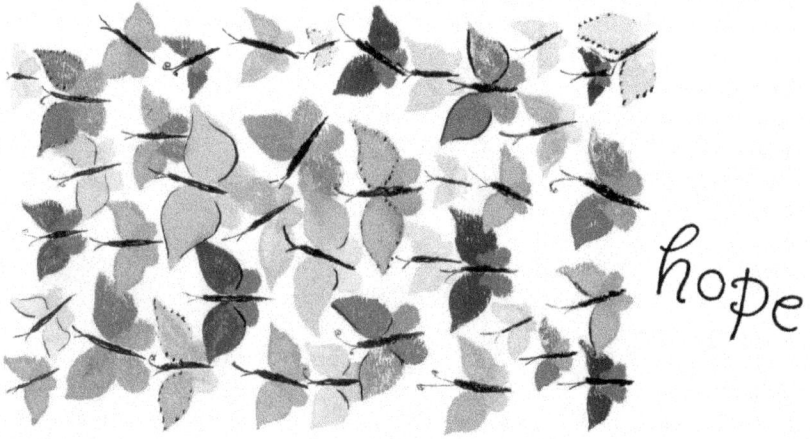

Thank you Kara . . . I can have hope again . . .

III

Part Three

After all of this time I knew . . . I had Lyme . . .

23

I Finally Test for Lyme

April 13, 2023

I had an appointment with my local functional medicine doctor today. I decided I want to do the test for Lyme disease.

Recently, Tim and I accepted help from a benefit through his work. They have been wanting to help us for many years now, but we always said no before. It just didn't feel right when we didn't know what was wrong. We felt, too, that we could give up things first before accepting help from anyone. So we did. But this has gone on long enough. Russell suffered because of our losses, while Tim and I have just been surviving and he now suffers from PTSD because of his wife's health decline. The benefit will help us pay off our medical debt and pay for the right testing for Lyme disease. The comprehensive tests are very expensive. We are so *grateful* for this help . . . it has lifted a huge weight off us.

* * *

A few months ago, I posted a video concerning my health on a public health group on *Facebook*. A moderator of the group contacted me and directed me to a *Facebook* page called *RISE ABOVE LYME (Support, Education, and Advocacy group)*. She felt I most definitely have Lyme disease or some other co-infection like Bartonella or Babesia. She helps people all over the world by finding proper testing and directing them to local Lyme-literate doctors.

I contemplated testing with my out-of-state functional medicine doctor first, but she uses Labcorp and I was told that is not effective enough for Lyme. Her labs were out of network for me, too, and insurance would not cover them. Blue Cross apparently dropped Labcorp, which is odd because they used to cover them before. *Maybe there is a reason for this*. I am glad I called my insurance company first, otherwise I may have done the testing through her.

The Lyme group moderator recommended testing through Vibrant or IGeneX. I have not been a part of any health groups since trying to rewire my limbic system, but this group has been very helpful in finding the correct testing. My out-of-state doctor felt that my original negative Western blot confirmed that I do not have chronic Lyme, and she told me that a lot of her patients with Lyme went into remission when candida and parasites were not taxing their immune system. So, at that time I decided *not* to do the testing through Vibrant with my local functional medicine doctor because I was being told resolving the other infections would put me into remission, even if I did have chronic Lyme disease.

A few months later I changed my mind and went through the Vibrant 2.0 testing with my local functional medicine doctor. The Lyme group moderator *stressed* that it's okay to start with her since she can order the test, but to take it to a Lyme-literate doctor to read the results. She told me that most functional medicine doctors do not train through ILADS and won't be able to read the results *properly*. She said it isn't *their fault*, they are just trained by the CDC criteria, which is outdated and misses a lot of positives.

I'm just not sure yet. My local functional medicine doctor went through the results with me and said I only have IgG (immunoglobulin G) levels of the Lyme Borrelia burgdorferi and that meant that I did *not* have chronic Lyme. I was informed it is a *past* infection that my body dealt with.

"I am happy to see that this is *not* chronic Lyme disease." She continued in more detail and by the time she finished I was more confused.

I also had an IgG level for a herpes virus, and she wanted me on an antiviral supplement for that. Why would I treat the herpes virus if it only has an IgG band, but not Lyme? My understanding is that they are *both* past infections according to the IgG level. So why treat one but not the other?

According to my local functional medicine doctor, I do *not* have a *current* Lyme infection, but I am shocked to see that I *did* have it . . . *Did this happen at the acreage, and maybe all of the therapies I have done got rid of it? Maybe that is why I am still sick, because my cells still need healing from the past infections?* I always thought that when you had a positive IgG alone it meant you *do* have chronic Lyme, depending on how high the bands are . . . especially in the *presence* of symptoms. I have read how it harbors in your tissues and can embed itself into bones, organs, and even your brain.

Before leaving, I told my local functional medicine doctor about my improvement with food-related reactions and migraines. I feel it's mostly from the lowered ferritin. She felt this could mean the oxidative stress levels are lower. I told her I even have a little sugar once in a while, and I don't have any issues with allergic-type reactions or hot feelings from it.

She said, "Just be careful, because that can increase oxidative stress."

I'm trying *really hard* to tell my limbic system that it is okay to have a little sugar sometimes. I know she is just trying to help, but those words stick with me and now I feel like I'm making myself sicker if I have just a tiny bit of sugar. The mental anguish is awful. *I don't want to make myself sicker.*

* * *

My acupuncturist is getting the live blood analysis in a few weeks. If I test positive through Vibrant, he was hoping to use what we see in *my blood.* That way he can help other patients when comparing what he sees in theirs. But I don't know if the *old infection* results will be any help. I am still planning on bringing him the results to get his opinion. Live blood analysis is pretty controversial in diagnosing things. A Lyme-literate doctor wouldn't accept those results alone. That's why I felt the need to pursue testing through Vibrant.

The Lyme group moderator asked me to send her the results when I got them. She was convinced I would need a Lyme-literate doctor. I really don't want to have to start all over if I don't have to.

My local functional medicine doctor seemed very convinced this is a *past infection* and ended with, "We can close the idea of this being caused by chronic Lyme."

She suggested that I may still have aluminum in my brain, causing the oxidative stress levels and *especially* limbic system impairment.

I have been having the strangest episodes of my tongue turning blue, as if I ate food coloring. I showed both functional medicine doctors, my primary care provider, and my acupuncturist. They all believe it could be *aluminum* detoxing out of my system. This is a very troubling thought.

It scrapes off, so it *isn't* vascular. It has been happening at random. I will be doing usual things, and the first thing I notice is that my mouth tastes metallic-like. When I look in the mirror my tongue is dark blue . . . as if I were chewing on the end of a blue pen and it exploded onto my tongue. It's actually a really disturbing thought to me that this could be *aluminum*. I was diagnosed with aluminum toxicity years ago through a blood test . . . I would think that would be cleared by now. We even went through my supplements, which are very few right now, and none could have caused this. The only thing different that I have started in the last couple of months is glutathione injections, but I have done these in the past with no blue tongue. I don't tell anyone these scary things that happen to me, except my doctors and close family. Just like I didn't tell anyone when I was passing arm-length wormlike things in my stools. It would just sound crazy to everyone, or too disturbing . . .

Who knows what most people think about me anyway . . . but I have learned it *doesn't matter anymore.*

I have been on many different supplements on and off while working with these doctors. Sometimes I felt there were too many. My out-of-state functional medicine doctor told me that they have a lab that tests

220

supplements. A lot of supplements that people bring in are found to contain contaminants like heavy metals, and some don't even have the vitamin inside of it that is advertised. *Thankfully,* throughout this process, I have only been on vitamins studied by third parties to ensure quality. I have used NutriDyn, Metagenics, and some brands off of Fullscript. It made me wonder about the prenatal supplement I was on years ago. It was an over-the-counter brand, and about a year after my pregnancy it was being recalled for high traces of heavy metals. I was very upset about that when I found out.

I was told by my acupuncturist that you even have to be careful where you purchase a red light. We chose a red light that was approved by the FDA, but he said some patients would come in with worse symptoms after using *"healing"* devices purchased off *Amazon.* My acupuncturist has a device that detects radiation levels, and one patient's device was emitting *three times* the amount of radiation that one X-ray produces. That was very upsetting to me. People are suffering enough already, and then they have to worry about what supplements or devices they purchase to avoid further damage . . .

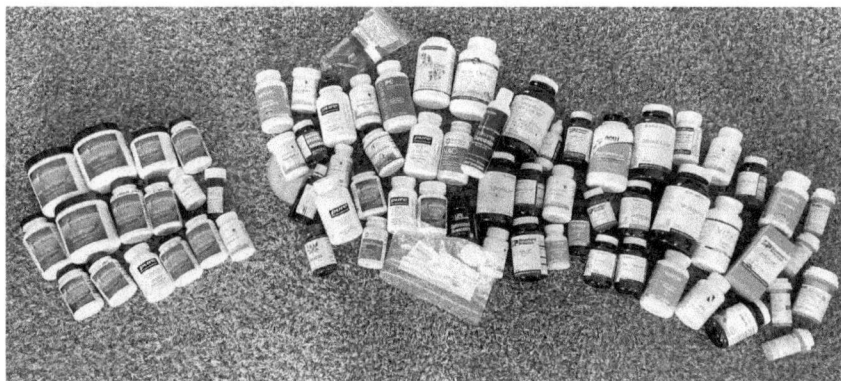

It scraped off like ink. I have tried a lot of supplements over the last five years, and my tongue has never turned blue . . .

I have been doing so much with limbic system rewiring. I pretend I am well.

I do things that I enjoy like painting with Kara, illustrating my *Boomer* book, grounding, deep breathing, visualization, prayer, ignoring my symptoms, finding joy, and having less *fear* around introducing foods. I have even been eating some gluten and sugar on and off with no issues.

I still experience troubling symptoms. When I talk about my symptoms to anyone, I don't hang around it long. I get it out if I need to, and then I move on so that I don't dwell or experience too much stress surrounding it. I have been having more night sweats lately, lesions on my legs, abdominal pain with no trigger, back pain, and feeling like fighting an infection. I still feel like I get recurring fevers, especially when triggered by the extreme regressions with acute illnesses. I have increased buzzing sensations during certain times of each month. The buzzing drives me mad sometimes. It's in my feet, head, and even internally, like a tremor. It feels like I am hooked up to an electrical current at times.

Some things have improved since lowering my ferritin. I feel that my local functional medicine doctor was misled that it was from inflammation. I don't blame her as it seemed very difficult for everyone to pinpoint, including the local hematologist. The hematologist that worked with my out-of-state functional medicine doctor was *sure* it was from the blood transfusions, but my local one was unsure, and it is difficult for insurance to cover out-of-state lab orders. Out-of-state lab orders will be covered by insurance for some, but in my case it wasn't. It seems obvious at this point that it was being caused by the retaining from the blood transfusions. It makes me sad that it was like that for so long, hurting my organs. My blood is much thinner too. It's so much better. I don't have near as much ear ringing, light sensitivity, and vestibular migraines. I feel the excess iron was causing more oxidative stress on my system.

If this is the case, my out-of-state functional medicine doctor was correct about this and there was a *reason* I still needed her. Sometimes it makes me question other things. Like, are we sure I don't have chronic Lyme?

* * *

For now, I will see what my acupuncturist thinks. I might still take the Vibrant results in to show him. Originally, I felt like I should put a close on it, like my functional medicine doctor suggested . . . but there is too much of an internal voice telling me *NO*. Even if *it is* a past infection, perhaps my results and the live blood analysis will help my acupuncturist help other people in some way.

I don't know if I will send my results to the Lyme group moderator. It all depends on what my acupuncturist thinks. *Honestly*, I *trust* his opinion the most and will pursue a second opinion with a Lyme-literate doctor if he thinks the testing shows a positive. Some people might think it's funny to *trust* the opinion of my acupuncturist above others . . . but he has been the most intelligent, most dedicated person that I have met, with endless suggestions . . . he is still at the top of my list, even above the doctors I met at Mayo.

My local functional medicine doctor still thinks that most symptoms are coming from limbic system impairment alone. I do agree in *some ways . . . but n*ot so much the recurring fevers . . . but s*ome things, yes.*

24

Now I Know for Sure

April 27, 2023

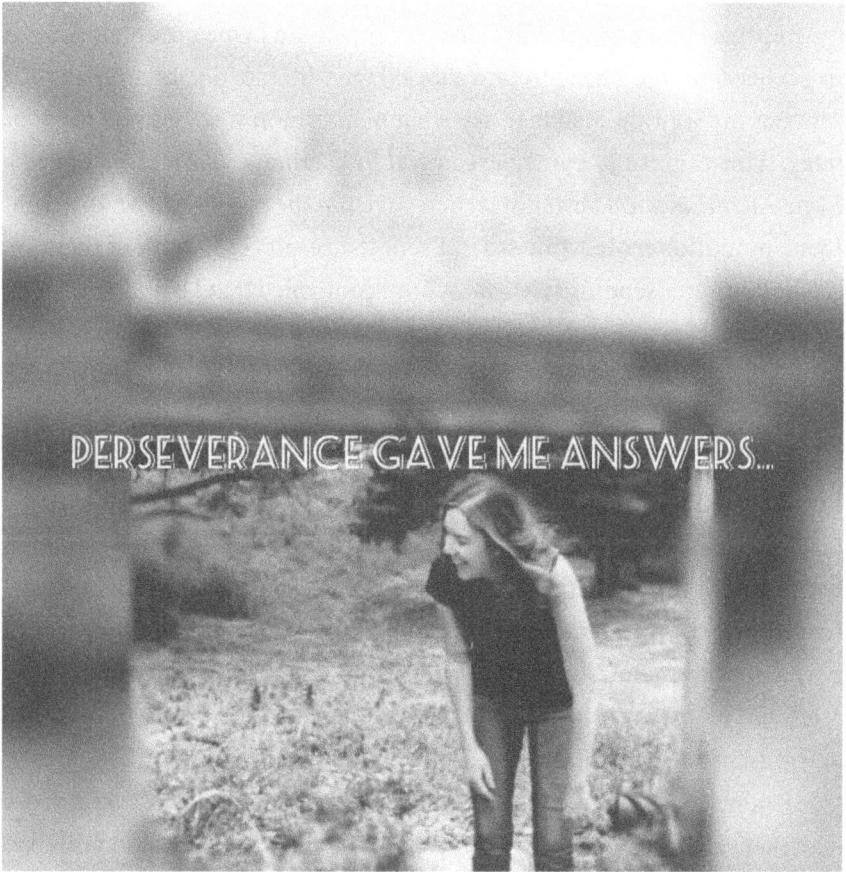

After all of this time I knew . . . I had Lyme . . .

I saw my acupuncturist today. While there, I showed him the results of my tick-borne panel through Vibrant. He really feels that I *do* have chronic Lyme based on these results. Later, I did the live blood analysis, and he called an hour later saying that he thinks he *found them . . .*

Spirochetes in my blood? I'm so confused right now. After being told by my functional medicine doctor that my results meant that it is only a *past infection,* my mind is racing again. My acupuncturist has always been my biggest advocate . . . but I know that live blood analysis cannot be diagnostic for Lyme disease.

225

After this appointment, I decided to contact the Lyme group moderator to get her opinion. I need to find a local Lyme-literate doctor after all . . . I sent her my Vibrant results to see what her opinion was. *She said the same thing.* This is chronic Lyme based on *ILADS criteria. She told me* I need a *Lyme-literate medical doctor* and then gave me the names of two different Lyme practitioners in Minnesota. I sent the results in to both of them.

Not long after sending the results, both confirmed that I have Lyme. *After all this time I knew . . .*

* * *

I could get in with a Lyme center in Minnesota on May 2. I spoke with the health coach through the Lyme center, and she told me that this can often happen with functional medicine providers because of the CDC criteria for Lyme. *I just can't believe this.* After all of this suffering. The concerns of both my acupuncturist and the Lyme group moderator were right. *"Most functional medicine doctors will miss it because of the CDC criteria. It is outdated and misses so many positives . . . "*

My new Lyme health coach had chronic Lyme disease for several years. The Lyme doctor who will be treating me said his wife and son both had Lyme as well and that is why he became a Lyme-literate medical doctor. He studied through ILADS. The clinic that I will be going to offers SOT therapy for Lyme disease, which is ironic, because I recently found out about SOT therapy through an experienced Lyme doctor out of Georgia on TikTok. I wasn't even searching for it. My phone probably *heard me* talking about Lyme disease over and over again . . . I plan on keeping him in mind if we ever hit a wall, or if I ever need help with my cells or guidance on testing later on.

I cannot be mad at my doctors . . . they have helped me with other conditions and diagnostic processes for other genetic factors. They *suspected* I had Lyme disease. *I am mad at the system.* I went undiagnosed with these conditions for so long because of how the system is set up.

I have had good doctors that were trying to help, but the system makes it nearly impossible. I feel if they could all come together, we could build a better medical system to help patients with a faster diagnostic process and better chances of healing.

The cost of everything and the battle between insurance companies sets people back. We have spent *so much money* throughout this process because a lot has been trial and error, and often insurance companies deny coverage.

I am so *grateful* for this health benefit. Because of the kind people who donated to our health benefit, we have been able to afford the right testing and the right doctors to get my diagnosis. I *hope* this is the *last* diagnosis I have.

With the band levels of Borrelia burgdorferi on the Vibrant testing, I quality for SOT (*Supportive Oligonucleotide Therapy*) from Europe! It can be quite expensive upfront at $2,600–$5000 per SOT, depending on where you go. The treatment works every day for up to six months after injection and there are follow-up appointments included. The cost is an entire treatment plan, not just the SOT. We are blessed to go to the Lyme clinic In Minnesota where the treatments are more affordable for us. *The SOT is injected intravenously, spreads throughout the body (including past the blood-brain barrier), embeds itself into the Lyme bacteria, and will disrupt its ability to replicate. SOT has a stealth-like ability to avoid destruction by the immune system and existing bacteria.*

I *hope* that with the help from our health benefit we can at least start treatment. If I had waited much longer, the test would have been expired and I wouldn't have been able to use it for an SOT. You are approved for SOT therapy for up to six months after the test was completed. I would have had to spend more money on another test if I had waited much longer for a second opinion.

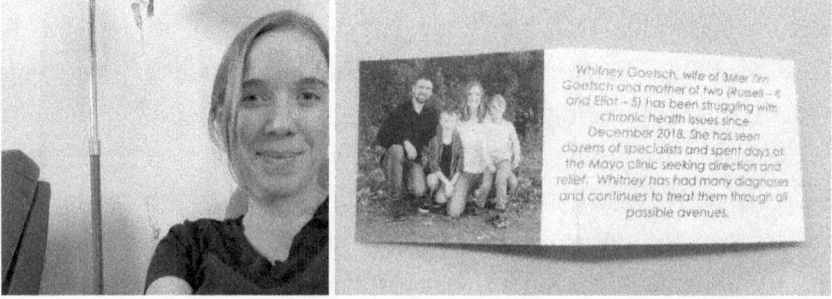

Because of this health benefit we were finally able to afford proper testing, and I have a diagnosis of Lyme disease and an appointment at the Lyme center in the future . . .

I have been very ashamed about having to accept help from others . . . but we have done this for so long on our own and many things were delayed because of the cost. Insurance does not cover enough for people with chronic illness . . . especially those who go through alternative care to find the underlying causes. This disease should have been caught years ago. It *should* have been treated. I should *not* be where I am today. I should *not* have been gaslit over and over by doctors. I should *not* have been cut into when I was dealing with something as serious as Lyme disease. *But* this is the *reality* that I face . . . and so many others. *It was missed.*

I am so *grateful* right now. I am so *grateful* that I listened to that small voice inside of me. *At least I finally know what is wrong with me . . .*

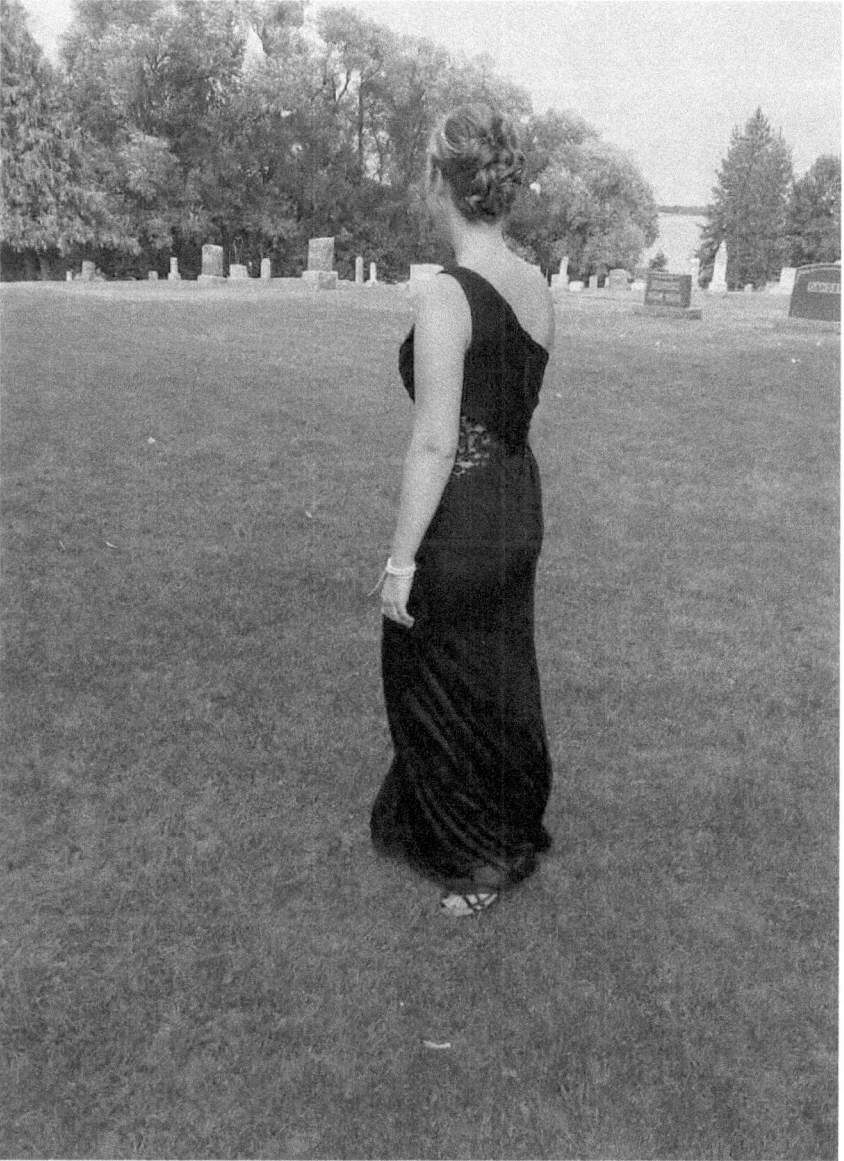

I remember now . . . it happened at the wedding. We pulled the tick off the back of my leg and crushed it on the pavement. I still remember how the blood smeared against the concrete. My life changed very rapidly after that tick bite.

* * *

I remember now . . . I *remember* the red tick that was pulled off the back of my leg at the wedding in Minnesota . . . just a couple of months before my heart symptoms began. *I forgot.* I never connected that tick bite, because I didn't know how serious Lyme disease symptoms could be. I always just thought it was a possibility because of how much my symptoms matched . . . *but I remember now.*

I wonder how long I have really had Lyme. I suffered so much as a child with recurring illnesses, and the GI issues worsened in my early 20s. My health drastically regressed after the tick bite in 2018, but I had issues even before then . . . was it dormant and the recent tick bite woke it up? Or other strains on my immune system like the mold or heavy metals? I will *never know,* but I do know that *I am not crazy.* I do know that this was *not all in my head.* I do know that it was *never* somatoform disorder.

I knew and I listened to that voice. I will always wonder if that voice was actually *God's voice* and not *my own . . .*

I begged God to give me the answers so many times. And *sometimes* when you hear that small voice it is *not yourself* but *God* leading you in life.

25

The Gaslighting Has to Stop

May 5, 2023

My visit at the Lyme center was absolutely *euphoric*. Everything was confirmed. I do indeed have chronic Lyme based on my level of IgG bands alone for Borrelia burgdorferi. Lyme affected my nervous system mostly, resulting in neurologic Lyme disease. I qualify for an SOT based on the level of these bands.

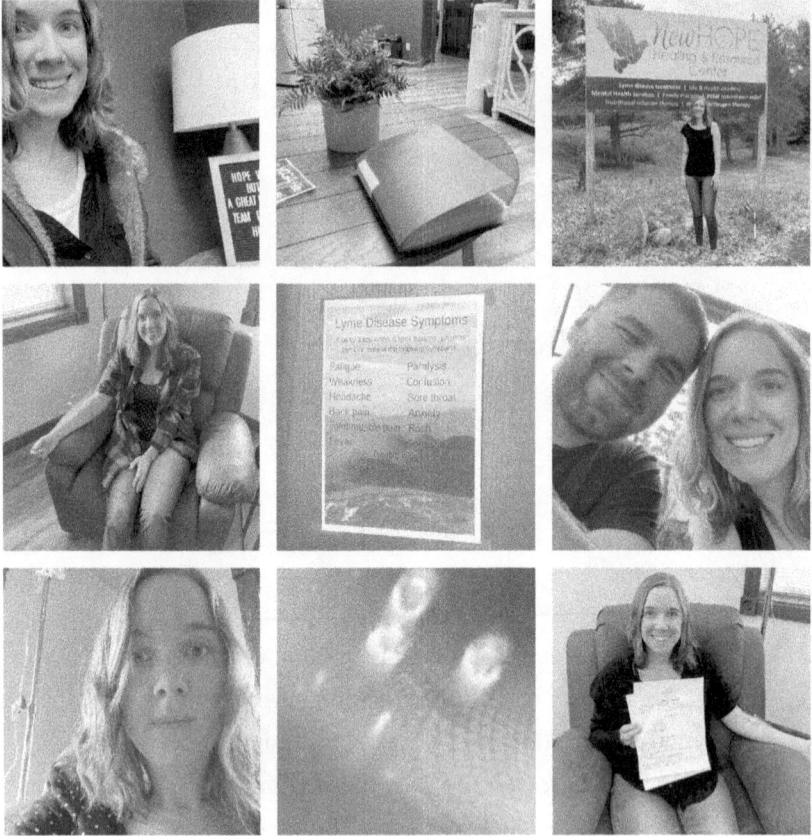

My symptoms were finally validated . . . I wasn't crazy.

It's a good thing we went when we did, because you can only qualify for SOT therapy if the tests have been done in the last six months. My Lyme doctor has also given me the clinical diagnoses of Bartonella and Babesia based on a clinical picture: my history, the rashes, and the symptoms. He was very kind to me, and I am so happy he is my doctor. He reviewed my huge medical binder and all of my skin lesion images and stretch-mark-type scars that were in odd places on the backs of my legs. He said those are signs of Bartonella, especially in my situation. I didn't get any stretch marks at all with my pregnancies, and the rashes were in odd places where I never gained or lost a lot of weight in a short time frame. They occurred

232

not long after a cat bite and looked like Bartonella rashes.

My memory flashed back to when I was a preteen. We had two cats that had just given birth to a litter of kittens. The grey cat was my grandmother's and was very unfriendly. I went downstairs to feed the cats, and the grey one was attacking my cat. I foolishly tried to separate them, and then the cat turned on me. I remember the way its yellow eyes widened and its ears flatted back on its head. She deformed herself in a creepy way and almost looked possessed. She growled like a lion and sprinted at me while she dug her sharp teeth into my leg and wrapped her clawed paws around my calf, leaving deep scratches all the way down to my ankle. I took off running, and she finally turned her back on me when I ran up the stairs, but not before I fell when I got halfway up. My grandma heard the commotion, and I started to cry when I got up the stairs. She cleaned and bandaged my deep slashes and promised she was going to drop that cat off in the middle of the field. She never did, but she did take it back home.

Not long after that, I got all of these weird ugly marks along the backs of my legs. I always thought they were stretch marks, but I was not prone to them and didn't grow super quickly in a short period of time. It makes me wonder now if that was the original infection and then it went dormant. I will never know.

* * *

All of my symptoms were explained to me in a way that I could finally understand, and I have such *hope* for my future. When I spoke with the health coach, her first symptoms had been burning and later buzzing in the feet. *Odd, that was the same for me.*

Prior to the chronic health issues, I remember that my feet would burn so badly I often had to run them under cold water before bed. Then they would turn purple when I stood for too long and would itch. Later, at times they were so freezing I had to put them under a heat pack. But the burning was awful.

The first symptom I had that sent me to the ER was buzzing in my feet.

It felt as if I were standing on a vibrating cell phone. I always thought it was a hormonal imbalance. My health coach asked me if anyone had ever explained why the buzzing sensation happens.

"No," I said.

She told me calmly, "It's from the Lyme or co-infections attacking your brain."

She continued, "When that happens, there is so much inflammation in the brain and the nerves respond from the attack."

This was very disturbing to me. Memories flooded in . . . *Tim, please just squeeze my head. This isn't normal. It's like something is attacking my brain!* My constant thoughts of . . . *something is really wrong with me . . . get out of me . . . this isn't normal . . .* flashed in my memories. For a moment I was back in the trauma of when it all began. When I experienced these symptoms, it always felt like something foreign attacking me. It never felt safe.

* * *

This experience has forever changed my life. It was the most euphoric feeling to be validated and have my symptoms explained to me. I was told that my story of gaslighting by the medical community is, unfortunately, the same type of story they hear from most of their patients. *Something has to be done to change this . . .*

My health coach was absolutely wonderful and gave me so much *hope.* She was also a mother of young children when she went through undiagnosed Lyme disease and treatment. I see myself through her and she inspires me to *heal.* She is so caring and supportive, and I don't think I could have asked for a better health coach to guide me in this journey. She believes fully that she has been *cured* of Lyme disease and that I can be too.

I finally feel like we have our answers. My biggest concerns right now are if the disease has caused any organ damage or permanent nervous system damage. She told me that most people with Lyme build up heavy metals, mold, fungus, GI infections, and other toxins because their body and immune system is struggling with the burden of the Lyme bacteria. When the body becomes overrun with the toxins and infections, it puts a *burden* of buildup on the immune system, which begins to struggle, causing a *perfect storm* for free radicals to run rampant, causing oxidative stress damage, mitochondrial damage, and damage to the nervous system and cells. *Waves* of emotions flooded into me as each picture finally fit into place. This makes so much sense. I learned so much from my other two functional medicine doctors, but now the root to the source of my body building up all of the other toxins is finally uncovered.

With all of the other diagnoses, I always felt a sense within me that *these are not all of the answers. There is more.* In this moment, I do not feel this way at all anymore. Not at all. Not today. I was able to do a vitamin and glutathione infusion while I was there. I felt more energy for three days. I also felt *waves* of emotions after my visit at the Lyme center. I would laugh and I would cry. When I drove to my acupuncturist's office later, I didn't even have to wear sunglasses.

I showed my Lyme doctor the live blood analysis video. He said the specimen in my blood did resemble spirochetes, but because of little research they can't be 100% sure if it was Lyme bacteria or a different co-infection or parasite. He said if they could use this form of testing along with other forms, they may be able to diagnose Lyme more effectively . . . but there is little research, so they use Vibrant or IGeneX mainly. Lyme also likes to hide . . . it may not always show up in a live blood analysis.

The SOT therapy I will be doing comes from Europe. Most testing and treatment done in Europe is covered by insurance and the diagnosis process can be much easier. But not here . . . not in America. No wonder many people travel to Europe when suffering with chronic illness. Most probably have underlying Lyme or co-infections. The plan is to do SOT therapy first and later methylene blue. He also has many other treatments, from herbals to antibiotics. They have HBOT and PEMF (pulsed electromagnetic fields) therapy too.

SOT is more expensive, but it is easier on the body. There is a warning that when you do SOT for one strain, it can cause the other more dormant strains to stir up and cause problems. But then they also have a chance of coming out of hiding and being caught in blood work. My out-of-state functional medicine doctor's words came into my head. *"You don't want to be on IV antibiotics. They destroy your gut and mitochondria."* I still have very bad feelings toward antibiotics because of her strong feelings against them. I believe her concerns, but Lyme destroys your gut and mitochondria too. It's not like she never used antibiotics for her patients at all. She did, but very rarely. She always felt the Lyme would go away when we treated candida. *But it didn't . . .*

I looked at the list of herbals the Lyme center offered. I have tried a few of them through my out-of-state functional medicine doctor. I really do want to avoid antibiotics if possible. Some of the medications, too, that he suggested can be hard on the liver and kidneys, like Malarone. He would have to monitor my levels if we chose to try that.

*　*　*

We are so blessed to have the funding from the health benefit organized by my husband's coworkers. The burden is so much lighter on Tim, and it saves us from terrible financial turmoil. It will take a lot of SOT treatments and other means to repair my cells and mitochondria. The benefit won't be enough for everything, but it can at least get us started and I am so *grateful*.

I am being told that SOT is one of the better treatment options available for Lyme and co-infections. Most cannot afford it. This makes me so sad. It is so unfair that everyone cannot have the same treatment options. It is not right. It is not humane. Insurance should be covering these lifesaving therapies. Something needs to change, but how? The CDC doesn't even believe chronic Lyme disease exists, so most of these therapies can't even be covered by insurance. I am understanding that SOT for Lyme disease is not yet FDA approved, partly because of lack of CDC approval concerning the idea that chronic issues from Lyme can be coming from a persistent bacteria. I understand the concern with long-term antibiotics, but some people truly do have persistent bacteria causing the chronic issues and need treatment.

* * *

Everything is falling into place. I finished the therapeutic phlebotomies for now. We have the money from the health benefit. I came across the SOT video just a few weeks before discovering the Lyme center, and they just happen to have the same treatment available at the one location nearest me that had an availability. *Thank God* I posted that video and listened to that small voice inside of me.

Thank God for my acupuncturist and for my Lyme group moderator guiding me and pressing me to get a second opinion. The only upsetting thing is that *it took so long.* I have a long road ahead of me. It can be very hard to heal from Lyme, and when you treat you can become worse before having any relief. Some of these issues with my pain could be damage from the Lyme. It's not over yet. But I have my answers. It took four and a half years to get them. I had so many unneeded surgeries that more than likely made the infection stronger. God gave me enough reprieve from my pain to cancel the surgery and look further into Lyme. *Thank God* I questioned further. It would not be a good time right now to have a surgery, even if I am in pain.

I am trying to figure out how I will tell my functional medicine doctors. I don't want this to happen to someone else. No wonder my limbic system is still impaired and I still have high oxidative stress levels. If I would have continued to think all of it was my limbic system, I would not be having this relief now from the lowered ferritin levels. I would have stayed stuck there, and who knows what could have happened over time with that retained ferritin and such thick blood.

I feel that *God has spoken to me from the beginning.* He gave me all of the answers within the first year. He gave me *strength* and *perseverance* and got me through when I made mistakes in my diagnosis journey. He carried me when I felt I could no longer go on, and he still does.

I had to fight so hard for every answer and I always listened to that inner voice. I did ignore it for the first two surgeries, but I listened the last time.

I am not angry right now. I am ready to heal. I am ready to fight.
"Lyme isn't killing me, I am killing it."

May 5, 2023

I go back to the Lyme center next month to get the blood draw for my first SOT. We will do a small test through IGeneX for Bartonella. If the bacteria comes out of hiding, we will do an SOT for that as well.

They say there is a possibility of fetal transmission. There was a study done on a pregnant dog where they infected the mother, and out of her brood several of the puppies had it while others did not. My Lyme doctor said his son had it and he had never had a tick bite. My health coach also has a son who has it. My thoughts go to my neighbor who had a son with Lyme and he was treated alongside her. None of them found out, though, until their children were experiencing symptoms.

I never want my children to suffer like me. *If I had to suffer for that many years just for them to get help right away, it was worth it.* I think of my mother, too, and all of the similar things she is going through.

The Lyme doctor I see has a suspicion I may have had Lyme my entire childhood. As a baby, I almost died of spinal meningitis. My mom found me unresponsive in my crib and had to rush me to the hospital. They found brain swelling, and I was kept in the hospital for several weeks. My mom and dad were told that I may be blind, deaf, or mentally incapable to care for myself. By God's grace, I had a miraculous recovery and the only struggle I had growing up was with math and dyslexia.

I remember every time my siblings and I would get sick, I would always be sick the longest. Stomach bugs were especially challenging for me because when my family would get sick they would be better in around 24 hours while I would go weeks with ongoing symptoms and vomiting episodes.

I can remember one time when I visited my family in Hill City for the summer. Those times were my best memories of childhood. My aunt was such a wonderful mother and I always admired her determination to allow us kids to have happy memories despite her pain. I remember going all over to the different amusement parks or lakes, and at the end of the day her feet would be four times the size they were when she woke up. She suffered with rheumatoid arthritis, and I could tell she was in pain, but she always pushed on for us. That summer we all got a stomach bug, and everyone recovered quickly except me. I was throwing up after almost every meal. When I went home, I continued to be sick for two more weeks. It lasted about a month total, and that's when my dad told me that my aunt was worried I was suffering with an eating disorder called bulimia. I laughed at him when he told me this. No, I was just sick.

I can't even remember if I was brought in to the doctor when I had these ongoing problems. I'm sure it was mentioned, but my dad was gone all week for work and my mom wasn't with us anymore during those years. My grandma was always so tired, so I didn't want to bother her with more concerns, and when Dad got home, he had so much on his plate already. I usually didn't want to burden him with my issues. Eventually I did get better, though, and the vomiting would subside. Lyme can go dormant for several years and only causes problems if something wakes it up, like a huge stress on your immune system. I won't ever know exactly when I contracted it. But I did.

My Lyme doctor told me that more obvious symptoms of Lyme cases, transferred in utero, usually start between the ages of five and ten. That would be childhood onset. I can't imagine a child being diagnosed with Lyme disease. There is a certain mentality of a child when they find they have a disease. It is incredibly scary for a child, depending on the personality. My Lyme doctor told me that some children's symptoms are very mild, and it's best to treat them before it gets worse.

Sometimes I wonder if any of the blood transfusions I had after my hysterectomy contained any additional Lyme or co-infection bacteria. That could make sense as to why my health has declined so much since then. When I did my phlebotomies, they had to throw them away because each was listed as a *therapeutic phlebotomy*. I asked the lab techs if the blood donated at that location was cleaned after donation.

239

They said, "No . . . most places don't clean it. There are some facilities that do, but it's not common."

How scary. My Lyme doctor said many patients contracted Lyme after blood transfusions and it really is an unsettling thought.

Since we removed mold, heavy metals, candida, and parasites, I really *hope* that the Lyme treatment will be easier for me. I *hope* I don't go through extreme *herxheimer* reactions and I really *hope* SOT is all that I need for the co-infections too.

May 6, 2023

I am *grateful* for:

- God
- *perseverance*
- my husband
- my children
- warm weather
- the Lyme center health coach
- the Lyme center
- health benefit
- family
- my mom
- Tim's mom
- friends that keep in touch, near and far
- my Lyme doctor
- my sister's new baby
- *Boomer* books

May 9, 2023

I just completed my blood draw for the SOT and Bartonella testing. I really love the nurse, the health coach, the counselor, and the receptionist that I have met. They are so kind to me. I also received another Myers' cocktail, vitamin C, and glutathione infusion. My migraine symptoms are much better after the infusion! I wish I could do these weekly, but the cost is high right now.

I will come back in a few weeks to receive the first SOT for Borrelia burgdorferi. If I test positive for Bartonella, I will qualify for that SOT as well. Bartonella can be very difficult to catch and is often diagnosed using a clinical picture. But to quality for SOT therapy you need a positive lab proving you have it. We may try using methylene blue and red light therapy primarily to treat the Bartonella if it doesn't show in testing.

Everything is falling into place. Even back home . . . a vitamin infusion center is opening at my *safe space*—the new clinic where the doctors that helped me the most are located. The doctor I see off and on that used to work with my acupuncturist is opening the clinic! It's so nice to know that I will have the option to utilize these therapies somewhere that I feel safe. I cried happy tears when I found out they are opening the clinic this summer! Just in time for my first SOT! God is lining everything up just perfectly.

Both medical doctors at this clinic have been involved with my health issues from the beginning and have been strong advocates throughout my journey. I will feel so comfortable there. I am just so very *grateful* for how this is coming together. I know that most with chronic illness struggle to *trust* or feel safe with any doctor. *There are good doctors out there.*

I also took a scary step and asked for our church to add me to their prayer list. I never felt comfortable with asking this before because I didn't have a diagnosis that would make sense to anyone. I feel like I need to do this now . . .

From now until June I am doing the sauna, red light, grounding, vitamins, and diet. I have also been absorbing myself in my *Boomer* books. It helps pass the time in between appointments and takes my mind off my daily pain. I love drawing the illustrations for my books and coming up with the stories. It brings me joy that I never thought I could feel again.

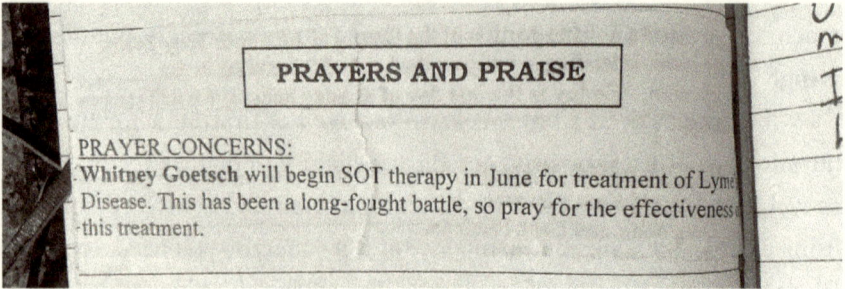

PRAYERS AND PRAISE

PRAYER CONCERNS:
Whitney Goetsch will begin SOT therapy in June for treatment of Lyme Disease. This has been a long-fought battle, so pray for the effectiveness this treatment.

May 10, 2023

Waves: A Memoir of Perseverance in Battling Chronic Lyme Disease. My story will be told. I will help others. *My story matters* too. *Our stories matter.*

26

I Want to Heal

We went back to Alexandria and I did the first SOT for Lyme disease. Two SOT therapies are often recommended for one infection. I was very nervous at first because of some of the side effects I was reading about on the paperwork. I was assured that the more serious side affects are an affect from SOT therapy for cancer. The symptoms are usually pretty mild after an SOT for Lyme disease. You can expect some *herxheimer* reactions from die off. It was recommended that I do more IV glutathione and detox methods through sauna, red light, and Epsom salt baths. I am familiar with these methods and I am familiar with die off. I have done many of these therapies before.

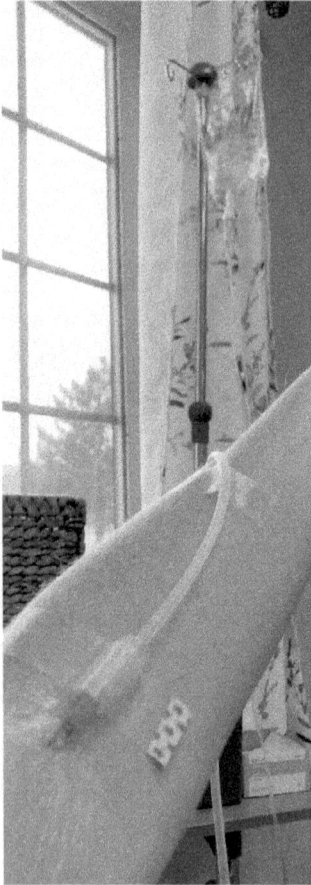

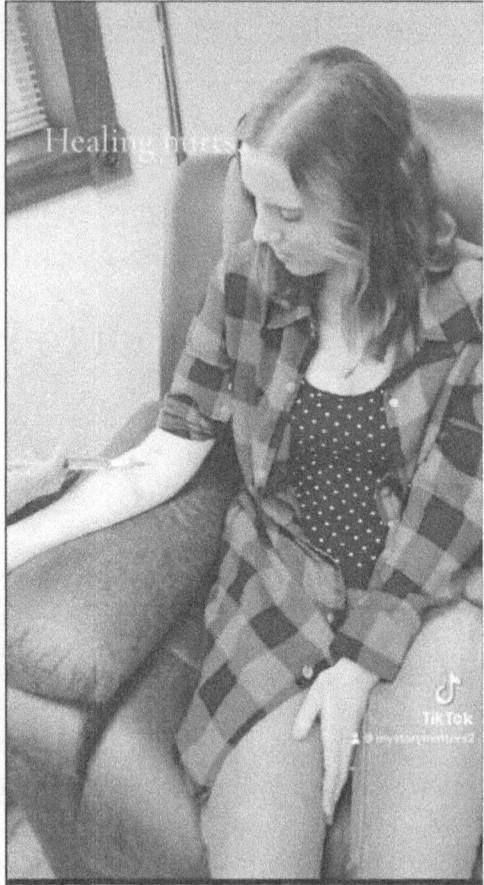

"Get out of me . . . " I screamed.

When the spirochetes die off in your body, it can stimulate an immune reaction. With antibiotics the *herxheimer* affect is usually more severe. They are still researching exactly why these symptoms occur. Some research papers I have read say it is because of the overloaded toxin released by the spirochetes, resulting in a cytokine spike. Other research papers say it's because of your immune system's response. Some say it's because of increased inflammation.

I struggle with injection anxiety because of bad reactions to other procedures that were done in the past. Once I overcame that *fear,* I did okay . . . *Be with me, God.* That night I did have body aches. My legs hurt the most, which I find interesting because that is where most of my skin lesions are at. I had to take an Epsom salt bath and slept with my heat pack and acupuncture mat under my legs.

* * *

Later that week, I met up with my neighbor's son who has been in remission from Lyme disease for several years. He still has some mild symptoms. He suffered for a long time in his late teens and early twenties with chronic migraines and other neurological symptoms. I showed him all of the paperwork and told him everything I had learned from the Lyme center.

I specifically asked him if he experienced the buzzing sensations, and when he said yes I told him exactly what my health coach told me. *"It was the Lyme attacking the brain . . . "*

With tears in his eyes, he told me that no one had ever explained the reason he felt the way he did when he was suffering. I could tell he was very *grateful* that day.

Later that evening, I pondered how I was placed right next to neighbors who had struggled with chronic Lyme for several years . . . *I do not think this is coincidence.* I feel God placed me in the right spot, and my purpose was to help put closure on what he went through. I was placed here to learn more from him and dig further as well . . . I just didn't have the right doctors at the time.

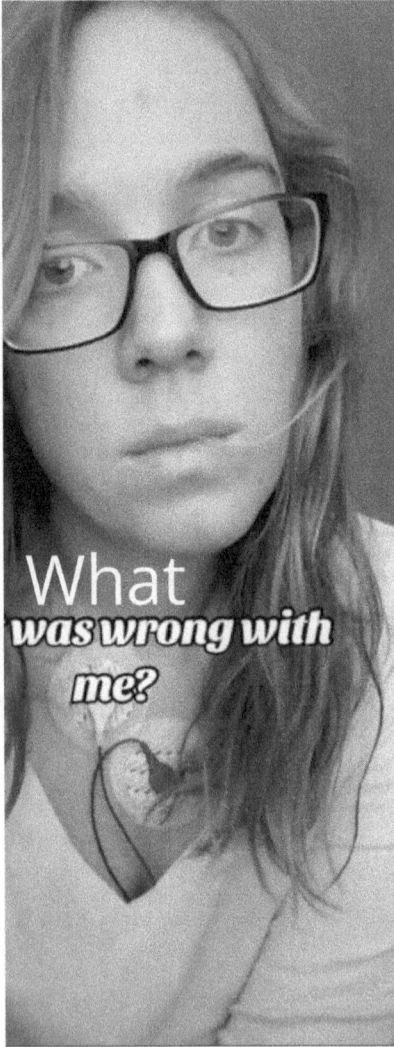

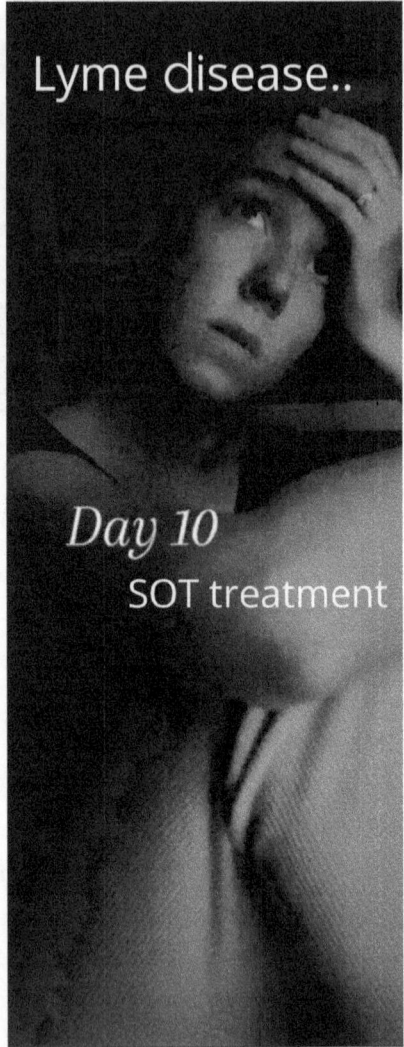

It only took four and a half years of suffering . . .

Later, I completed a biopsy to see if we could catch Bartonella. I somewhat regret the timing we chose. It was negative for Bartonella. After the SOT for Lyme, I began to notice the lesions resolving. When I did the SOT for Lyme Borrelia burgdorferi, the first symptoms I had were aching in my legs. I know I need to slow down, but sometimes I feel on high speed because I want to reach some form of remission *before* my children grow up. *I want to heal.*

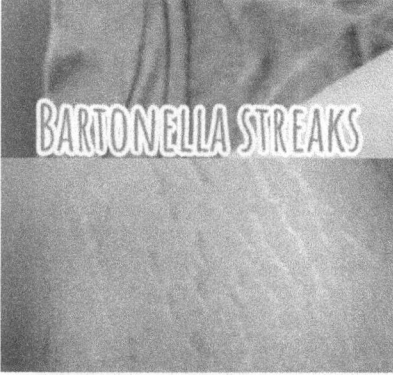

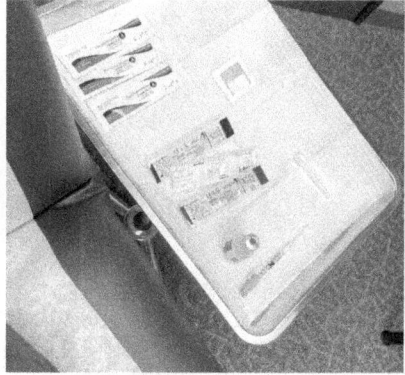

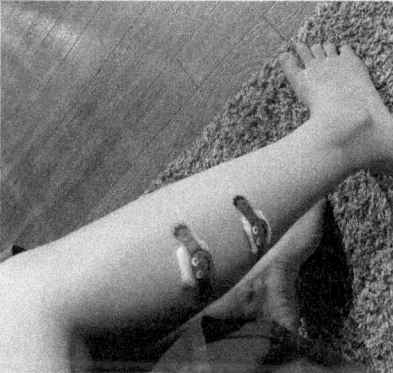

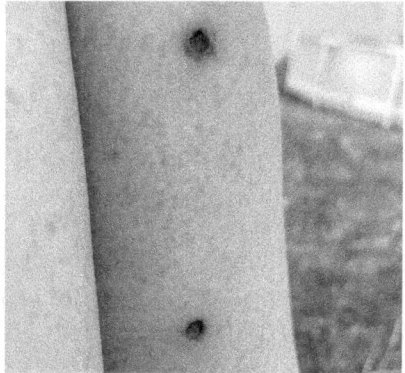

Bartonella can burrow deep inside of the body, into the brain, the bones, and tissue. It likes to hide.

27

I Don't Want My Loved Ones to Suffer

July 21, 2023

I had to take my mom to the ER recently. This is the first time I have been back since my last ER visit years ago. It was odd not being the patient. My mom was experiencing symptoms very similar to my own. Her entire head was buzzing, and the back of her neck and face would go numb. They did a CT scan of her head to check for signs of a stroke. Thankfully, there were *none*. The ER doctor felt there were mild signs of fibromuscular dysplasia in her imaging. We discussed the recent antibiotic that was prescribed to her by her primary care provider, doxycycline. She was put on this a few weeks ago for two weeks for a suspected case of lingering Bartonella. While she was on the medication, her vision and other symptoms were improving drastically, but not long after she got off she was having trouble again. We wondered if the issues she was having that day could be related to her past infection of Bartonella. The ER doctor ran labs and said there were no signs of her fighting an infection. He did say that Bartonella can do similar things to the arteries, *but* he did not feel that she had it.

Her primary care provider did not feel that she had this condition, but followed up with the ER requests and she was referred to a specialist for the suspected fibromuscular dysplasia.

The specialist reviewed her scans and felt that she did *not* have this condition, but they would do a repeat ultrasound in one year. We are *grateful* that even the specialist is not concerned . . . but something is *still* very wrong with my mom. We decided to proceed with Lyme disease testing for my mother through the Lyme center.

July 29, 2023

Tonight Tim told me that he feels *dead inside*. Later, he said he didn't mean it. The result of the latest Lyme test is what caused this moment of *despair*. I know he has struggled with these feeling since the beginning of all of this and tries so hard to hold it together . . .

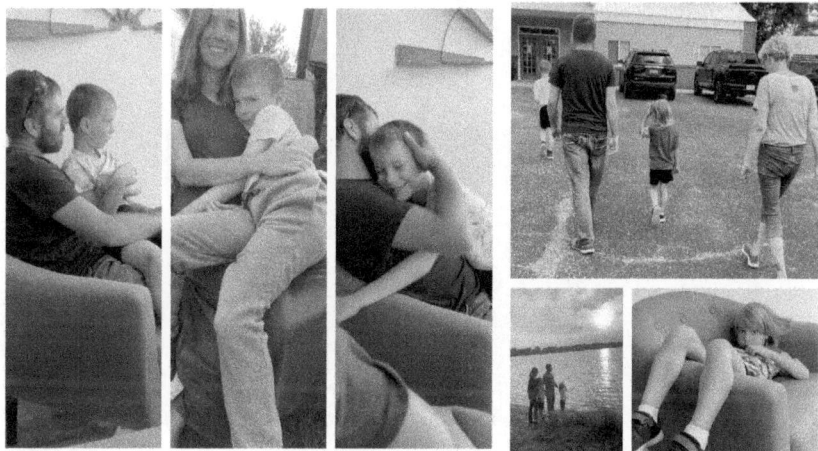

Lyme disease doesn't care who you are. You can be a mother trying to raise your children. A father trying to provide from your family. A grandmother. A child. It does not care who you are or what you are trying to accomplish. It can rip apart your body and many parts of your life. Lyme disease takes so much from you and gives you back a life full of isolation and pain that affects you in many different forms. You are left fighting an invisible invader that is trying to take your life.

We did additional testing for Lyme disease. My mother was *positive*. She

specifically has a CDC positive because of the anaplasmosis. *I knew it
. . . my mom has Lyme disease and Bartonella.* My thoughts go back to
her diagnosis of fibromyalgia in her 30s, her mood disorders that did not
respond well to medication, and her regressing health conditions now. I
clearly remember a story she told me. When she was a young girl, she fell
into a bush and went up to her bedroom where she noticed ticks crawling
all over her. She picked them off one by one and threw them out of her
bedroom window. *How long has she had it? Did the Bartonella infection trigger
a dormant Lyme case and awaken it?*

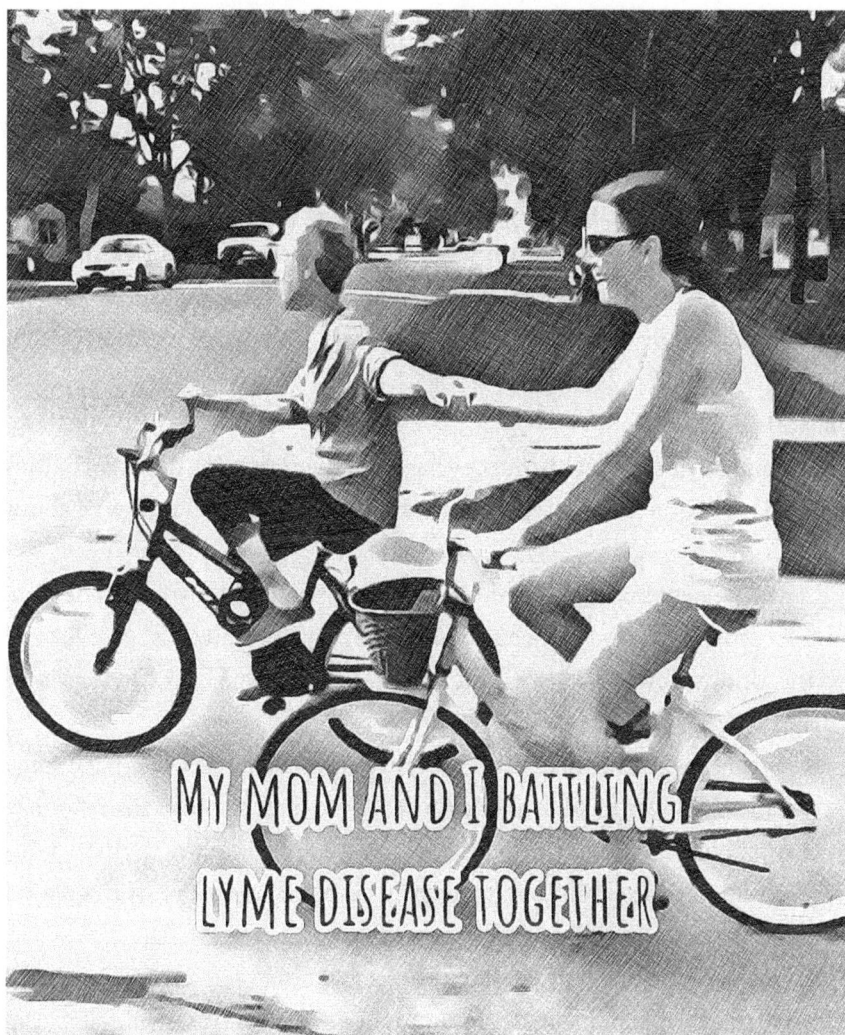

My mom tested positive . . . I knew it.

Tim had one very low IgG band. The Lyme doctor said this is a negative. *Thank God.* There is some ongoing research concerning Lyme transferring from partner to partner through sexual transmission, which is partly why we tested him. My Lyme doctor said he has never *seen* a case like this, but it is still being researched as a possibility. It's possible he may have been exposed, but his body fought it off.

I often tell my children that Lyme disease and other diseases do not affect everyone in the *same* way. There is more than one factor that caused *my* health decline. It was the *perfect storm,* not just Lyme alone. A *healthy* immune system that is *not* overburdened *can* overcome Lyme. That is why many are affected differently by it. The best thing you can do is not *fear* the disease but be educated on what to do if you *ever* get a tick bite and educate yourself on the proper testing and treatment methods. *I do not want them growing up in fear.*

July 30, 2023

The entirety of my health journey has been spent fighting different battles with most people every step of the way. Maybe they feel that way about me too . . .

I always knew that Tim tried his hardest throughout my health decline, and he still does. He has been to almost every appointment. He listens, writes things down, and tries to understand . . . but I know I *overwhelm* him.

Sometimes when I think of the last few years of struggles, I do have some resentment. It was hard to mention things to Tim because his response was usually one of anger or panic, which was hard on my own nervous system. Sometimes I felt that his nervous system was more dysregulated than my own . . . but I knew that he was experiencing PTSD.

There were times when I experienced a moment of grief, and he would often turn away from me and said he could not hear it. He would just keep going to work and making the money to pay for my care, because that is all he could control. I didn't need him to *fix* everything in that moment. What I really *needed* was an *embrace.* But he has always been a fixer, and not being able to fix me tore him up inside. I went to bed so many nights crying in isolation. I often wonder if he did too.

I had concerns on and off as to if *he even believed me.* He always said he did. But . . . I know none of this is his fault, even his responses. He has always been there for me and tries to understand, and I will forever be *grateful* for that.

This experience has been very traumatizing and overwhelming for him too. In chronic illness, spouses go through ups and downs like this. And I have come to understand that this is hard and loved ones deserve grace, too, in the difficult moments.

I still go through ups and down of feeling like I cannot fight any longer. I try to *remind myself that I was just diagnosed with Lyme.* I just did one SOT. Results are not instant. I try to remind myself that I have a long way to go yet to heal. But I get so *angry* and I don't want to fight against any forces anymore. Sometimes it makes this healing journey very difficult to know that my life circumstances have been so difficult for my husband and others to bear.

When I get really angry about my circumstances, thoughts like "*Everyone would be better off with you dead*" invade my mind.

My life still feels very out of my control. I can't get through without God carrying me. That's when I think about "*Footprints in the Sand.*" I loved that poem my entire childhood and even asked for a huge picture of it to hang up on my wall as a wedding gift. My entire life led up to this moment.

Everything makes sense now after the Lyme disease diagnosis. I don't want this quality of life for *anyone.* I don't want my loved ones to *ever* suffer like I have. And if I had to go through this hell so that they never have to it was worth it.

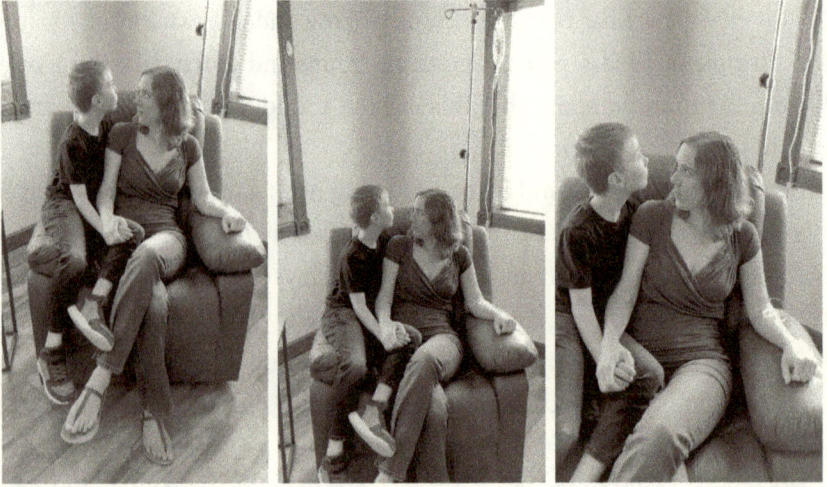

If I had to suffer for all of those years in order for my loved ones to be diagnosed and never go through the same experience that I have . . . then all of the pain was worth it.

28

I Can't Live in Fear

August 1, 2023

When my mother's results showed a CDC positive for Lyme and anaplasmosis, and a diagnosis of Bartonella, I questioned my Lyme doctor about the concerns with her arteries. He said that both Lyme and Bartonella can affect the arteries and veins because of inflammation building over time. Similar to how it has affected her vision . . . It may not be the *only* factor, but I *hope* we have caught these infections soon enough.

Not my mom too . . .

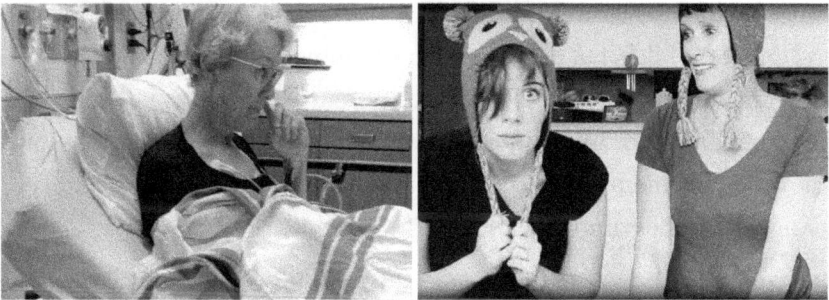

I don't know how I would have made it without her . . .

Her veterinarian also recommended that she rehome her cat, Eddy. She said they can treat Eddy with the medication to try and kill the Bartonella, but unfortunately there is no evidence that it will fully eradicate it. In my mother's condition, and with her compromised immune system, the concern is that any potential fleas from Eddy could pass the bacteria to her *again* as *a weakened host*. Since she is already having such complications from the disease itself, the risk of keeping her cat is too high. I expressed my concerns about Eddy passing this disease to the next caretaker *if* the antibiotic did not eradicate it. She told me that most cats actually carry this bacteria and people who don't have compromised immune systems *do not* usually contract this from their cat. She said it would be safe to rehome him. Because my mother is already dealing with intense infections that are lowering her immune system—Lyme specifically, and *Bartonella* as the triggering factor—the risk is too high for her to keep her cat.

My veterinarian was very saddened with my mother's case.

She told my mother, "It is not often you hear of something like this . . . but Lyme and Bartonella can be absolutely devastating."

My mom has had Eddy for thirteen years, and in that time frame he never bit her. It was an unfortunate accident when he did. He thought my mom was a dog. It is unlikely that Eddy would ever bite my mom again, but the flea concern is challenging, especially because of her condition right now.

When I told my mom the situation it was very difficult. I could hear her voice breaking on the phone, and it was not an easy decision to make moving forward. My mom followed the one-month recommended treatment for Eddy, but because of her declining health she could no longer keep him. This was a very difficult decision for my mom as Eddy has been her companion for many years. It was *not* a decision made lightly, and I know that my mom has cried many times because of the loss of her pet . . . along with her declining health.

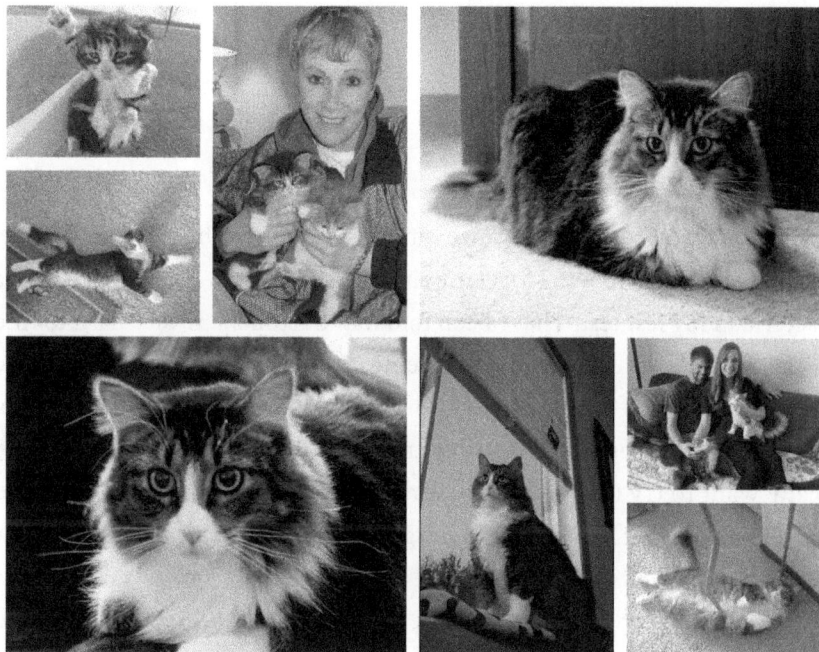

You experience a lot of loss with Lyme disease and co-infections. I never wanted my mom to experience it too . . .

August 1, 2023

I am *grateful* for:

- forgiveness
- *hope*
- help
- my mother
- more support, I am not alone
- love
- answers
- nice weather
- fewer migraines
- less light sensitivity
- fewer night sweats

- fewer skin lesions
- fewer headaches
- less buzzing

August 28, 2023

I haven't noticed major improvements yet since the first SOT. I am unsure what to do moving forward, since they could not find the Bartonella bacteria in my last test. I have been told that Bartonella is very hard to find because it likes to hide. My doctor mentioned doing another small panel to perhaps look at different forms of co-infections since the Bartonella is not showing up. He suggested possibly trying antibiotics for the Bartonella. I really want to try to avoid antibiotics. He also says sometimes you need more than one SOT for Borrelia burgdorferi to penetrate further into the cell membrane.

We have limited funds. It is upsetting how fast money went toward testing, and we had a lot of medical debt that we had to pay off on top of this. The test we really want to do is a comprehensive co-infection and Lyme panel through IGeneX, but it's $2,500. This test covers so many different strains and has been the most accurate test at catching the co-infections. But if I do this test it gives me very little money moving forward to do more SOT therapies. There is also a window of time after a test until it expires and is no longer good to qualify for the SOT.

We have all of our answers, but now we feel stuck because we have used so much of our finances in the past and we have little to put forward for these treatments. I don't want my husband to be burdened financially again or work himself to death just to pay for tests. We discussed what we could cut out financially in order to afford my care. He mentioned maybe putting Russell's Tae Kwon Do on hold. *No.* That is the one thing that brought him enough joy to get out of his slump after losing our house in the country. I won't take that from him. It is his only social activity that he is able to do with other homeschoolers right now. I have heard way less of his grief over the loss of our home and have not found a single drawing of the yellow house since he started Tae Kwon Do.

* * *

We were unable to get the homeschool group to move to Volga because they could not find a director. *I cannot do it.* I am not well. We found the perfect location at our local church right across from our house. It has so many classrooms.

Our pastor ran the idea by the consistory members and they were in approval of the location. The pastor and his wife have been so incredibly kind to us. The church people are incredibly kind . . .

The main director loved the church space, and if we could only find a local director it would happen. But we could not make it work this year. I decided that this may have happened for a *reason*, perhaps we need another year where we can heal first.

Unfortunately, I am not instantly healed after my first SOT. I cannot yet take on that roll.

* * *

We decided to become members of the church, and Tim is attending Bible study. It's helping him so much. Because of how kind everyone has been, I decided it was time for me to ask if I could be put on the prayer list for my recent diagnosis of Lyme disease and treatments. It has been several weeks now since I asked to be put on the list and several weeks since my first treatment. I know everyone means well when they ask me if I am feeling better. Sometimes I feel embarrassed that I asked to be on the prayer list because I don't have much difference since my treatment. It's hard to explain that when Lyme goes undiagnosed for this long, it can take many months or even *years* to heal the damage. I feel embarrassed sometimes, or like I'm failing, when I have to tell people that *I am still about the same.* Some days I am worse, depending on if I have had an acute illness or if I've had a recent treatment or flare. But I know I am not a failure. I just feel stuck right now, and I don't know the exact path to take moving forward.

The burden of the expense is so high I just want to run away from it. The thoughts of *A funeral would be cheaper . . .* repeat in my head. *Stop.*

* * *

When I tried the methylene blue, I started to have severe side effects. There is a suspicion that the dose was too high for me, resulting in serotonin syndrome. It sure felt like serotonin syndrome. I had that years ago from anti-anxiety medications. It was measured then by a 24-hour urine test by a neurologist. When the medications were out of my system, the extreme symptoms went away. The same thing happened when I went off the methylene blue.

Recently, the world got so bright and fun-house-like again. I kept feeling tunneled and out of body. I swayed a lot, experienced ticks, tremors, and what felt like minor seizure activity. I missed another funeral because of this. Another one. I missed an entire weekend with multiple family members. I had to stay home and recover. Once the medication left my system, I began to feel back to my baseline. It is hard to measure if it was serotonin syndrome or not. If it *was not,* then it was a *herxheimer* reaction. I could not function like that. I couldn't be around my kids like that. It makes me nervous for what lies ahead of me if this is what die off feels like from Lyme and Bartonella.

During these symptoms, I still had to be a wife, a mother, a daughter. I mostly masked my pain because that's what you do a lot in chronic illness. For the most part, your pain cannot be helped and you just live life in and out of a state of not knowing if something is normal, a *herxheimer* reaction, or a medical emergency. It's great fun. Not really . . .

It took me a while to *trust* trying Malarone for Babesia. I was on that short-term because of a change in my treatment plan. Right away I had more sore throats, swollen lymph nodes, and night sweats. I have noticed, since being on Malarone, that I have a lot less night sweats. I may have to retry taking it again at some time in between SOT treatments.

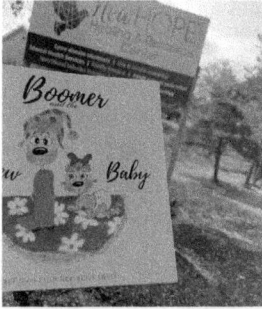

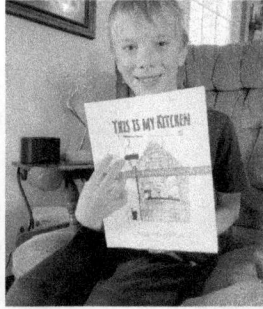

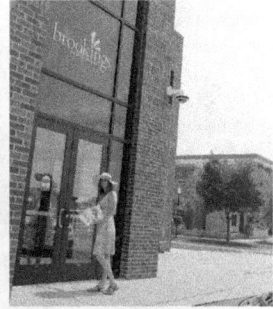

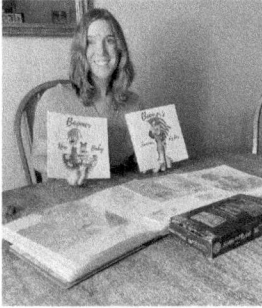

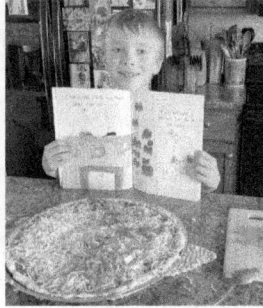

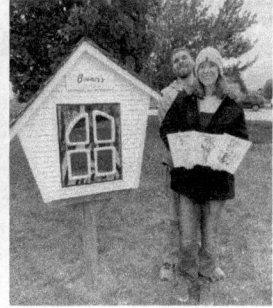

I find joy in the small things and am grateful for the talent God gave me to pursue my dreams . . . Tim is helping me pursue them . . . I am forever grateful.

I often wonder if this nightmare will ever end. I find joy in the small things. The time I spend with my children, my *Boomer* books, Russell's books, homeschooling, friends, going to Tae Kwon Do practices, or the Children's Museum. But I struggle with an empty feeling inside from lack of progress. *But then I remember, I just started this journey.* I think that is a limbic system impairment for sure. I have had so many disappointments after starting a therapy and not having the expected results. I *fear* I will *never* have those results and continue to live in this endless cycle. I distract myself by investing my time in my artwork or projects. Recently, Russell and I painted our little free library that Tim built us for our front yard. It was very healing as we decided to paint it the same shade of yellow as our home in the country.

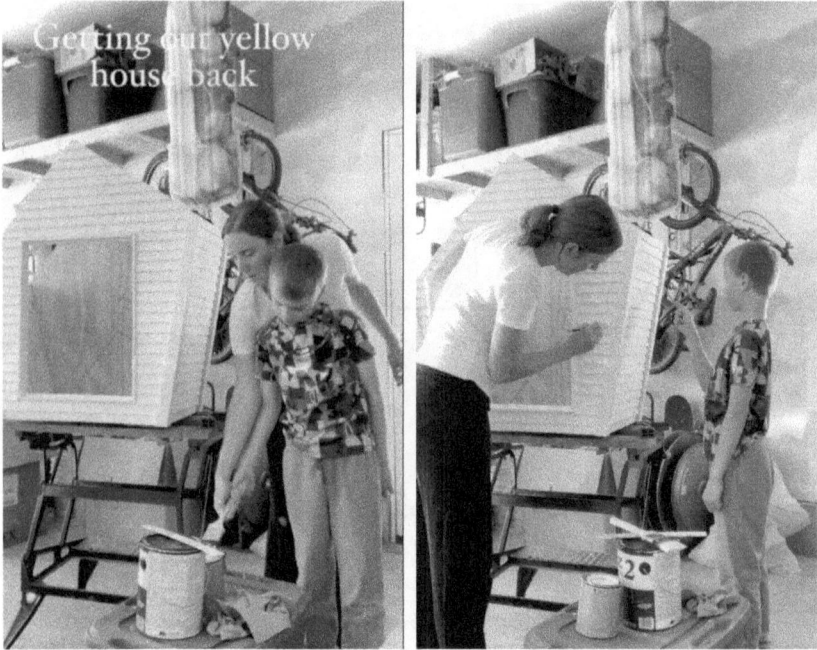

Getting our yellow house back . . .

I recently decided to let my functional medicine doctors know that I had a second opinion and was diagnosed with Lyme disease. Both of them seemed okay that I had a second opinion and just want me to get better. My out-of-state functional medicine doctor did suggest some other therapies with her to resolve this, but I just want to be somewhere local right now.

It's so nice going to the clinic in person and having support group meetings with local people. My local functional medicine doctor asked if I noticed any issues with beef. I assumed she was talking about alpha-gal syndrome, which is going to be evaluated. It's more difficult getting this specific test done out of state so I am trying to find an allergist open enough to consider testing me for it.

I honestly can't tell if my issues are coming from beef. Perhaps they are, and it was more difficult before because my body was reacting to everything. Maybe it will be easier to pinpoint. I do notice severe stomach upset sometimes after eating beef, but other times I do not.

I am just *grateful* right now that no one is upset with me for getting a second opinion. Neither of them ever made me feel like they would have responded in that way, but it's always hard for me to know. I just want them to be able to help other people like me. My local functional medicine doctor, too, always said she is open to learning from others. Hopefully they can all learn different things from each other.

* * *

August 29, 2023

For the last year, I wake up at night with my eyes completely fused. I press above my eyes and all of this hot fluid comes out and my eyes burn. I really *hope* this is related to the Lyme bacteria and goes away. Sometimes I worry my eyes are being damaged more from the Lyme.

I have a repeat MRI scheduled to see if there is an explanation for this. We can't do contrast because of previous reactions, so I will do the MRI on a T3 machine. I should probably go to the eye doctor again soon too. I've just had so many appointments, but I know it's important because of the inflammatory eye disease, keratoconus. Sometimes Lyme can cause damage to the eyes. The only thing shown in my past MRI is a small syrinx in the spine. Many neurosurgeons told me this was idiopathic, like the microadenoma of the pituitary. I have read that a syrinx often forms from a disruption of CFS fluid, due to inflammation of the spine . . . Lyme can do that.

My MRI of the brain and spine came back unchanged from the last scans. I did an MRI of the abdomen as well. It showed signs of improvement of the fatty liver at the time, but later, when I had an ultrasound, the liver was fatty again. Odd.

* * *

My mom was recently contacted by the CDC concerning her Lyme disease and anaplasmosis diagnosis. She has a positive CDC case. They told her that two weeks of doxycycline would heal her. Well. She did two weeks of doxycycline two months before we tested her, and it sure didn't *cure* her. *What kind of clown world do we live in?* So many are suffering. So many go undiagnosed because of failure in the CDC testing diagnostics and treatment guidelines.

After I was diagnosed with Lyme disease, the CDC announced that there was an uptick of Lyme cases this summer. In previous years, whenever spring would roll around, I would take my kids to the campgrounds and the nature park. But this year, people on the local weather group were warning people about how bad the ticks were at the local nature park. One day I went outside to save a baby bunny from my dog. I picked it up with a glove and dropped it because there was an engorged tick on its back. *A tick on a rabbit, in my small square backyard in town, where there is little foliage and dying grass everywhere.* I haven't seen a wood tick in years, but right after I was diagnosed I see them everywhere. Terri also told me the new acreage they bought is crawling with ticks right now and they have pulled a bunch off their clothes. *I'll be right over to visit . . .*

I remember I can't live in *fear*. I can just be *educated*. Instead of worrying and not being able to enjoy nature, I can practice preventative measures. My Lyme doctor goes on a camping trip in the boundary waters of Minnesota where there are acres upon acres of woods and wildlife. Prior to going, they prepare by hanging all of their clothing on a line and, while using gloves and a garden sprayer, he coats all of the clothing, the tent, and the equipment with the spray Permethrin. They allow this to dry fully prior to their adventure, and it can last for several weeks. Permethrin helps repel the ticks, it excites their nervous system and the ticks either drop off you or they die. The spray is safe to use as long as you don't touch it while it's wet. I have also been recommended Ranger Ready Picaridin as a decent on-the-go spray. Certain essential oils can be helpful, such as lemon and eucalyptus, but I have been warned that they may not be as effective.

Always do your tick checks while adventuring and before turning in for the night. If you do find a tick attached, removing it *properly* with a tweezers is important. Always make sure to remove the head. You can place the tick in a Ziploc bag and send it off to be tested, or you can place the tick in the freezer and watch for symptoms and then send it off—whichever you choose. *Never* remove a tick by dousing it with essential oils, vaseline, or by burning it. This can cause the tick to regurgitate into your body, raising your chances of disease transmission. The same situation can happen if you squeeze a tick too hard while trying to remove it with your fingers, which is *why* a tweezers is recommended for removal.

The best thing for tick prevention in your yard are guineas, chickens, and ducks. They will eat up those bugs, making it less likely to find one crawling on you.

There has always been a *rumor* that *only* certain ticks—like the *deer tick*—transmit disease, but that is just *not* true. I was told by my Lyme health coach that even *"common"* dog ticks can carry disease, they have seen it acutely in their practice. My Lyme center sends ticks out to a lab often to be tested. Dog ticks can carry Rocky Mountain spotted fever, other deadly co-infections, and *sometimes* Lyme. For years, we have been told that only *certain* states have Lyme, but there have been several cases where a person contracted Lyme in a state that is not *supposed* to carry the disease. I was told that alpha-gal syndrome mostly occurs from a Lone star tick and that those kind of ticks are only in abundance in the southeastern and south-central United States. The tick that set off all of my severe symptoms and alpha-gal syndrome *was* in Minnesota. Ticks *can* transmit disease even if they are only on you for a short time. The tick that caused alpha-gal syndrome for me was only on my leg for a brief amount of time in between taking pictures at a wedding. It's possible that that tick bite also woke up the dormant Lyme bacteria in my body.

A controversial possibility is that one can contract Lyme disease from a mosquito or spider bite. Bartonella can be transferred by certain flies, not just cat bites or ticks. How can you possibly *hide* from every bug? But it's still *terrifying.* I used to live in the world and just live, but now I am terrified of getting these diseases from a bug. The diseases are really that bad, though, and sometimes a common bull's-eye rash does not even show up if infected. The signs may not be obvious. I did not develop a bull's-eye rash after my tick bite in Minnesota, and I have *never* had one with any tick bite.

Recently, the CDC quietly released information on their website admitting that chronic illness can occur from Lyme Borrelia burgdorferi. So basically *chronic Lyme*. For years they have been saying it *doesn't exist*. Chronic Lyme has been a rejected term in American medicine. I read the information. The biggest thing I notice is that they are leaving out that these chronic issues can be coming from a persistent infection. This is a *big* problem because when people get diagnosed with a chronic condition after having been infected by Lyme, they will not be given proper treatment if there is still bacteria present. I know of many people who have completely gone into remission, or claim to have healed fully from chronic Lyme, when they were able to do long-term antibiotics, herbals, or SOT therapies. Insurance companies will continue to deny longer-term treatment for patients, making the high level of suicide remain a concern.

After I was diagnosed, I watched a documentary called *The Quiet Epidemic* (see List of Resources). It was very disturbing as there was one woman who was treating Lyme with antibiotics, but she was denied further care because of the CDC guidelines on the length of treatment and insurance policies. They found spirochetes in her spine even *after* completion of the CDC duration of antibiotic therapy. *She died.* I think of her face often and what she said in the video. *She didn't want this to happen to anyone else . . .* so she had to share her story . . . even on her deathbed . . . Her eyes looked so empty and defeated.

The Quiet Epidemic (see List of Resources) discussed the removal of the two most sensitive bands from the standard Western blot after making a vaccine for Lyme in the late 90s. Removal of those two bands was done because if everyone got the vaccine, they would *always* test positive for those strains. The vaccine failed and caused a lot of debilitating side effects, so it was withdrawn from the public. They *never* added those bands back into the standard Western blot. My Lyme center says that the standard Western blot misses over fifty percent of positive Lyme cases.

The stories from my Lyme center and my support groups are unsettling.

"I just want to be normal again . . . " one patient cried.

I saw myself in her. My Lyme center has had patients come in with Parkinson's disease, multiple sclerosis, fibromyalgia, many different mood disorders, and autoimmune diseases like lupus and rheumatoid arthritis. When they test these patients for Lyme they are *all positive*. I think of my aunts, who have suffered most of their lives with autoimmune conditions. I think of my own mother with fibromyalgia and thyroid conditions, who later was diagnosed as a CDC positive for Lyme through more elaborate testing. *How many years has she been suffering with spirochetes destroying her body?*

The story that really affected me, through the Lyme center, was a patient with Parkinson's. He was treated for Lyme with SOT therapy and his tremors and shakes *went away*. *Lyme* is the *great imitator* and the *real epidemic*.

* * *

The previous understanding concerning *chronic* Lyme was that there is no *cure*. You can *only* reach remission, and you can heal certain areas of the body, giving you a quality of life back. Some claim that as long as you take care of your immune system you can stay in remission, while others claim that certain factors can bring you out of remission, such as certain viruses or other therapies that affect the immune system. I have fellow chronically ill friends who have had EBV (Epstein-Barr virus), COVID, or they received a vaccine and their Lyme turned chronic again. I often wonder if, in these situations, it meant that the person was still harboring an infection, which turned the disease chronic again.

There is research right now that SOT therapy could be a *cure* for Lyme disease. But with the expense and amount of SOT therapies you may need to achieve complete eradication of the disease from your body, it may not be attainable for many. Just because you do one SOT for Lyme disease does not always mean an instant cure will occur, because there may be other strains present to target. I *hope* that one day there is an affordable *cure* for all, and I believe there is *hope* for everyone to be cured from Lyme disease.

* * *

There are several other conditions that a chronic Lyme patient can have that can keep them in a chronic state of illness. Common secondary factors in chronic Lyme include the buildup of mold, heavy metals, fungus, systemic candida, gut infections, and viruses, because of the state of the immune system. These toxicities to the body cause free radicals to run rampant, resulting in high levels of oxidative stress and damage to the cells and mitochondria. These conditions result in a chronic blanket of diagnoses like POTS (postural orthostatic tachycardia syndrome), MCAS (mast cell activation syndrome), and CFS (chronic fatigue syndrome). Do you see what they all have in common? *Syndrome.* As I mentioned earlier in the book, a *syndrome* is *a group of signs and symptoms that are known to go together but don't have a clear cause, course, or treatment plan.*

Because of the way our medical system is set up, if you are diagnosed with one of these *syndromes,* you are set up for failure to achieve any other answers or treatments. The medical system fails in chronic illness. The system is not set up to help people like us . . . *it needs to be changed.* The blanket label of *syndrome* needs to be lifted. Each one has a different cause.

Sometimes the cause can even be structural, like CFS (cerebrospinal fluid) leaks in the spine or brain. I couldn't believe the amount of people in my research groups who were diagnosed with POTS and ended up needing spinal fusions because their fluid was leaking out of their spine into their brain. It was misdiagnosed over and over again. It's almost dangerous to get diagnosed with a *syndrome,* because then all investigation for anything else is closed and you are left to live in that state with only salt water and compression socks as a form of therapy. *I am so sorry for any of you going through this.*

* * *

August 30, 2023

My sister recently found out that her aorta is dilated. She has Marfan, which is a connective tissue disease. I was tested for Marfan and the result was negative. I am worried about what is going to happen, but I'm trying to stay positive. I am trying to be here as much as I can for my sister during this time. It's hard that this is happening when I am not yet healed. I am just starting to treat my infections and I may feel worse before I feel any relief.

I feel more pressure to be healed because so many people need me. *I want to be there for everyone.* I have friends and family going through hard times. I want to be there for everyone, but my body limits me. I have no control over my body, and this causes deep anger inside of me . . . anger that I am trying to let go. I know that I cannot hold on to this anger when I am trying to heal, and I know that I cannot give myself a timeline to heal, but it is still difficult to be stuck here.

* * *

When I left the clinic for Lyme disease I was given a hotline number for suicide. I always knew POTS patients had some of the highest risks for suicide, and now I know that Lyme patients do as well. With POTS, your life is compared to the condition of late stages of kidney dialysis, COPD, or heart failure . . . this makes many people choose to end their life. Lyme has a high suicide rate, too, because of the extreme suffering for the patient and their families, financial burdens, lack of care, or disbelief by the medical community or loved ones . . . which leads to hopelessness . . .

My biggest *hope* right now is that my *Boomer* books can take off. They are sweet. The illustrations are cute. Kids will love them. My dream is that one day *Boomer* makes it as a loved children's book series. I would love to watch *Boomer* as a cartoon series or even on the big screen. *Boomer* is simple and I know he could be loved. It would be so fun to see *Boomer* toys and clothing someday. I *hope* that could happen for us. I can't do book signings yet, though, or public advertising. *I am not well enough.*

My *hope* is that someday I won't need any financial help from anyone anymore, including my husband. Then I can afford to do the tests and treatments I need without feeling any guilt. If I achieve my goals with my *Boomer* books, and when I'm healed, I want to find a way to help others going through this too.

The only thing you truly need to live a normal, happy life is your health. Most don't realize how important your health is and how much losing it can impact everyone around you. A house is just a box that you can lose in an instant. Material things don't matter. Where you live or what what your yard looks like really doesn't matter . . . *as long as there is no black mold growing all over.* The only things that really matter are people and health.

I just don't want to burden Tim any longer with the financial strain of this. That's when those thoughts creep in again. *"A funeral would be cheaper."* *No . . . stop those thoughts.*

* * *

September 1, 2023

I am sad and tired. It's 1 a.m. and my nose just started bleeding and I'm spitting out blood. Maybe the parasites from Lyme are dying in my brain. Everyone tells me they are living in there. *"Your brain is inflamed"* or *"The Lyme are in there."* My head has sure felt squiggly today. It sounds crazy, I know. I recently read an article about a guy that ended his life after treating Lyme disease with antibiotics for years. He left a suicide note asking to autopsy his brain. They did and they found Borrelia spirochetes all over inside of his brain. *I'm scared.* How many different Borrelia strains are inside my brain? If that's the case for me, I just want them to die already.

I have Lyme disease and so does my mother. My entire family has suffered because of what Lyme has done to our family. My very pregnant sister has an aorta dilation that will require an open heart surgery. Tim is dealing with his own stressful family situations and we are running out of money for my Lyme disease treatments. Bartonella won't show up in my tests, so I might end up being on long-term antibiotics. *"But don't forget to be grateful and have positive thoughts, because if you do not then all progress is lost."*

I hope that my children will remember the happy times and not the times when I have been overwhelmed. I hope that they someday get the healed version of their mommy.

* * *

October 6, 2023

I woke up this morning in pain. I sat down at the table and started to frost my older son's 9th birthday cake. I couldn't help but think to myself how *I am still here.* Because *I didn't give up* I am *still here,* frosting my son's birthday cake. It matters. You matter.

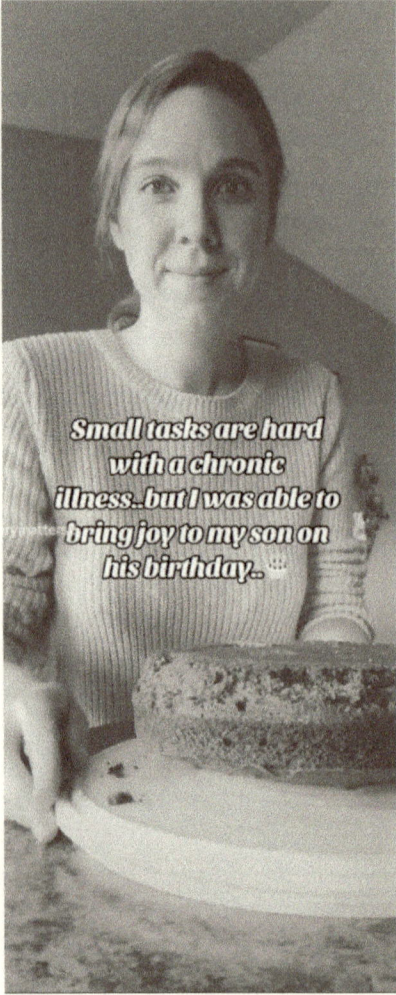

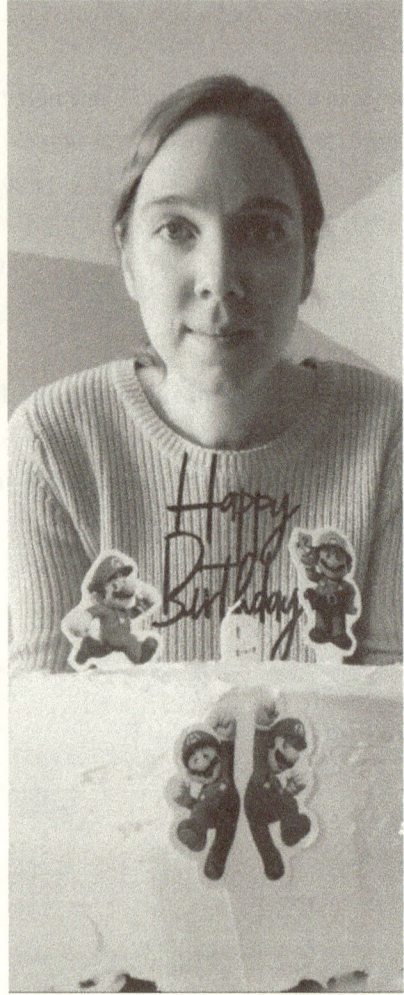

I am still here . . .

December 5, 2023

I was able to be there. I was there for my sister when she delivered her baby. I cut my niece's cord. The experience was so beautiful. My niece is a light in our world that has been full of such darkness for so long now. *New life. New hope.* I am so *grateful* I was able to be there. Oftentimes when I go through a milestone like this . . . or even a birthday party for my children .

. . I think to myself how *grateful* I am to be here. If I would have given up and taken my life in the darkest of times, I would not be able to be present now and experience the light . . .

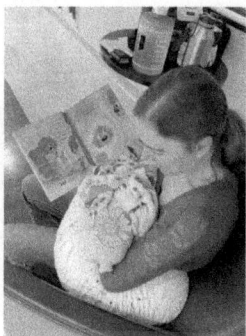

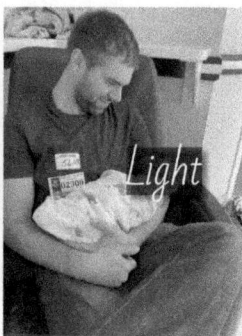

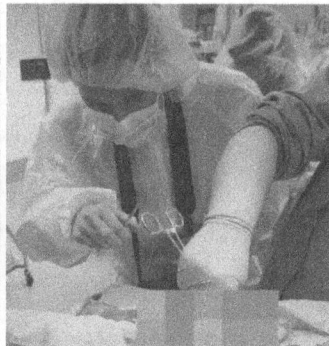

She brought light back into our lives . . . when we had been clouded in darkness for so long.

Wee Wee,

I don't think I will ever have the right words to express How Grateful I am for our relationship & how close we have gotten especially over the last year. Your strength to be there for me even when you are fighting your own battles does not go unnoticed, & I am eternally grateful!! Having you in the delivery room with us ___ is a feeling/moment I will never forget. The memories we were able to share together I will cherish forever.

She ___ is so lucky to have such a strong, caring, loving, selfless auntie to look up to. I can see how much light she has brought into your life in the last 4 mo. I got you this gift as a daily reminder of how much you are loved & appreciated & to always remember your bond with her & to most importantly Never give up! Thank you will Never be enough for all the selflessness over the last year.

♡ you forever   - Asha

29

There Are Still Ups and Downs

January 1, 2024

I recently published my fourth *Boomer* book. The Christmas edition brought me so much joy in illustrating, despite my physical health. Christmas is my favorite holiday, and I always look forward to this time of year.

I had two SOT treatments for Lyme Borrelia burgdorferi. Each SOT was $2,700. We went through our benefit money very quickly, but I am so *grateful* that we even received this help. Without it, I may have still been stuck back and forth between my functional medicine doctors or doing another surgery. I am still not noticing major improvements. I have had an improvement in aura migraine and heart palpitations with eating and I have less night sweats and less skin lesions.

Last month I did experience a pretty severe long-lasting migraine. It felt like a seizure or stroke. The abdominal pain has been getting worse again this month. I get air hunger from it and feel very foggy. Depending on where it is at, it almost feels like someone is stabbing me. The pain has progressively gotten worse throughout my kidney region and radiates down to my lower back. It has been discouraging. The biggest *herxheimer* reactions I feel from the two SOT therapies are depression and rage. The SOT injection kills Lyme for six months after it is injected. So right now, as I type, it is killing Lyme.

I did two co-infection panels. One through Vibrant and a smaller one, with different Lyme strains, through IGeneX. Vibrant showed the co-infection called ehrlichiosis. Long-term issues from this infection can affect the central nervous system, cause migraines, cause nervous system dysregulation, and can affect the kidneys and abdomen. It sounds like me. It's interesting how the co-infection did come out of hiding. I tested negative for this co-infection in past testing through Vibrant. This could be why I am struggling more with pain, because when you kill one bacteria the other ones can get angry and cause more symptoms.

My doctor said that it is not common to see ehrlichiosis causing chronic issues, but it can happen. We decided to do the IGeneX panel because my doctor is concerned that I may have another strain of Lyme. He also says there is no SOT for ehrlichiosis. If my next test shows nothing significant enough for an SOT, then I will be doing antibiotics.

I have spoken to many others like me in my support groups. I attend a support group through the Lyme center and their stories are heartbreaking. A patient traveled all the way to Germany for stem cells after treating Lyme with an SOT. It was very costly, over $10,000 for stem cells. Later, this patient was diagnosed with Bartonella. The stem cells were destroyed because the Bartonella was missed. The missed infection destroyed all of the new healthy cells. My heart just broke hearing this. It's hard for me to hear others suffering. It's almost harder for me to hear others suffering than it is to experience my own. I feel deeply for all of these people. *I will never forget their faces and the desperation in their voices . . .*

* * *

I have had ups and downs these last few months. I feel positive, then hopeless. My moods have been all over the place. I experienced such highs after my diagnosis and treatment opportunities, but then I experience such lows when I realize this is not going to heal quickly. For five years, I had such hopes when other things were diagnosed and with all of the promises that I would heal. I feel like I'm starting all over again, and sometimes it feels like it will never end. *You were just diagnosed. Quit it, inflamed brain!*

A few months after my last SOT, for some reason I sobbed and hyperventilated in the bathtub for several hours. I think everything just hit me. *I have been sick for five years!* There was so much false *hope* from other doctors concerning the other diagnoses, and loss for what to do moving forward. I cried over how many experiences I have missed with my children. *Russell was four and Eliot was one. They are nine and six now . . . I missed so much . . . I can't get it back.* I cried over the loss of my uterus. *My chance of ever having more children was stolen from me.* I cried over the crippling pain. *I can't do this anymore. Get this out of me!* I cried over the battles I had with food when I would go into allergic reactions eating most things . . . the *fear* that brought. *I can't breathe . . . I can't breathe.* I cried over the damage to my eyes . . . *Everything is so bright . . .* I cried over the impact this disease has had on my hearing. *The ringing is so loud I can't even stifle it with my screams . . .* I cried because I don't understand . . . *Why did this happen to me?* I suspected later that these extreme emotions could be coming from die off. But in all reality, I feel that I am finally starting to be able to properly grieve from this trauma.

I try to redirect my mind . . . I am *grateful* that I can drive short distances when I am not in a flare. I seem to be able to eat more foods. *The crippling pain, though . . .* I try to give myself grace when I fall to pieces and remember that I can do better tomorrow. I give myself grace when I fall back. I hold myself in an embrace . . . and tell myself *it's okay . . .*

* * *

My Lyme doctor suggested I see an ENT for my chronic sinus-type headaches. He reviewed my most recent MRI and, of course, everything looked *normal* structurally. He saw a lot of mucus and said it could be from silent reflux. We did allergy testing. The biggest thing that showed up was mold. *Not surprised.* It was one of the same types of mold I had in my body at high levels. Mostly from food or from the soil. Harvest can stir it up.

Great . . . we live right next to the soybean plant. But I know the problem really isn't the occasional mold exposure. The problem has been retaining it because of the state of my immune system from having Lyme disease. I still feel traumatized by mold, though. *Who wouldn't be?*

My allergies concerning common foods were *none,* but food often has mold on it. So if I react to any of these foods it's most likely the *mold,* not the food, causing it. He is still suspicious that these silent reflux-type symptoms and sinus-related issues are from an allergy to something.

I left a blood vial with the nurse to see if they can possibly test me for alpha-gal syndrome. *Alpha-gal syndrome (AGS) is an allergic condition in which people are allergic to alpha-gal, a sugar found in the tissues of all mammals except humans and other primates. It is also known as mammalian meat allergy, alpha-gal allergy, red meat allergy, and tick bite meat allergy.* My doctor felt this was an unlikely possibility because my throat does not close up after eating beef. *I used to feel like it did . . .* He was concerned that insurance would not cover the test because I do not show extreme anaphylactic reactions after eating beef. There have been many times in the past where I *have* experienced these types of reactions. I eat beef almost daily and, even after fixing other underlying factors, I still have extreme GI discomfort. In the past, there were too many foods that were causing reactions. I couldn't often pinpoint the food, especially when something as simple as the air seemed to trigger reactions. I don't know if I have this syndrome, but I do have Lyme, and it is time we investigate it. Hopefully insurance will cover the test. If I do not hear back from them then the test was not covered by insurance.

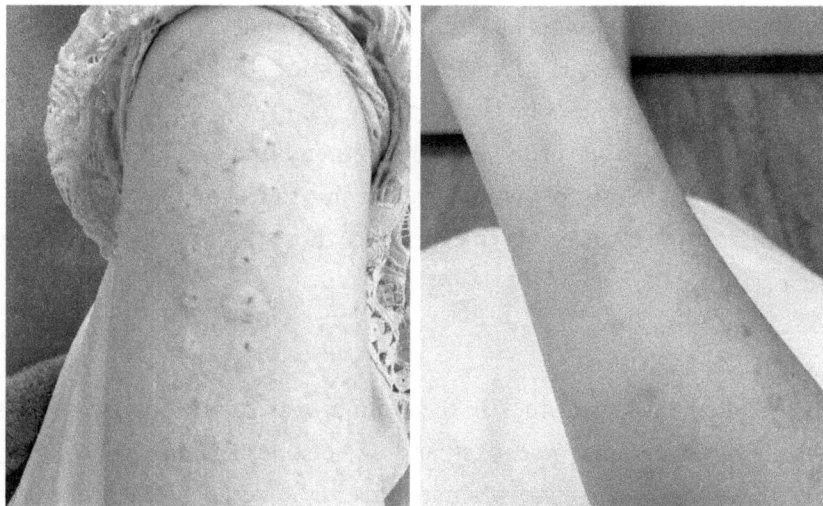

mold . . .

I cried Sunday when I opened a letter from church. It was money donated to me for my health expenses. I feel so unworthy with how dark my mind can become. I love God. I am not angry at God like I was during the first year of my illness. But sometimes he feels so silent. I cried more when I wrote the church a thank you letter. I included my poem and tried to explain my situation in the best way that I could. I never expected the church to help me . . . I never asked them to. I am so *grateful* for their kindness. Even the smiles when I make it to church on Sunday. They want to see me get better so badly. So many do. I feel it's hard to explain how long something like this can take. And I often feel like a failure when I have to respond that *I am no better.*

January 1, 2024

We had a very nice Christmas holiday this year. No one got sick over the holidays, and we got to do a lot of things this year that we have not been able to do in a long time. It was nice to be together and open gifts. Around this time of year, I am always somewhat reminded of a new year passing since my health regression started . . . but I refuse to let that take the warmth and happiness I have always felt around Christmas.

When I was a little girl, I remember lying under the Christmas tree and looking up, mesmerized by the bright lights. It was always so magical, and I always felt so warm and so happy. When I first became sick around Christmas, I didn't think I would ever be able to feel that *joy* again. But I do, and now my children get to experience those things with me lying by their side.

January 27, 2024

I feel like I have been stuck in the twilight zone for the last two weeks. I started to experience mid-back and GI episodes again. I feel so foggy and it takes my breath away when it happens. Sometimes it feels like I am being stabbed with a hot knife all over. And I can't breathe well for a while afterward. I was able to see my family, too, but unfortunately, they started to feel unwell halfway into the visit. My most recent flare developed after I contracted influenza. It's not their fault.

I had terrible chills, a fever for two days, and buzzing (in my teeth) tremors. I had terrible leg, back, and neck pain . . . and a headache that felt like a brain aneurysm. I am dealing with the aftermath now. I have had heart rate episodes in the 150s while just sitting. I feel like I am in a constant state of recurring fevers. Amanda had to take me to urgent care one day because of the episodes. They even did an EKG because of my heart rate. Oddly, my levels actually *showed* something wrong. I was severely dehydrated and some liver enzymes were flared. There were other blood levels that usually indicate an *infection* that came up abnormal too. My glucose was all over the place. But they saw nothing acute in the ultrasound of my abdomen. Just fatty liver. My bilirubin was elevated again. They attributed this all to fighting the infection, on top of my underlying conditions.

I thought I was going to die again. I visited my safe clinic several times, getting IV fluids for the dehydration flares. Since the acute illness, I have been dealing with hearing issues, stiff neck, buzzing sensations everywhere, and episodes of high heart rates in the nighttime again. A few days before the onset of this flu, I had started azithromycin and methylene blue. I had to go off of everything because I was just too sick. My mom got it, too, and it was terrible for her as well, but she didn't have the long-term issues like me. *Why does this keep happening to me? It's as if I am having fevers all of the time.* I had been bedbound for many days, crying out to God. *Be with me.*

Then something good happened. I had been so torn over the decision to do antibiotics for Bartonella and ehrlichiosis. I was so concerned that it would bring back the candida that I had worked so hard to eradicate. The last Lyme test also showed a different strain of Lyme that was positive but was just under the cutoff by one level to quality for SOT therapy. *Really . . . I screamed inside.* My friend who goes to another Lyme clinic told me there *is* an SOT for ehrlichiosis. I met her through TikTok and she has helped me so much. I emailed my doctor.

"Sure enough . . . " he said, "There is one!"

He missed it, because previously there was not an SOT for ehrlichiosis. It's funny how you meet the kindest people online that care enough to reach out to you even though they hardly even know you. I am *grateful* for all of them.

I'm not too thrilled that he missed this information. I could have been treating ehrlichiosis a lot sooner. But I feel pretty emotionless right now, and I'm in too much misery to be angry. Why waste any of my energy on anger? Instead, we changed treatment plans and I will be doing an SOT for ehrlichiosis. The bummer is that I have to wait two weeks to get the antibiotic out of my system before going in for the blood draw.

I can tell Tim is more stressed than normal. With Eliot and I being sick, and me being on bed rest again on and off, his energy is hard to be around. He came into our room while I was resting and felt that that was the best time to scold me about not putting a DVD away. I just kind of looked at him. *Really? . . . I am on bed rest . . . again.* Sometimes I wonder if he ever thinks before talking. *"She is going through enough right now, this isn't a big deal, it can wait"* or *"I can take care of this myself. I am just going to let her rest and not make a big deal over small things."*

But no.

I get frustrated because I feel like if I had *cancer,* or something more understood, people would show more compassion concerning my struggles. *Especially* during this kind of flare. The *worst* kind I ever go through. But with Lyme, you just get treated normally most of the time. And I can't really blame him or others. I have been sick every day now for five years. I'm sure the *flares* get old.

It wasn't a big deal, but I just can't deal with anything right now. I try *so hard* every day and struggle with small tasks and short-term memory. I used to get so hurt and angry toward people when they were insensitive, and I would wish they would feel this way for just one day. But then I stopped doing that because I was worried I would manifest those thoughts into reality for someone I love. I just get so tired. Small things are small and there is no reason to stress someone who is going through something big with a small problem.

I can't stand up for very long now. I feel like this when I overdo it for a few days. It's a terrible feeling that I am unsure if I can ever properly explain. I think it is from increased oxidative stress. During this time, a girl I used to follow on YouTube died by self-assisted suicide. She had Lyme and Bartonella. This really makes me sad. When someone old dies and they have been suffering, everyone is *grateful. They are finally at peace.* If you are young and suffering, everyone just wants you to hang on and keep being strong. I can understand the feelings that she felt. I know no one in my life would ever approve of letting my suffering end in that way. Part of me imagines how peaceful it was for her. After all of those years she spent taking all of those medications and supplements to end her suffering, and then one pill finally brought her peace as she was surrounded by her loved ones. The other part of me feels very sad and wishes someone could have healed her on Earth and not just in heaven. I also picture myself in her place, and I wouldn't be able to swallow the pill because I want to live.

"I researched assisted suicide many times and was hopeless . . . but then I achieved remission, and you can too." (From a fellow Lyme Warrior.) This repeats over and over again in my head.

January 30, 2024

When my sister called, she said that she has to have open-heart surgery for her aorta. Thoughts flashed through my mind of my dad in the hospital bed after his aorta tore unexpectedly. I held my father's hand as he passed away. *But this won't happen with my sister.* It has been caught, and it will be a different scenario, with her life being saved and she will heal.

Journal Entries from 2010-2011

September 22, 2010: Every night I dream of you. When I awaken I have to distinguish between reality and my dreams. The dreams of you are so real to me. They are somewhat frightening. I dream that you come back to life in the hospital room . . . that you are still here with me. You came back to life so much that you were walking. When I wake up I am so excited and overcome with joy. You are back! You are here with me. But then I start to remember . . . the funeral . . . seeing you connected to all of the tubes in the hospital room . . . your death. I remember how cold you felt in the coffin and I wish I had never touched you. And then, I am hit with dread, pain, and sadness. You are really gone. The dream goes so far to mess with my mind that it is explained to me how you came back to life even though I saw you in your coffin. These dreams play with my mind and when I awaken it takes me a long time to distinguish between what was real and what is not. Maybe my dreams are trying to tell me that you are living again in heaven. But I am filled with a void, an empty space. I wish that I could have you back again Dad.

September 7, 2011: Today means that one year has passed since the death of my father. The man who was my protector. I miss my dad every day. Some days worse than others. I don't think that I have ever really dealt with his loss . . . how does one "deal" with something like this? I guess I just keep myself busy. Keep moving forward with life. I know it is what he would have wanted. The song from his funeral still plays at random when I am doing wedding things. "I miss his blue eyes . . . every time . . . I close mine . . . " The song played when I was at the store two days ago, waiting to pick up lipstick for my wedding. I wonder if

283

it is a sign from him saying he is still with me even though he will not be able to walk me down the aisle. When I sit here and really think of my dad and how he is gone, I feel such powerful sorrow, loss, and longing. I still cannot come to terms that he is really gone. I cannot believe it. I wonder how many years will have to pass before I can accept it? I have a feeling that years won't change it.

When my sister started having similar symptoms to my own, I originally thought maybe it could be Lyme/POTS onset (because of fetal transmission since my mom has it) *but,* before dragging her down that road, I suggested she get an echocardiogram first because of what happened to our dad. Not *everything* is Lyme disease . . .

I had many echos of my own in the past and they were always *normal.* But I wanted her to check that first before going down a winding path like me. Sure enough, her aorta was dilated and she was diagnosed with a connective tissue disease called Marfan. Now we know what caused Dad's tear . . .

She navigated the rest of her pregnancy with this diagnosis, and I attended as many appointments with her as I could. This has brought us very close together, and I want to be here for her to help her heal. I can be here as a listening ear for her. I understand the grief she is experiencing with a sudden traumatic change in her health. I pray every day that we have found these issues early enough, so that surgery can bring healing and a good quality of life when it is stabilized.

When she told me she had to have open-heart surgery in just a few months, it put even more of an urge inside of me to heal faster. But I know there is no time frame in healing. *I need it to happen now.* I have always wanted to be here for those who need me, and I need to be able to heal to help the ones I love without fighting my body every step of the way.

30

No More Toxic Positivity

March 4th, 2024

If I could go back to this time again . . .
when my body was free from pain.
I would run along the trees
Escaping from these chains.
My body would no longer trap me
Locking me tightly here.
Where pain is overwhelming
I cry out for healing to be near.
A life without suffering
Could this subside?
My legs could carry me again
Instead of keeping me trapped inside.
But for now I will look at memories
And escape in that form.
What was once a whisper
Has turned into a storm.

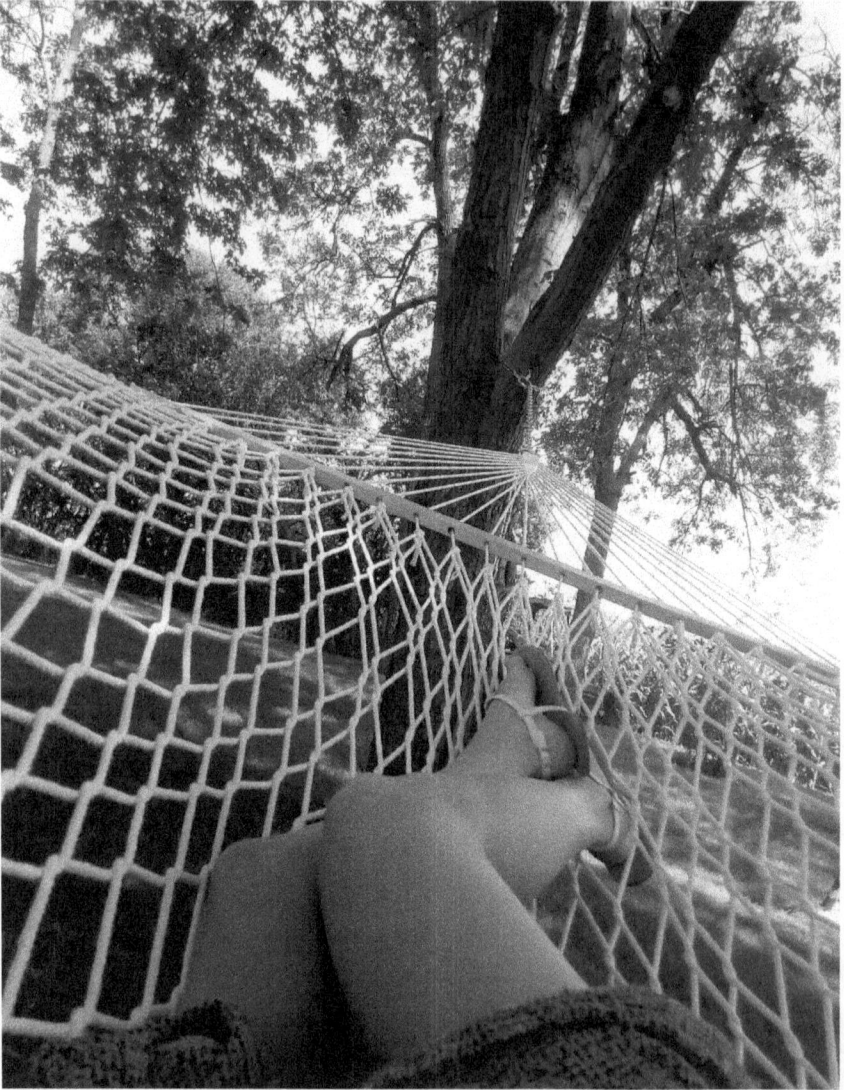

Trapped . . .

I caught an acute illness two more times since December. I needed fluids and got them at my *safe place.* I still avoid the ER like the plague and have not been back to one since the day I was sent home with a sheet on anxiety/somatoform disorder and was refused IV fluids. That was several years ago. There were many times that I felt I *needed* to go to the ER, but I couldn't emotionally deal with another hit like that. Instead, I chose to suffer at home. It amazes me how so many things have circled back in my life since being diagnosed with Lyme disease. All of the doctors who advocated for me in the beginning have now opened a safe place for me to go to get acute care.

* * *

"It has been nice to no longer be treated like I am 'crazy.' No longer being gaslit by medical doctors or treated negatively makes a big difference when trying to heal from medical trauma. I know you are not supposed to, but there is a huge stipulation with having a mental health condition. When I view mental health conditions, I do not have those feelings. I believe people suffer with these conditions because of imbalances of the chemicals of the brain or microbiome that they cannot control. They can suffer with unexplained debilitating symptoms. Imbalances may have occurred from trauma or even underlying illnesses or toxicities. But doctors do treat you differently if anything mental-health related is indicated in your chart. The first time that anxiety was written on my chart, any other symptoms of acute or chronic issues, like POTS, were brushed under the rug. All they could see was anxiety. I think I made it worse for them because I challenged that thought for a long time. I was not a submissive patient. I still strongly believe that if our medical system was different and looked at underlying factors as a cause to unexplained anxiety and depression, many could get better. For now, I will continue to go to my 'safe place' for acute care, and I no longer have to fear being treated like things are all in my head. My present doctor makes things easier, but I understand the battles she has as well . . . and I am so grateful."

* * *

It took me about four and a half weeks to recover from influenza. About a week after recovering from that, I got a sore throat illness from Eliot and fought that with night sweats for several nights. Then, right near the end of that illness, we got COVID. I have been feeling very fatigued from the last three infections, and some symptoms are popping up similar to what I experienced after influenza. So far, COVID has not been as bad as the last viral infection. I am on a lower dose of methylene blue and peptides for Bartonella. I have been tolerating the low dose much better. Hopefully, being on this will help improve the acute issues affecting the oxidative stress levels and cells.

I am becoming increasingly concerned with the amount of recurring acute illnesses that I am getting. I know it makes it harder to heal and raises oxidative stress levels. It's so stressful for others, too, to have to constantly worry about exposing me to things. I cannot imagine how exhausted they feel having to worry like that. I am just glad that no one does it on purpose. The last two issues really were no one's fault. I am not mad at anyone. No one was hiding illness. Illness happens in life, the problem is my condition and the fact that it is very hard on me to get sick right now. My children are at an age where they bring everything home to me. They are not a burden, the chronic illness is.

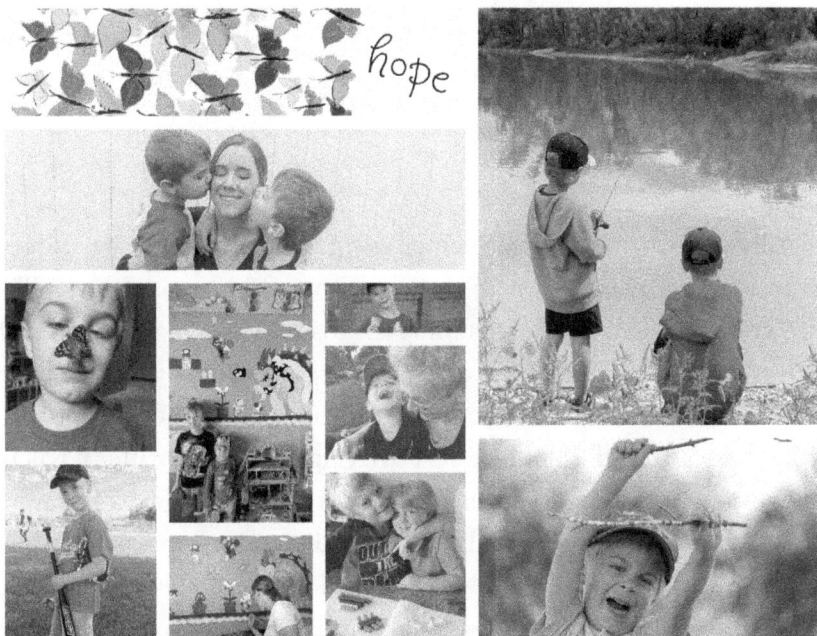

Being a mother is not a burden. The chronic illness is. They are the ones that keep me going even on the hardest of days. Being a mother is an honor and chronic illness can steal a lot of that away. The worst days can feel like valleys that I have to crawl through . . . but my children are my greatest achievements and I persevere because of them.

I have asked my chronic Lyme group what they do in these circumstances, and a lot of them say they have to tell people to wear a mask if they are suspicious of any illness, and if they start to have symptoms they leave. It seems very drastic. I don't know what to do. No matter what I do or what I avoid, my kids catch things and I always get it. I am their main caretaker.

I will be happy if I have a few months of no illness after this. I honestly have not had over a month at a time for at least a year now of not catching something acute . . . even in the summer. I don't know what has been happening since COVID, but I catch everything. When I do, it's very bad and I am in and out of the doctor's office with acute concerns or in need of fluids.

I have been doing vitamin C and glutathione infusions as often as I can, but it's almost $300 a time. I can't afford any more right now.

* * *

I finally made it to the Lyme center again for the blood draw. It took an entire month because there have been complications in Europe. The farmers are on strike and are ruining the roads by digging them up with their tractors. The people from the SOT place have been having to deliver the SOT to a certain location themselves. It does make me nervous, because if the strike affects the blood or SOT arriving in a timely matter it will be destroyed. I pray over all of these Lyme patients' blood and SOT draws.

While at the Lyme center, I also did an additional test for co-infections and Lyme through IGeneX. It was half off and is the exact test we have been wanting to do. Every test has given me an answer. They were not wasted. We also got money back from our insurance company from our last two tests. We were able to cover this test with the money we got back from our insurance company and the donation from our church. *I am grateful.*

I go back in about three weeks for my next SOT for ehrlichiosis and will be on methylene blue in the meantime.

I have been working on my *Boomer* books and have two more in the process of publishing. I also decided that it is time to tell people *my story.* My story about my journey with chronic illness and diagnosis.

March 1, 2024

My Lyme health coach often says, "Not everything is Lyme, and it's important to make sure you are safe while healing."

She has had several patients call her, asking if Lyme can cause heart race and chest pain. *Well sure . . . but so can a heart attack, so it's best to rule that out too.*

So with this in mind, I recently saw the general surgeon who was recommended to me by my primary care provider last year. I went for suggestions for the recurring pain and fatty liver issues, not to inquire about surgery. In the past, she performed my colonoscopy and later ordered the hida scan and gastric emptying study. She suggested I do an ultrasound of the kidneys if the pain persists, but she wanted me to first check with my Lyme doctor to see if he has a specific specialist in mind for these issues. She suggested this because my Lyme doctor suspects it is the Lyme and co-infections causing my pain because of how the bacteria can sit in the kidneys.

She felt it's best to ask him if he knows of anyone for my specific issues. It's very easy to discuss things with her. I feel very open to be able to talk with her about my diagnosis of Lyme disease. She believes me and, in her words, Lyme was the *original "Long COVID."*

I had a hard time keeping it together emotionally at this appointment. Between my primary doctor and her, I am overwhelmed because they are so *kind* to me. *No gaslighting . . .*

She also suggested physical therapy if the pain does not improve after my next therapies for Lyme disease. She is suspicious that if this pain is not coming from the Lyme or co-infections, it is possible that when I had all of the internal bleeding it caused scar tissue that fused things together. I didn't realize this, but she told me that when you bleed into your abdomen, even the blood can irritate the organs, causing scar tissue and fusing of organs. That could explain some things . . . I have had so many internal cysts rupture and even if I do not still have some internal bleeding, when I had the injury, my entire abdomen filled with blood and then later a hematoma formed. I can't imagine how much scar tissue I may have . . .

My acupuncturist is probably right too . . . he says I am breathing wrong. I have had to hold myself a certain way for a long time because of the pain or severe symptoms. Maybe physical therapy would help me be able to move my body easier. I often feel so stiff.

A part of me wonders . . . if we could have found the Lyme first and never had surgery, would I be where I am at today? If I could have just stopped getting acutely ill would my body have been able to heal faster? But I cannot think like that because I cannot rewind time.

* * *

I went back to the Lyme center and had my blood draw for ehrlichiosis. What I like most about SOT is that it can break through biofilm, while some antibiotics cannot. Lyme survives by hiding in the biofilm, bone, brain, or cells, and can even encapsulate itself in tissue. I am on methylene blue at a lower dose again and peptides. I will have to stop them next week and then, in two additional weeks, my SOT should be here from Europe. With the strike going on I *hope* it arrives safely.

Everything takes so long. The wait time to get in with a medical specialist can be from two months to up to a year. It can take months to get in with a functional medicine doctor. Each lab that you do can take several months to get back, and then the treatments take time to arrive. So many people are so sick, and the system cannot keep up with them. Chronic illness is growing every day and there has to be a way to stop it.

March 6, 2024

Last night Russell brought up the dreams that he used to have of the black fox. He told me that it has been a long time since he has had any dreams like that. I asked him what the fox looked like. He said it didn't have a face, his face was a shadow. *A shadow . . .*

This really bothered me. I asked him how he knew it was a fox if it didn't have a face. He said it was because it had two black pointy things on his head.

I have never told Russell about my dream, and he has not had a nightmare about the black fox in two years. This really bothered me, and I had a hard time sleeping. I couldn't stop thinking about my own haunting nightmares of the man with a shadow for a face, and now I found out that my son had been dreaming of it as well.

March 19, 2024

I saw my acupuncturist recently. I have been experiencing episodes of cold sensations rushing up and down at the base of my spine, accompanied by pins and needles and sometimes a burning sensation. Sometimes it feels like cold water is being dripped down my back. I don't like this as it feels like nerve issues. This has been happening more recently since the fevers went on for so long.

He did acupuncture on the area and also gave me some breathing exercises to do at home. I know that he is right. My breathing is not right and hasn't been since all of the air hunger episodes and trauma began. He also helped me with a referral to do pelvic floor therapy and scar tissue manipulation with a trusted physical therapist. He warned me that it may be painful . . . *great*. I feel this is the better path to try, though, rather than having a surgery ever again. I remember this physical therapist from when I tried therapy for the uterus prolapse and felt that she was very helpful then.

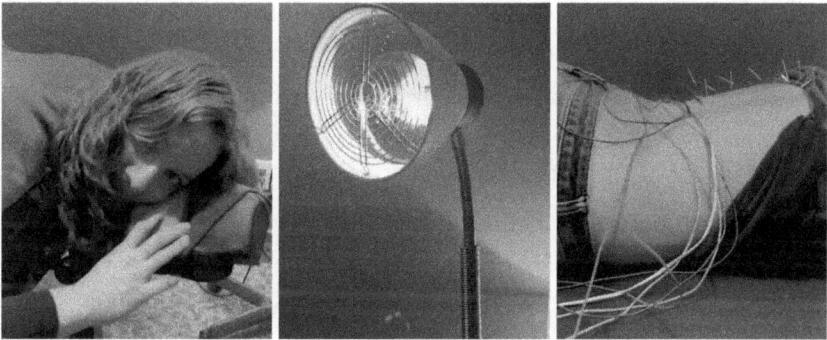

Please allow my nerves to heal . . .

March 19, 2024

My results came back from the Lyme center. I tested positive for tick-borne relapsing fever. We finally know why I have been having such regressions with illness and feelings of fever over and over again. Knowing this, I feel so at peace right now. The strains that cause this issue are from *different* Borrelia strains, *not* from Borrelia burgdorferi. My Lyme doctor feels that this is why I have not had significant improvement after the first

SOT. We were targeting the main beast, but *not* the right strain that causes tick-borne relapsing fever. There are some strains of Borrelia that he can see in my testing that could be responsible . . . but they are not specific enough to point to which SOT we need to use. We cannot guess, because if we guess wrong it would target the wrong strain.

Next week, I go back to the Lyme center and I will be doing one small blood test for these specific strains through Vibrant. Thankfully, our insurance has been covering part of our testing through Vibrant and IGeneX lately, and we were able to get a significant amount back from our insurance company to complete more testing. Insurance covering these tests is a *huge* step in the right direction.

If this testing shows the correct strain and we are 100% sure on it, we will do an SOT. If not, then we will have to either take an herbal or antibiotic path. Everyone's path in healing from chronic Lyme is different. Some are easier than others. Some people are very confident in antibiotics, while others claim that antibiotics caused them harm and had better success with herbals. This creates a difficult terrain for those suffering with Lyme. *Should I go with antibiotics or herbals?* My situation is proving to be challenging. I want to do SOT therapy to heal. I have been told SOT is easier on the body and actually *kills* the bacteria more effectively and does not force it into hiding. The cost may be too much for us. I have stayed on the same path, despite not having significant improvement. Because we persisted in testing, I have been able to see on paper what is causing my issues. There is great healing in that alone. A lot of times, the answers do not even show up on paper for others.

* * *

A few days later, I received a phone call from the ear, nose, and throat doctor. I was surprised to hear from them as it had been several months since I had seen them. They informed me that I tested *positive* for *alpha-gal syndrome*. I could not believe it. I had suspected the insurance had not covered my testing because of a lack of a clinical picture. But the office had just failed to call me with my results. They forgot.

I almost laughed on the phone when she told me that I should always carry an emergency EpiPen with me wherever I go. It has been *five years* of me dealing with extreme anaphylactic episodes that were blamed on panic attacks. *I am still alive.* Instead of laughing, I cried. I was overwhelmed with all of these answers coming together. I have been in a state of highs and lows since my Lyme disease diagnosis. I can put together more pieces just in this last week than I have been able to in the last five years. This syndrome can be reversed by eradicating the tick-borne bacteria from the body and repairing the overactive immune system. My ENT doctor's nurse has confirmed this, as they have seen reversal in alpha-gal syndrome before. I can at least refrain from red meat products for now and move forward on my treatment to heal from chronic Lyme.

In the past, I have done so many things with my diet. I have tried all-juicing, grain-free for months, oxalate-free, histamine-free, gluten- and dairy-free for years, and I even tried carnivore. I was mostly consuming organ meats and bone broth . . . *nice.*

There was a time when my local functional medicine doctor did some testing, looking at levels for allergic reactions. The blood test showed I *wasn't* having responses to *anything* I was eating, but I continued to have debilitating stomach pains. This shows how *sometimes* the tests just don't pick things up. Throughout my experience, several tests have been very unreliable.

Because of these results, at one point I even tried *ignoring* my food reactions to continue practicing limbic system rewiring. Food has been a huge battle for me. At least I have some idea on what to avoid for now.

* * *

I saw my acupuncturist again after the diagnosis of alpha-gal syndrome, and we decided to try an acupuncture therapy called SAAT (*Soliman Auricular Allergy Treatment*). I had found information through my Lyme group about this therapy, and many claimed it helped them reach remission for this specific syndrome. My acupuncturist found a PubMed medical journal that showed that this therapy resulted in a 96% rate of complete remission of AGS (alpha-galsyndrome), lasting months to years. That is a huge percentage and I am very hopeful that this could help me.

I feel that the other factors, of course, are important—eradicating the tick-borne bacteria and avoiding the foods until the inflammation and food allergy is closer to remission—*but* this therapy sounds promising and is an easy procedure. I will go in once every couple of weeks for the therapy. It's funny how, throughout all of this, it always comes back to my acupuncturist helping me . . .

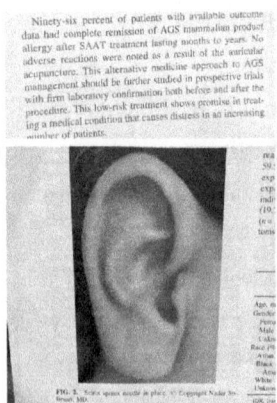

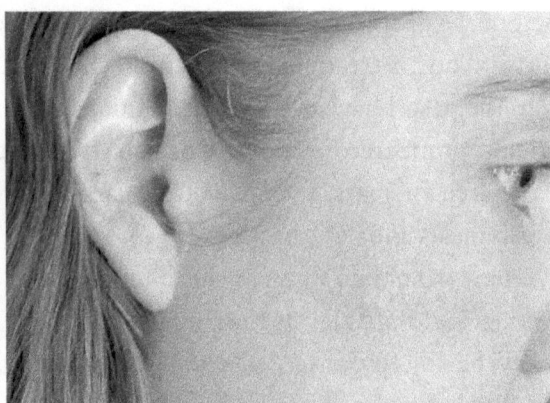

SAAT (Soliman Auricular Allergy Treatment) for AGS (Alpha-Gal Syndrome)

The biggest improvement I have noticed since cutting out beef products and incorporating the SAAT treatment is that my debilitating upper abdominal pain is mostly gone.

March 20, 2024

I have had many suggestions from fellow Lyme sufferers who claim to be healed to try a Rife machine or magnetic treatment facilities. My neighbor used a frequency device, along with other therapies, to put Lyme in remission. One of the kindest people I know gifted me a frequency device in hopes that it could help me. I will forever be *grateful* for her care and dedication to those suffering with chronic illness. It always surprised me how *strangers* could care about me.

I have also been hearing a lot about the celebrity from *The Bachelor* who suffered since childhood with Lyme disease. Because Lyme and other toxins built up in her body, she ended up losing her hearing and needed a cochlear implant later in life. Her family did a GoFundMe for her and she traveled all the way to a facility in Germany to put herself into remission. She was there for an entire month and did a lot of different therapies. One therapy specifically raised her body temperature, while others were focusing on removing heavy metals and rebuilding her microbiome. She was on different antibiotics, herbs, and supplements as well. I looked into the clinic . . . $70,000.

In the media, I often see celebrities who are suffering with Lyme disease, and they claim to spend around $10,000 a week on therapies to help put the disease in remission. Common people cannot afford these luxury treatments, and if they somehow manage to and they fail, they are left to pick up the pieces while still suffering, with *added* financial turmoil.

By the time people are diagnosed with Lyme disease, they have often already gone through most of their savings. It is an unfortunate reality.

A conversation between my son and myself:

"Mommy . . . someday I am going to get a mowing business and when I make all of this money I am going to get you better."

"Oh honey, that money is going to be yours."

"No, Mommy . . . I just want you to be better. I want my mommy to be better. You deserve to be better. I don't know how you feel, but I can't imagine being sick every day for five years."

"Oh honey, you don't need to worry about me . . . you keep your dreams for you."

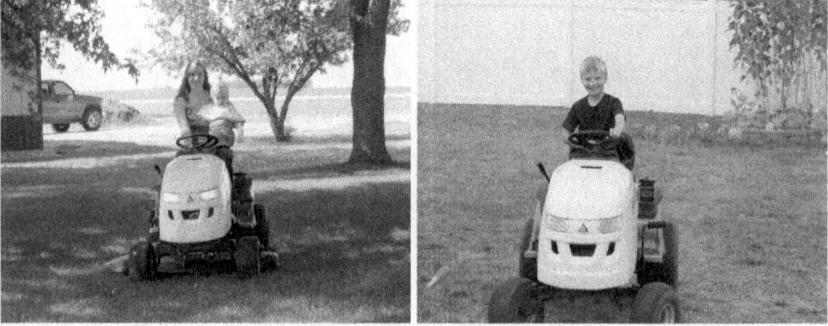

"Someday I'm going to get a mowing business . . ."

March 29, 2024

I just did my first SOT for ehrlichiosis. My *Boomer* sales have helped to afford parts of my care. Tim recently repaired and sold a vehicle in order for me to be able to get my SOT treatment. He may feel that I don't appreciate these things, but I do. I just feel very bad that he has to exhaust himself in order to afford my treatments. He works so hard already.

Recently, the Lyme center took three vials of blood to see if we can catch the specific Borrelia strain that is causing the tick-borne relapsing fever. I am relieved that we have a treatment in progress for the co-infections, and a path to move forward. I *hope* they catch it.

* * *

A fellow Lyme Warrior told me that the chances of remission go down with every year of being misdiagnosed. It is a very *troubling* thought. If I have had this disease since birth, would my likelihood of reaching remission be very small? If it happened during childhood that is not much better. If it happened five years ago, I feel I would have a better chance.

She went on to say that she has tried everything and, unfortunately, is submitted to this life. She told me her statement was in no way meant to diminish my *hope* or *strength,* and we all need a *cure.*

I think of her often and pray for her. She has been going through this longer than I have, and our symptoms are very similar. I hear the cries of those *suffering*, and I wish I could help them all.

* * *

While doing my treatment, the nurse said they were talking about why SOT works instantly for *some*, but *not* for *others*. I brought up my situation. My Lyme doctor responded, "Your labs have been far more complex than others."

It brought me back to when my brain health specialist said I was the most complicated immune case he has ever seen. *Lucky me.*

My wonderful nurse also brought up that when they do SOT therapy, they often see other strains pop up and other symptoms. This 100% is what has happened in my case. My recent results came back showing several Borrelia strains, and I qualify for SOT therapy again! I even had a positive IgM (immunoglobulin M) level. We will have to do herbals or antibiotics for some of these other strains because we don't have the funds to do all the SOT therapies.

The plan right now is to continue treating the multiple Borrelia strains and co-infections. My timeline has shown how true it is that other strains will come out of hiding when treating. The strain that is causing the tick-borne relapsing fever recently revealed itself as Borrelia turicatae. We will be treating that with an SOT. I have multiple strains that popped up in my most recent tests, and we plan to start out with herbals for those strains.

Later, we will reevaluate if I need another SOT for Borrelia burgdorferi since I had an IgM level show up this time. Seeing the positive IgM brought me back to my appointment with my local functional medicine doctor a year ago. *Would this result have presented as a positive diagnosis of chronic Lyme disease?*

After the SOT for Borrelia turicatae, we will evaluate how I am feeling and decide if I should do a second SOT for ehrlichiosis. I *hope* that by then my symptoms have improved and I will not need further SOT therapies.

My symptoms have changed since starting treatment, and more recently

I have more nerve pain, body aches, and a general increased feeling of fighting infection. The infections are surfacing. I feel my body fighting. I see the levels popping up in testing. I *know* that I have Lyme and I am *telling* it to *GET OUT!*

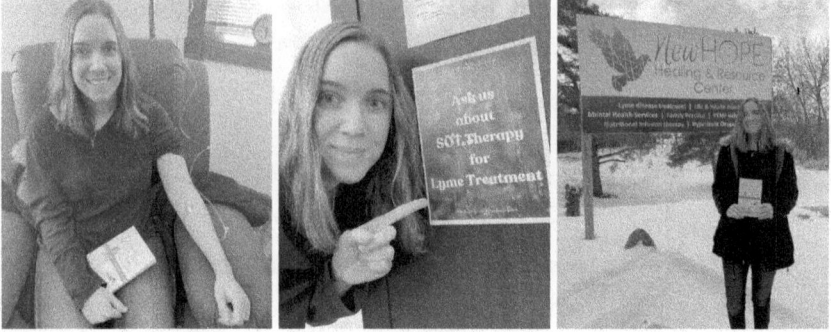

hope . . .

* * *

Western medicine is mostly about symptom management, so with a condition like my own we originally go into this battle with expectations for instant results. Because that is often what we experience with common illnesses, that is what we expect after treatment. It can be a real struggle to accept that these issues can take months, years, or decades to repair. So, throughout that time, it is so important to find any way you can to get through the low times.

Symptoms:
   If I am not experiencing the symptoms associated with a migraine or a fever, I experience the aftermath of those episodes. I struggle with eye pressure and brain fog. The eye pressure triggers often from pressure or heat changes. These symptoms will onset often after a hot shower or even

from something as simple as the wind. The pressure changes affect me. It's hard to explain it, but it is as if air is pumped into my head right behind my right eye. I experience visual disturbances and eye floaters. I still have buzzing and tremors, especially during flares.

Because of these symptoms, I often struggle to feel present. Sometimes I feel like an outcast in society, especially when I try to involve myself in normal social gatherings and struggle to do simple tasks. I struggle with communication and lengthy conversations. I begin to stammer a lot if my symptoms trigger, which makes social gatherings very difficult. Because of this, it can be difficult to involve myself in normal social situations.

I deal with post-concussion symptoms daily. Besides conversation, triggering events for me are also bright lights, overstimulating environments, loud noises, and stress. Sometimes I wonder how inflamed my brain really is.

I still struggle with facial flushing, even after eating my "safe foods." Sometimes I get sore throats and mild air hunger too. I don't remember what it was like to not experience symptoms of some sort after eating.

I experience POTS flares, mostly after acute illness, but the POTS syndrome has been a lot more manageable. At times I am bedbound for several days or weeks because of an acute illness, due to the increased tremors or dizzy sensations or lingering recurring fever onset.

I don't have a lot of resilience with exercise or being active in general. My body will crash from doing simple tasks, and I cannot schedule a full day of visiting numerous people or going to several places. If I do a lot of chores, I begin to struggle with air hunger and vertigo. I will experience gagging and nausea if I overdo it. Sometimes I will get fevers or swollen lymph nodes, depending on the amount of physical exertion I use. It's frustrating, and I will scream at my body to work from time to time.

I have nerve pain and extreme stabbing sensations in the mid-back area where my kidneys are located. After this happens, I also feel a lot of air hunger. I experience burning, ripping, scraping, pins and needles, and cold-water feelings in my back.

More recently, when I am flaring, I know it's because of the Lyme being

killed in my body and I internally scream, *"If you don't like it, then get out . .
. "*

I learned this technique from my health coach, who also battled Lyme
disease. Instead of yelling at my own body, I try to encourage it to kill
the Lyme. I know that may sound silly, but I truly believe your body does
better when you can internally tell it what to do and target your anger
toward the invader instead of yourself.

My Lyme health coach said that the immune system can struggle for
an entire year after the bacteria is eradicated. We are still working on
eradicating the bacteria in my case, so I have great *hope* for my future. I
know that I have a long way to go yet with healing, but I have had *some*
improvements that I am very *grateful* for.

Some improvements I have had:

1. I can ride in the car again without an episode
2. I tolerate more loud noise and bright lights than ever before
3. I have not fainted for several years
4. The POTS syndrome is more manageable
5. I can ride a bike for exercise
6. I can tolerate the heat in the sauna
7. I experience fewer stroke-like episodes and less migraines
8. Skin lesions have improved
9. I can visit longer without certain symptoms popping up
10. I can tolerate the heat outside better than the years before
11. I sleep better
12. I have less night sweats
13. I have less night terrors
14. I feel good while swimming
15. I have less air hunger

* * *

For a long time, I experienced a form of toxic positivity surrounding my symptoms. I never felt like I could fully express how I was feeling, in an honest way, without it being blamed on my thoughts or limbic system alone. I no longer have to feel this way with my current health coach. I can tell her anything and not feel like I am failing.

I felt like a failure all of the time when I expressed that I was still dealing with a lot of the same issues, or new ones, even after completing past protocols.

When my providers started to feel that it was my limbic system mostly causing my symptoms, I felt like I couldn't be honest about how I was really feeling anymore. I am naturally a very positive person and keep to myself. When I was experiencing pain and expressed it to others, it was very real. I understood what the doctors were trying to do, but because of this (and because of my own thoughts surrounding how I needed to be more *positive*) I ignored what I was *feeling* and attempted to heal my limbic system on my own.

I did this when I had my iron infusion and my surgery. I could feel that the iron infusion was going wrong, but I was trying to tell myself it would heal me. Instead, it actually hurt me. I did this before I underwent my surgery. I didn't feel right about it, and I kept having internal worries that I did have Lyme disease. I ignored that internal voice because I was trying to have a *positive* outlook. I ignored my true thoughts concerning the retained ferritin and missed Lyme disease . . . I began to blame myself for failing my protocols because of my limbic system. I began to feel like a complete failure.

As the year has gone on since my diagnosis of Lyme disease, it's unsettling to think about how much we missed because I felt pressured to always be positive. We missed the tick-borne relapsing fever, which was a very uncontrollable factor in my scary regressions after falling ill. It was finally caught after a regression from an acute illness. I remember specifically telling one of my functional medicine doctors how concerned I was becoming with these flares from acute illness. She said that everything looked good in my immune and cytokine panels and that I needed to worry less. She said I was going to get sick, but my labs showed that my body was fighting it. In a way, she seemed somewhat annoyed because she couldn't see anything specific on paper. I wondered if she was annoyed at me or just the fact that we couldn't find anything specific in my labs. When I expressed my worries, she wanted me to focus more on healing my limbic system . . . but *I already was.* I was throwing up and having unbearable pain after the fever illness that summer, and I didn't know what else to do because *positive* thoughts and grounding was not stopping the vomiting and pain.

I went to see my brain health specialist for these episodes and he had a lot of suggestions besides HBOT. The day that I arrived, though, his demeanor had changed from the passionate *I'm going to help you* energy, to *a lot of this may be resulting from your limbic system.* I found later that he had just gotten off the phone with my functional medicine doctor. I had given him permission to speak with her because he had some suggestions for supplements for the cell damage. I told him I didn't want to do anything outside of my doctor's permission, and that was why he originally had called. It was hard, because after he said this my entire mind frame going into the chambers was *Do I really even need to be here if it's my brain that is keeping me sick?* He still did think I could possibly have Lyme.

Near the end, the situations started to bring me back to the times when I was being told that all of my issues stemmed from anxiety alone. I never intended to have so many people involved in my situation, but not everyone could help me in the same way, and it was recommended by my out-of-state functional medicine doctor to try these therapies. I tried everything 100% and was always very dedicated to my protocols and therapies, which is how I went about limbic system rewiring as well. I still practice limbic system rewiring. I felt, at this time, that I needed to separate myself from all of the different opinions because I couldn't even understand my own thoughts on it any longer.

So I stayed home on my own for some time, practicing grounding, limbic system rewiring exercises, and positive thoughts. I lay in the grass daily with just a bathing suit, trying to force the Earth's energy to heal me. I felt worse doing this for some reason. I redirected every negative thought relating to my symptoms to a positive one. I would force myself out of the house with my kids, informing my symptoms that they would no longer prevent me from living. I would run to the bathroom and vomit, all while completely ignoring my symptoms and my *fear* surrounding them. I would come out of the bathroom acting like nothing happened. I smiled and tried to be a normal person in society, while internally feeling like death.

I even looked into some brain trauma programs that included visual stimulation for resetting trauma of the brain. I could not find something in my area. So I used YouTube at home. I did sound therapy through YouTube, and I even did a session with my mom. I was on the phone off and on with someone who practiced energy healing. That didn't work.

I spent a lot of time in the sauna listening to Christian music and meditations. I had lost so much weight from the vomiting episodes, and it was during this time frame that I decided to see my acupuncturist again. It had been months since I had last seen him because I had disconnected myself from everyone. I wanted to try to heal my limbic system on my own, and I wanted to be able to hear my own thoughts again, instead of the thoughts of others.

When I sent my results off to the Lyme center and was told I was positive . . . even then I had doubts and kept thinking it must be my limbic system keeping me here. Because that's all that I kept hearing. Eventually, I was able to *trust* that I even had Lyme disease and I proceeded with treatment. I think I was just so exhausted from the internal battle of it all.

I don't feel like people suffering with cancer or other illnesses go through this. It is not common for their providers to bring up the idea that the mind can be keeping them sick. It is common with chronic illness though. I believe that the mind has a huge impact and, yes, the brain can be stuck in certain patterns, but my mind was blamed too often, missing several diagnoses, and I was tired of hearing it.

I wanted to include these feelings here because I see a lot of others struggling in the same way. I understand the difficult predicament that doctors face as far as figuring out if it's a mental health disorder, limbic system impairment, or a different underlying factor keeping their patients chronically sick. I understand they feel they need to talk to these patients in a specific way because of the repeated trauma that has caused PTSD. But it was a very difficult thing for me to feel that I could not fully express how I was feeling over time. I felt like I couldn't be honest any longer concerning how I was feeling, and I buried my symptoms while my body suffered.

This was *my experience,* but others' are different. I have read many books where practicing limbic system rewiring completely eradicated the conditions because the immune system was no longer being hindered by chronic trauma and stress.

I am sure it was *not* any of my doctors' intentions to make me feel like I couldn't express myself honestly. I clearly remember all of the times when my functional medicine doctor's eyes filled with tears. I remember *every* time one of my specialist's eyes filled with tears. They cared for me and wanted to see me better. Each did the best they could do for my situation, and none of them were forcing me to ignore my symptoms. They always said there *could* be more than one cause besides my limbic system. But this is just the way I began to feel because of everything I was learning about the limbic system, and I blamed myself for being stuck there.

Now—after being diagnosed with Lyme disease, tick-borne relapsing fever, and alpha-gal syndrome—I am very glad that I persisted, but I sometimes feel the damage could have been less had we found this earlier. I always knew from the beginning that there was more to my health issues.

I no longer blame the limbic system alone, because doing so in the past resulted in damage to my body. The pain that I have experienced since the summer of that first fever flare has now resulted in chronic back and nerve pain. I now have to debate whether I need to try an opioid medication for this debilitating nerve pain. Because of the feelings I had about my own mind causing my issues, I gaslit myself while experiencing the extreme vomiting and pain, and over time it resulted in these present issues.

I have been told the Lyme and co-infections are likely the cause of the nerve pain that I experience today. I don't know the level of nerve damage that I have or if it can be reversed, but I am doing everything I physically and emotionally can to try and reverse it.

I don't feel that anyone has the right to tell a person how they feel, and I do think that, at times, being told to be *positive,* despite what you are going through, can result in negative consequences. I feel it is important to practice limbic system repair for trauma, but ignoring my symptoms is something I will no longer do.

Presently, I no longer have to battle these internal struggles because I now have a Lyme health coach who battled all of this herself. She listens and guides me and encourages positivity channeled toward defeating Lyme. I will forever be *grateful* for her.

31

What is Your Name

August 28, 2024

I feel them crawling all over me.
I cannot escape them.
The lights are so bright.
Only the darkness relieves my pain.
They are all over.
Outside of me.
Inside of me.
Tremoring.
Like an angry demon.
The tremors circulate to my very core.
All the way to the bottom of my feet.
The roads move.
The world moves.
I am swaying as if I am on an invisible boat.
All while I am still . . .
Grounded.
I can only scream inside.
Who are you?!?
I hear a tiny whisper.

And now I can see it.
It says, "I am Bartonella."

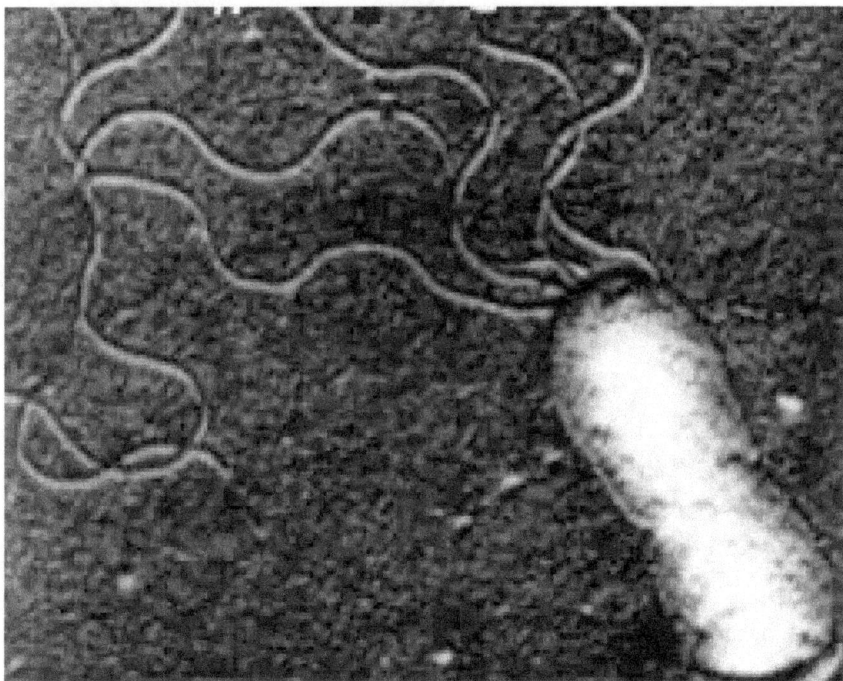

After a year of treating Lyme disease, Bartonella revealed itself in testing.

I knew it all along and now it has finally revealed itself to me. I can see it and now I can kill it, the beast inside of me. I finally have its name. And its name is Bartonella. *I tested through the Lyme clinic in Georgia using MDL (Medical Diagnostic Laboratories). The infection revealed itself, finally. I guess I needed this doctor all along to help me in this journey. The day I came across his TikTok was not just a coincidence, but a God moment.*

32

Persevere with Me

Most people do not know that I am sick, or they don't understand it. Tim is usually the only one who can tell when my symptoms are acting up in public. It must be the look in my eyes or how I start to stammer or slur my words. Overstimulation can still trigger episodes for me. It took me a long time to go to family events again because of that.

I have always been a very *private* person, especially concerning my health struggles, which began in December of 2018. I was always taught that you do whatever you can to take care of things yourself *first*, which is what we did for two years by making a lot of financial sacrifices and losing our home. But the sacrifices we made were at the expense of my husband's mental health and that of our son. I didn't ever want my son to experience that kind of loss again because of my pride.

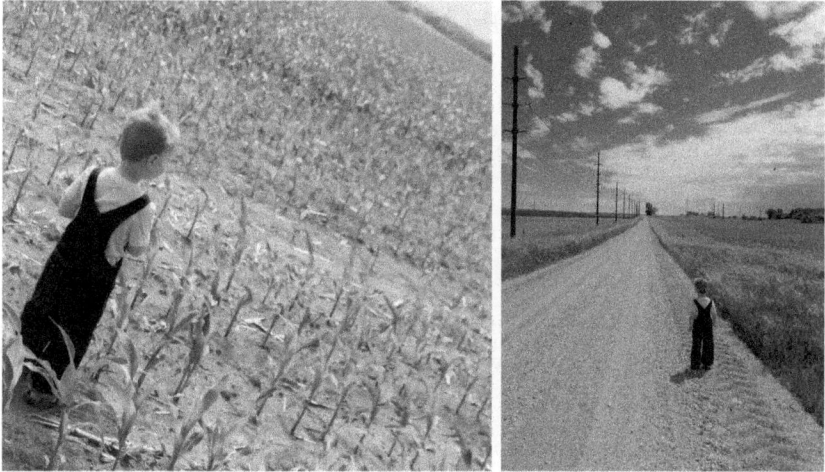

I put my pride aside a long time ago because I didn't want my suffering to affect my family negatively ever again.

I didn't start to tell anyone the details of my illness until we did our GoFundMe in 2022. We didn't have all of the answers, but I did have POTS.

When I am in public I look *normal*. I am quiet and keep to myself. I hide the suffering because *I don't want to upset others*. I hid my issues as much as I could when I was around others because I didn't want to *ruin their day*, and I didn't want people to have to accommodate me.

I am starting to realize why so many people are so silent about being sick. I am open on my online health forum because I want to *help* others. I kept most things private for the longest time, until others insisted that I share my story. But honestly, in *real life* I am the complete opposite. If anyone asks how I am, I usually say *I'm fine* and I don't go into a lot of detail unless it's someone that I *trust*. The only people I share my suffering in detail with are those that may *try* to understand. But I *understand* the complexity of my situation and why they may struggle to *understand* it.

When I was growing up, I didn't have a support system like I have now. I always had to pick up all of the pieces myself. I felt very alone. Oftentimes, because of my family circumstances, I felt that I was the only one I could rely on. But after December of 2018, I had no control of what was happening to my body anymore and had to *accept* the help of others. At times, my health was so bad that I couldn't even get a dish from the cupboard. To onlookers, it may appear that I am lazy or entitled if I ask for help with simple tasks like this. It took a long time for me to be able to ask for help with those things, because if I did it would mean that I was having to accept my condition. It was a very scary situation to accept. Other days, my body allows me to do quite a lot of things, but I always crash for days afterward. Sometimes I even get fevers when I exert myself too much.

During this journey, one of the most challenging things has been having to *surrender* by *accepting* help and putting my pride aside. My *frustration* comes from my body failing me while I do *everything* in my power to take back my health. Regardless of how well I was taking care of my body and doing everything I was told to *fix* it, it was *still* failing me. I had no control over this.

Imagine how frustrating that must feel when you wake up in the morning and you experience heart rates in the 180s and then faint . . . just from standing. I didn't get dehydrated from ignoring my water intake, or from avoiding eating. I would have these episodes because my body was fighting something invisible that I had *no* control over.

I have *not* just been sick . . . I have been *dying* from an *invisible invader* that has slowly been *killing me* from the inside out. It's more than just being *sick*. I know that people have a very hard time *understanding* this, or maybe they feel I am not pushing myself enough. I *pray* they never have to *experience* what it feels like when your body is attacked like this.

Asking for help was never something that I was comfortable doing in the past, *but* when I could see how my children and husband were suffering I knew I had to put my pride aside and get help from others. If it was just me, I may have suffered in silence because, again, I do not like attention placed on myself. But it's not about me. I accept help because my family suffers when I don't.

In the past, I worried often about what people would think of me and the last thing I wanted was for people to feel sorry for me. I *worried* that many people would turn it into something else, like *me looking for attention*. I have always *loathed* being the center of attention . . . those who saw me try to do public speeches in high school would confirm this.

In all reality, if I was suffering with cancer I wouldn't have to feel this way at all. When you have cancer, the entire world walks together holding signs and and wearing T-shirts in the name of healing the disease. People stand by your side. People drop off meals. People don't expect you to push harder . . . they don't judge when you ask for help. People don't judge your choices in treatments. People don't think you are making it all up. But it is not like this with chronic illness. It is not like this with Lyme disease. Am I trying to compete with cancer sufferers and say I am far worse? *No.* I am trying to make the point that with Lyme disease and chronic illness you are often treated poorly because of a lack of understanding. Programs for aid with these conditions are nearly nonexistent. You are *alone* to suffer and it is up to you to *persevere* and sometimes, for the *sake* of your family, you have to *humble* yourself and accept the *help* of others.

It shouldn't be this way, but it is.

* * *

Why did I write this book? So that it could *help* someone, like *you*, who may be going through a similar situation. There are many people suffering in this life, and they are hanging on by a thread every day, not just *me*. I *did not* write this book to make people feel bad for me or to draw attention to *myself*. I *did not* write this book to publicly humiliate doctors or the medical system . . . I am just telling you the *truth* of what happened to *me*. I did *not* want to share my story. *I wanted to bury it in a deep dark hole in my past* . . . but it is *not about me* . . .

There are many of us out there who are *suffering,* and sharing my story may help others. My *hope* is that others will read this because they want some insights into the lives of the chronically ill, and that they will choose kindness moving forward if they know of someone going through a hard-to-understand situation.

313

Many of you who picked up this book are suffering with blanket diagnoses, and the only therapy offered is salt water and compression socks. You experience medical gaslighting, and you may have been abandoned by everyone around you. *Some of you want to dig for answers.*

More recently, as I have been brave enough to share my story, I have been met with more positivity than I could have *ever* imagined. I have helped *others* in reaching a diagnosis for certain health issues. Even being properly evaluated for POTS is huge if you are being told you just have anxiety. I have *helped* others get properly evaluated for Lyme disease, and many have left me *grateful* notes and shared their healing experiences because I chose to *speak* out.

Just like my dad always said: *"There are some things in life that we just can't control . . . it's not up to us. But . . . we can control how we choose to respond."*

I have chosen to *respond* by sharing *my story* with you as I continue to explore *all* avenues to improve my health through SOT therapy, herbals, red light therapy, grounding, infrared sauna, prescriptions, medications, and DNRS to heal from the trauma . . . I *hope* that you can fight along with me. Remember you *are not* Lyme. You *are not* a burden. Lyme is the burden on you.

Persevering . . . is a brave thing to do . . .
Persevere with me.

IV

Part Four

What is it like to be chronically ill?
It kind of feels like you are drowning.
It feels like waves rushing in, crashing into you.
Like a current you will never escape."

33

Caretaker's Perspectives

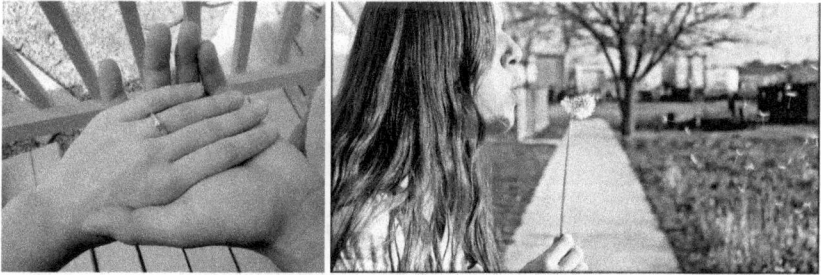

Having good support makes a big difference . . .

It is important to understand the struggles that caretakers go through in the experience of *witnessing* the regression of their loved one's health. This is for all of those who are going through difficult emotions from watching a loved one suffer:

You may feel out of control and hopeless because you want to fix their suffering. It may cause extreme distress when you realize you cannot fix it. Your feelings are very *valid,* and it is okay if you need to take breaks emotionally, seek therapy, or find other outlets that help with what you are going through yourself while being a witness to the traumatic decline. Your emotions are valid and important, too, and chronic stress can lead to health issues for yourself. Finding ways to lessen the burden can help.

Accept help from others, confide in someone about what you are going through, find times to go do fun things with friends, and find new ways of interacting with your partner if you are unable (at the moment) to do the things you used to do together. It's *okay* that you cannot fix it on your own for them. We don't expect you to. Practicing some of these methods when your partner is going through this can be helpful: Do grounding exercises. Meditate. Pray. Do small things that bring happiness. Your partner wants you to be able to feel happy, even during the lowest of times.

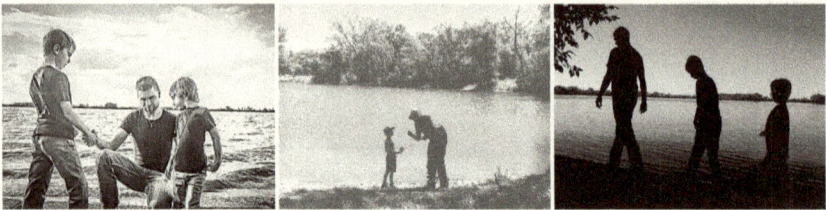

Timothy, thank you for being there for our children . . . it's okay that sometimes you needed their hugs more than they needed yours . . .

**These are the experiences and emotions that
my main caretakers went through:**

* * *

Timothy:

Sweetheart, I'm sorry I haven't read your book. It's not something I can do right now, and once we're past this I won't ever want to go back. Every struggle you faced and every pain you felt will forever be an example of my failure to protect you from it.

There are many things about the past five years I don't remember, and that is on purpose. I know the limits of what I can and can't handle physically and emotionally. What I can't handle, I erase from my memory. Call it what you want: weakness, cowardice. I call it survival for myself and my family. I worry every day that I've erased something important, something that could help heal my wife. I likely have. I worry I've missed that all-important clue to her survival because I couldn't keep it together for her. I likely have. I solve technical problems for a living, and I'm generally pretty good at it. But they're never really *my* problems. I have a much more muted emotional reaction to those phone calls when they're coming from work. But this, I'm simply too close to. It's mine, and it's irreplaceable.

I remember vividly everything that happened that first day. Everything from getting the frantic call from my wife until after we arrived at the emergency room. After that, our life is mostly fog. That first phone call came in while I was at work, fairly late in the morning for me. I was already dug in to the problem of the day, and a phone call from my wife wasn't out of the ordinary. My phone rang. I answered, but no one was there. Less than a minute later, it rang again, and this time I heard her on the other end sobbing, "Tim, you have to come home." I knew that tone. I'd heard it before when her father was passing away. Someone was dying, or had already died. My heart sank, thinking one of our boys was gone. She assured me the boys were okay, but something was wrong with her. She couldn't move her legs to get out of the bathtub.

I left work and started for home, a half-hour drive away in the country. I was more calm now, the box labeled "everyone is alive" was still checked. I spoke with her on the way to make sure I didn't need to call an ambulance. When I got there, she said whatever it was had passed mostly, but something still wasn't right. We decided to get her checked out, so we loaded up the boys and headed back to town. We didn't make it five miles and it came back. I got on the phone with 911 and they dispatched the ambulance. She kept telling me, "Go faster, you have to get there, I need to get there now." I remember weighing the options in my mind. I could go faster, but an accident would only make things worse for us and whoever else might be involved. I could stop and try to help her while we waited for the ambulance, but I wouldn't know what to do anyway. It was best to just keep going, fast enough to get there safely, and if it's not fast enough then it is what it is. I chose what I thought was the safest way forward for my

319

family in this crisis. It seems like I haven't stopped doing that ever since.

It might sound silly looking back on it, like I'm being overdramatic, but I don't think I am. I think those situations instigate poor decisions, which often make the situation worse. After that day, the list of things I was concerned about in life became much shorter. Generally, as a husband/father, the big check box is "everyone is alive." After that is just a long list of check boxes to move your family forward. Mine pretty much stopped at the first one for a long time.

As the months went on, it became increasingly clear she wouldn't be able to stay on her own in the country with our two tiny boys. Neighbors were close and were great people, but it just wasn't enough. With medical bills rolling in, we really needed the money too. For my sanity, and her health, we needed to let go of the country home that we were dreaming of only four years earlier. I spent all of that summer working overtime to pay bills, then working on the house at night to get it ready to sell. This all on top of her doctor appointments, etc. We sold the acreage and bought a house in town. Closer to work for me and close to people for her. We moved her mom into town as well. It seemed like we went through more that year than most people do in a decade. We did it, but it wasn't healthy. It took its toll on both of us.

At this point, we were seemingly out of options. Every specialist we had gone to had no good answers, and only some offered sympathy. We had reset our lives financially, for now, and I had plans for the future if we had to sell again. The house I had chosen was less than ten years old and was completely finished inside, but it lacked a finished garage and a fence. I figured we could probably make it another three years if my overtime held out, and by then I'd have the garage finished and a fence put up. The new house would be ready to sell again, and we should make a profit to get by for some time more. The first year in our new house, I worked almost 600 hours of overtime. We needed the money, for sure, but at times I think I used that as an excuse to avoid what was going on at home. The problems I had at work were solvable, if not by me, then by my other resources, my team. At home we had almost no team left. We were all but completely on our own now, just waiting for it to go one way or the other. Everyone was exhausted.

I remember the ride home from yet another appointment with yet another specialist. I remember coming up empty again, no better answers. She started crying and told me, "You're so smart, I've watched you fix everything that's ever broken and build things most people can't. You have to fix me now. You have to figure this out. Nobody else is going to do it. You have to do it. If you don't, I'm going to die." I was so angry by then. Not at her, but at the world and at myself. "I can't fix you, I just can't. You can't put that on me, I can't handle it. I'm doing my best to provide to you every resource we can find to get you better. That's my role here, and I'm killing myself to fill it. That has to be enough because it's all I can do." I think we both realized that day that we were on our own. She started researching and started reaching out to more and more doctors. She did it all herself. I just paid the bills when they came in. I was almost useless.

At this point, she had been sick for so long. It was obvious that most people had given up *hope* and thought it was silly for us to have any *hope* left ourselves. Close friends and family showed it the least, but it was there. I've had conversations I never thought I'd have with people. Conversations about whether I thought some of the doctors were right, and my wife was just crazy now. I never believed the root of her issues came from any sort of mental health disorder, but some symptoms definitely did. How could they not? Heck, I was having trouble with my mental health. I couldn't imagine what she was going through. Five years on, and just now I'm beginning to be able to answer my phone when she calls without panic setting in.

One thing I never expected to encounter was how many people were surprised that I hadn't left her. I guess I never realized that was an option. It had never entered my mind. I took a vow before God and over 200 of our closest family and friends to love, cherish, support, and protect her in sickness and in health, until death. Last I checked, the "everyone is alive" box was still checked. We had many conversations about how this all could be affecting our children, and were careful about what they saw and heard. At some point, there is no avoiding it for them, though, so we had to work

321

through that. She has always still been in there somehow, through all the pain and suffering. My wife is still there, and my children's mother is still there.

My overtime had fallen off completely at this point, so money was becoming a real struggle. Whitney could see the strain it was putting on me. She had wanted a health benefit a while ago, but I wouldn't allow it. I was too ashamed. But, as the debt piled up, I had to give in and allow our friends to put one together. We wouldn't be where we are today without that help, but it still bothers me quite often. I pray for the day we are able to pay it all back to our community.

With the money from the benefit we were able to afford testing we had been putting off for a while, one of them came back positive for Lyme. The Lyme diagnosis seemed at first to be yet another "we've got it" moment that would soon pass after chasing it for a while. But unlike other diagnoses, this one had tangible positive test results to back it up, and Whitney seemed to be very confident about it. As time went on, and more tests came in from other doctors that supported this diagnosis, I became sure we were fighting the right thing, but I was also terrified. I knew how hard this road was going to be and what the odds were. And here we are, still in it.

I cannot express enough how grateful I am for all of our friends and family that have supported and helped us during this time. Something like this tends to be a very effective, but heartbreaking, filter on the people in your life. It saddens me to think about those that fell away from us, and it amazes me when I see those that have showed up and embraced us in our struggle. I don't blame those that fell away. It was likely more than they could handle and I understand that completely. But, to those that stepped up and stepped in, you are truly God's people, and we can never thank you enough.

Another big shift for me, throughout all this, was my relationship with God and my feelings about faith in general. It's easy to become bitter when things like this happen, but then you're only more alone. I spent months thinking about why this happened to us, and I still don't know. But I do know it has changed us in some ways for the better. I know I am a much more compassionate person now than I used to be. I'm more honest with people and I'm more thankful when good things happen to us, instead of feeling like they were a well-deserved reward because of our earthly accomplishments. It seems like now, the more I look, the more I see him working in our lives. I don't know how this will all turn out for us, and I'd be lying if I said I wasn't still a little scared, but I trust more in his plan for us than I ever have before. He has a plan. Right now is hard, but I believe we'll be stronger for it.

This isn't my book, so I'll end it here. Sweetheart, I couldn't be more amazed at how strong you've been through this fight. This was—and continues to be—a literal fight for your life and livelihood. You've always been the stronger one of the two of us, we both know that. It isn't fair what you've been put through, you don't deserve it. I'm sorry I wasn't able to protect you from it.

I love you. I will always love you. No matter what. Forever and always.

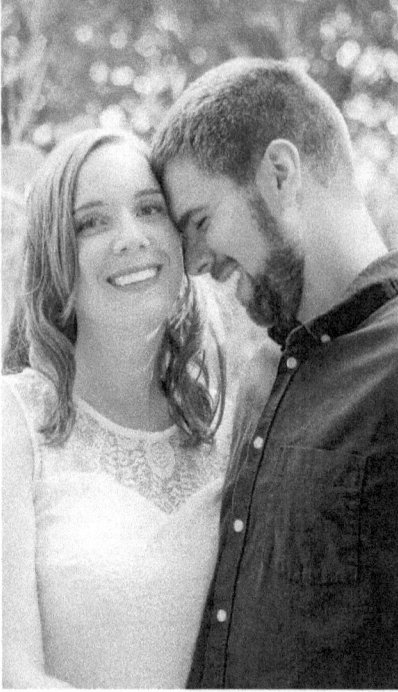

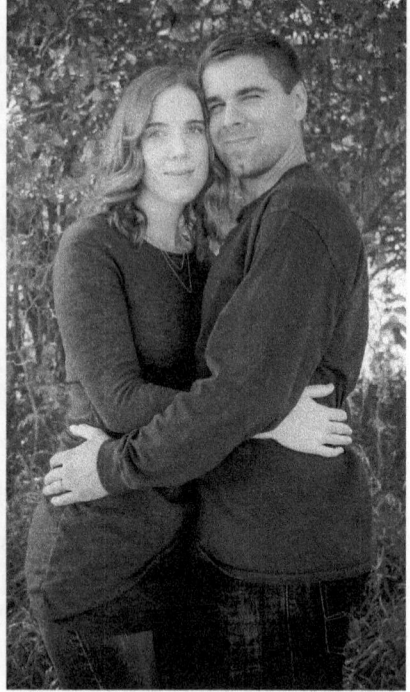

"Timothy, I love you. I will always love you. No matter what. Forever and Always."

* * *

Sandra:

When I first learned that my daughter became ill, it set off great worry within her and me. She experienced so many symptoms that would send her to the E.R. After many appointments with different specialists, the doctors would send her home with very few answers. She continued to struggle with unbearable symptoms and more E.R. visits, appointments with specialists, and she even went as far as taking a long drive to the Mayo Clinic for answers.

After a year of the ongoing suffering, she met with a functional medicine doctor out of state. She had many appointments and diagnoses through her that were hard to understand. There were a lot of suggestions for blood work and other tests since her diagnosis of POTS through Mayo. Many of these test results showed abnormal levels, and she continued with the recommendations through the functional medicine doctor that included supplements, diets, bio-identical hormone replacement therapy, and things that a young woman in her late 20s would never think to expect in order to just feel healthy and normal again. Some of these therapies did improve her quality of life, but she kept experiencing fainting spells from the repeated iron loss, and other symptoms continued to affect her quality of life.

She underwent a partial hysterectomy because of cysts and the encouragement that this would relieve some of her symptoms. But, unfortunately, this did not result in much benefit and because of the complications it made certain things worse.

At this point, I'm sure my daughter felt desperate just to feel alive again somehow. There were many times when she told me that she felt like she was dying, and all that I could do was let her know that I was there while hugging her as the tears ran down her face. I began to feel as hopeless as she did for so long. All I could do for her was listen and show my deep concern. There were many times she felt that no one believed her because her condition was ongoing, and with every attempt to get answers or improvements it caused a lot of despair. Not only for herself, but also for her family and loved ones.

The long continuance of her recovery meant more appointments and other treatments. One included a brain injury program that took her away from her children again for a week of therapy. Instead of going on trips or getaways with her husband, their "trips" were spent by going to therapies and appointments while I watched their children at home. This was very difficult for me, as her mother, to know that she was having to go through this.

This brain injury program gave her new *hope* to find improvement, but little progress was shown, and she was encouraged to look back into Lyme disease as a possible factor. Later, she found a facility that specialized in Lyme disease out of state which confirmed her concerns that she was dealing with Lyme disease. My daughter was diagnosed with Lyme disease after over four years of suffering in every way possible. Later, she was diagnosed with tick-borne relapsing fever and alpha-gal syndrome. It was scary to think that she had been having life-threatening allergic reactions and none of us knew . . . all from a tick bite.

With a treatment plan in place, she began to receive SOT therapy, IV infusions, prescriptions, and added supplements. Since the beginning of my daughter's health decline, I never thought it would go on for years. I thought it would be a simple fix and she would go on to be back to herself . . . the way I had known her as my healthy daughter. Little did I know that she would continue to struggle through ongoing years, but I had never given up on *hope* for her.

Because of these conditions, my daughter has been immune-compromised, and any virus or infection sets off flares of POTS and tick-borne relapsing fever episodes. She is continuing to seek help, knowing that Lyme disease can take years to recover from. Her struggle is very real, and as a mother of two young children there are many challenges for her. She struggles to function at a normal level, and at times certain things make her confined to her bed because of dizziness, heart race, tremors, brain fog, air hunger, and the list goes on.

The road of recovery is ongoing, with further appointments, tests, and treatments. During these times I have been helping in any way that I can, and that's the most important thing that I can do. I have watched her children several times while she and her husband travel away from home for these therapies, and I pray every time that one of them will bring her relief.

Because of her diagnosis, it brought discovery to my own health struggles. So many of our symptoms were similar and she insisted that I be tested as well. Shortly after her diagnosis, I was tested and diagnosed with Lyme disease myself. I am very fortunate that we caught this, and I was able to start treatments right away for the anaplasmosis. Little did I know I would end up with a CDC positive and be contacted by the CDC themselves concerning my diagnosis and treatment plan. We go through many similar symptoms together so we can talk, laugh, and cry together, knowing how much support we can offer one another. We now have a plan for treatments that will hopefully bring us relief, although I am just now understanding that it can take a long time for many to recover from Lyme disease.

It has definitely been a long journey for my daughter and our family, but we have new *hope* for a promising future, healing, and a positive outcome. Our *hope* is restored again with another avenue to try.

Watching your child go through something you don't have control over and seeing the frustration, the crushed hopes, the disappointment, and the pain can be contagious. After time, a loved one begins to feel the same, and I felt it as well in the journey, but I never gave up on Whitney and she never gave up on me.

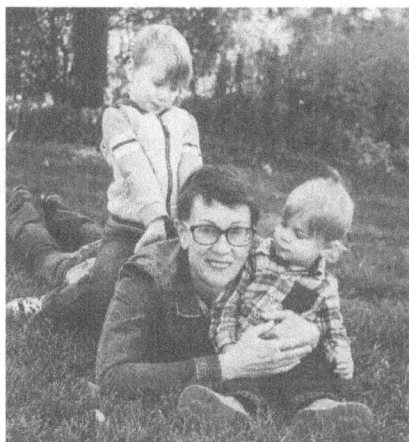

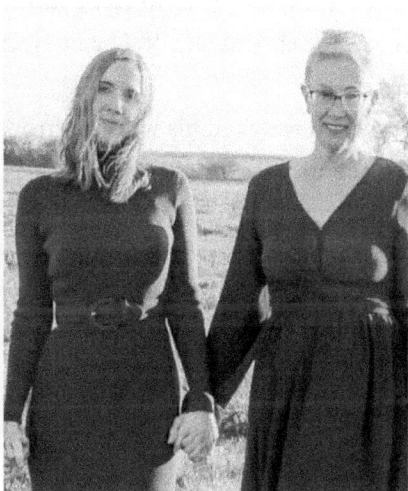

"Mom, I couldn't have done it without you."

* * *

Terri:

I was a "fixer" in my son's eyes as a young man. And to fail him is soul shattering.

I love my mom because _she solves my problems_

When my son called and told me he had to rush Whitney to the emergency room, my heart sank. Upon hearing him tell about the details of what took place, I found my heart racing and my mind revisiting the cloudy, dark, and numbing moment of helplessness one feels when you watch someone you love slipping from your grasp.

It may have been easier had I not experienced those feelings firsthand. Ignorance is bliss, they say. But ignorance will not help you survive the lifelong struggle for good health and the right answers.

In my experiences so far, I immediately start questioning if a doctor makes the statement, "It'll be okay, things like this are rare, odds are you'll be fine."

My son watched his wife go through a serious medical episode in which she had no control over her muscles, her body, and what was taking place. As he drove, he listened as she described to him what she was experiencing and what her body was doing. He thought for sure he was going to lose her right there in the car with their sons in the back seat as he tried to get her to the emergency room.

When the doctor was done with the exam, my son explained he just wasn't sure what to think when the doctor consulted with them and told them he felt it was a panic disorder. The doctor was very convincing in his diagnosis. There was a possibility he could be right, and it would be an easy answer, but something still didn't feel right. It is my understanding that the doctor told them that at this point they wanted Whitney to go on medication to help her with her alleged panic disorder.

Being very in touch with her body and how it reacts to situations and her surroundings, Whitney immediately expressed her disbelief of her diagnosis. Life experiences have created in her a strong sense of grounding and survival abilities, both emotionally and spiritually.

Whitney reached out to me about her diagnosis and how against the medication she was. Whitney had done some brief research and found many things about the medication that were not good. But, feeling she had no other option, she tried the medication.

I remember the phone call. "This stuff makes me go to weird places in my mind. It is no good for me. I can't stay on this, it's really bad for me. Please, I need someone to believe me. It isn't just in my head. There is something really wrong with me. After everything I've been through in life I've never had a panic attack or anxiety. I've always handled things, and now they want to write it all off as a panic attack. Please, I need you to believe me!"

I wanted so badly to be there with them to help them maneuver through this nightmare. To help them physically so they could rest, to support them emotionally and encourage them so they could think more clearly. I wanted to meet the doctors, question them, see their body language to judge for myself what quality of people were making these decisions. Not that I was superior in any way, but more to satisfy my doubts about what was taking place. But I couldn't. I was separated from them by distance and obligations of my own that prevented me from being there day to day. Telephone support seemed like a cop-out, an extremely weak means of support. I felt like I failed in every way.

I believed Whitney when she stated "it's not in my head, it's not anxiety or panic."

I, too, had gone through health-related things that were written off by the doctor as anxiety or panic disorder when, in fact, it was not. Anxiety does set in, however, when the people who are supposed to be helping you want to sedate you and ignore the symptoms you are explaining to them. The ones around you become convinced as they, too, tire, and in their despair the long road of true recovery feels unreachable.

I made up my mind that I had to be there. I had to find a way to make it work. I started making the three-hour trip to their house regularly to provide whatever support I could. All the avenues I had taken earlier in my life for health care, all the ideas, research and testing provided little help. I was out of resources and ideas. I was no longer the fixer.

While Timothy went to work every day praying he had a wife when he returned, Whitney spent hours, days, and weeks researching and pushing through her exhaustion, trying to find avenues of help. Many times going against the beliefs of the doctors around her, advocating for herself and many times being denied, let go as a patient, and refused by insurance. Whitney's mother spent countless hours and days being there, doing whatever she could to help. I was there as much as I could, but the distance limited my time.

Timothy had taken on as much overtime as was allowed to help keep ahead of the bills rolling in. Adding to his exhaustion of daily life duties, it proved to be too much for them to remain on their rural acreage that they all loved so very much. Leaving a home you love, in which you have shared and created beautiful memories, is emotionally exhausting and causes great grief—conditions the family was already plagued with due to Whitney's unexplained illness.

In the evening hours, Timothy pushed through his fatigue and got plans put in place for the acreage to be sold and a home in town secured for the safety of the family as a whole. Searching for a home proved to have its challenges. Fortunately, within months a home was found and the family moved to town. I was able to stay for a month to assist with what I could. The move was a family effort, involving siblings and great friends who helped in many ways.

This, however, did not end the couple's struggle to find answers. Several times during my stay, Whitney would have scary health episodes. I went with her to an emergency room visit and spoke with the doctor, explaining that these episodes are very real, with a racing heart and passing out. People cannot fake these things. The doctor seemed to be convincingly concerned, but to no avail. Once again, nothing was done. During one of the heart race episodes, we ran to the bathroom to find Whitney on the floor.

I asked Timothy if we should call the ambulance, to which he replied, "No, they won't do anything but send us home again anyway."

There had been so many trips to the doctor, only to be sent home with a pounding heart, feeling faint, weak, terrified, and hopeless.

I remember hearing, "They're supposed to be the ones who help, and they turn us away to deal with it on our own. If we can't go to the medical field for help, who do we go to?"

Every time a new test result came, we hoped it would be the one to cure. I still try to convince myself a new test result will be the cure. *Hope* has to remain.

It is an overwhelming feeling of abandonment, as a mother, to leave your children when they are being beaten down by life in every way possible. Watching while your children slowly slip away before your eyes and become a shell of what they used to be.

I am a woman of deep, rich, and strong faith, taught to me by my parents and many I have encountered throughout my life so far. Nothing has tested my faith more than parenthood and watching my children suffer. Their faith is strong, but the journey is ugly.

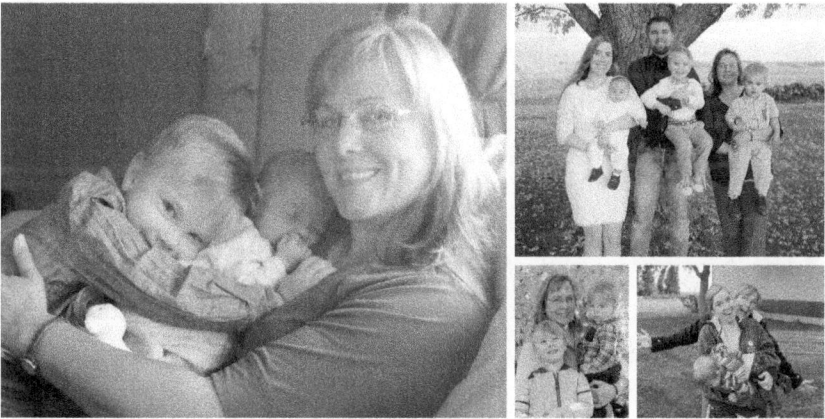

"Terri, you did enough."

331

34

So You Think It May Be Lyme?

Before finally being diagnosed with Lyme disease, I saw four gynecologists, three gastroenterologists, two neurologists, three endocrinologists, two infectious disease doctors, one internal medicine doctor, two hematologists, two allergists, one ENT (ear, nose, and throat) doctor, three surgeons, two functional medicine doctors, and five naturopaths. I went to one of the *top facilities* in the world at the *Mayo Clinic in Rochester, Minnesota*, where my diagnosis was *still* missed.

I was evaluated for many other diseases: multiple sclerosis, rheumatoid arthritis, lupus, hypothyroidism, cancer, Addison's disease, Sjögren's, heart disease, kidney disease, liver disease, pituitary disease, Chiari malformation, root canal infection, adrenal disease, mental health disorders, endometriosis, CFS leak, seizures, brain aneurysm, stroke, blood clots, fibromyalgia, autonomic nervous system failure, POTS, dysautonomia, reactive airway disease, porphyria disease, abdominal bleed, perimenopause, and many others.

Prior to diagnosis, I had undergone multiple CT scans, ultrasounds, multiple MRI scans, surgeries, spinal taps, sleep studies, echocardiograms, EKGs, at-home heart monitors, an upper endoscopy, a colonoscopy, a hida scan, a gastric emptying study, many blood tests, and other invasive testing. I was *not* diagnosed with Lyme disease until the spring of 2023, four and a half years after suffering from a tick bite. I was *not* diagnosed with alpha-gal syndrome—which is suspected to have occurred after the tick bite in 2018—until March of 2024. I suffered extreme symptoms of anaphylaxis from the mast cell activation syndrome and alpha-gal syndrome. I was told repeatedly it was anxiety. *I had no help.*

* * *

If you think you may have Lyme, co-infections, or other underlying factors common in Lyme disease—like mold, candida, heavy metals, or other gut infections—here are some things to start with:

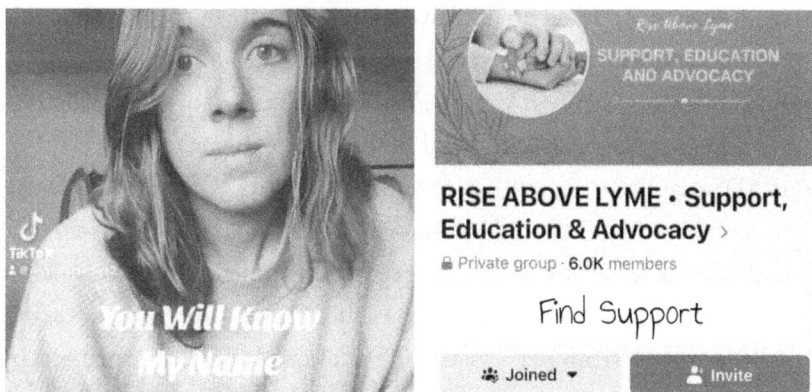

RISE ABOVE LYME · Support, Education & Advocacy ›
🔒 Private group · 6.0K members

Find Support

👥 Joined ▾   👤 Invite

You can find support and guidance on certain Facebook groups. I also have found emotional support on TikTok. Some may laugh about that, but people share their real stories using that platform, and it has helped me greatly in finding the correct questions to ask my Lyme doctor.

Could I Have Lyme?

- First and foremost, find a Lyme-literate doctor, trained by ILADS. I wish I had done that right away. If you can find one who also practices in functional medicine, that could also benefit you. That way none of the other factors get missed and keep you sick. Not all doctors are created *equal,* including Lyme-literate doctors, so check with your local support groups to help you find a good one in your area.

- Find a local support group online that can help connect you with the right doctors in your area. I joined *RISE ABOVE LYME: Support, Education, and Advocacy* through Facebook. The moderator of the group helped me find local providers and I chose the clinic that best fit with how I wanted to treat Lyme disease.

- Please visit the site of the International Lyme and Associated Diseases Society (ILADS). Fewer than fifty percent of people suffering with Lyme disease remember a tick bite. Standard Lyme disease testing, like the Western blot or ELISA test, misses a high percentage of positive cases, especially if you do not have a Lyme-literate doctor reading your results. Visit ILADS.org to read more about the above statistics.

- Proper testing through Vibrant Wellness, IGeneX, or MDL (Medical Diagnostic Laboratories) is vital in the diagnostic process.

- ILADS.org has a search bar that can help with finding local Lyme-literate doctors. You need to find a doctor who is *compatible* with you and who accepts your wishes and respects your boundaries. Some clinics offer antibiotics only, while other clinics offer a large variety of treatments, from herbals, to SOT therapy, HBOT, Ozone therapy, PEMF, and even biomagnetic therapy . . . healing from Lyme is a *long* journey,and you will be with your doctor for quite a long time. Choose wisely.

- Please accept any emotional or financial help offered to you. There is no shame in this. The cost of Lyme is high, especially the cost on your body if you cannot afford a proper doctor or treatment. It is okay to need help.

- Learn how to properly remove a tick and what to do with it. When you receive correct treatment soon enough after the infection, you *can* avoid long-term health complications. If treated early enough, you can avoid chronic health problems. Find more info at ILADS.org.

* * *

LYME AND CO-INFECTION SYMPTOM CHECKLISTS

SYMPTOMS	HAD IN PAST	NEVER HAD	HAVE NOW
Hearing loss			
Speech errors			
Unable to use the computer for very long			
Neck pain			
SWEATS WITH FEVERS			
Joint swelling			
NECK CRUNCHES OR CREAKS			
Chest or rib soreness			
Muscle pain and aching			
Joint stiffness			
Pain and achiness all over			
FEELING FATIGUED EVEN AFTER ENOUGH REST			
Blurry or double vision			
SHOOTING PAINS OR ELECTRICAL SENSATIONS THAT SHOOT AROUND			
Crawling sensations of skin			
Malaise (feeling "icky")			
Trouble remembering words or names			
Symptoms worse in 4 week cycles			
HEADACHES IN BACK OF HEAD			
Poor short-term memory			
Get lost, trouble with special orientation			
Symptoms get worse around your period			
IRREGULAR OR FAST HEARTBEAT AND PALPITATIONS			
HAND WEAKNESS			
PAIN IN JOINTS THAT MOVE AROUND			

Lyme Disease (bold items above are the most predictive of a Lyme infection)

SYMPTOMS	HAD IN PAST	NEVER HAD	HAVE NOW
New skin sores/ acne/rashes			
Wake up often			
RED LINES "STRETCH MARK APPEARANCE" ON SKIN			
Tender lymph nodes			
Abdominal pain and fullness			
Depression			
Blurry vision			
Pain in bladder/genitals			
Other urinary symptoms			
NUMBNESS AND TINGLING			
Ears sensitive to noise			
CONJUNCTIVITIS/EYE INFLAMMATION			
Anxiety and panic attacks			
TREMORS			
UNEXPLAINED RAGE			
Tender lumps under the skin			
SOLES OF FEET HURT ESPECIALLY IN THE MORNING			
Head congestion and sinus drainage			
TROUBLE FALLING ASLEEP			
MUSCLE TWITCHING IN FACE, LEGS, ARMS			
Ear pain and fluid in ear			
BOGGY SWOLLEN TISSUE/EDEMA			
SWOLLEN LYMPH NODES			
Eyes sensitive to light			

Bartonella (bold items above are most predictive of a Bartonella infection)

SYMPTOMS	HAD IN PAST	NEVER HAD	HAVE NOW
Easy bruising			
SEVERE FATIGUE			
Fevers			
Anemia			
AIR HUNGER (FEELING AS IF NOT GETTING ENOUGH AIR)			
Symptoms came on all of a sudden			
SYMPTOMS WORSE IN 3 - 6 DAY CYCLES			
Weight loss			
Shortness of breath while active or at rest			
Feeling lightheaded or faint/pass out			
DIZZY UNSTEADY ON YOUR FEET, TIPPY			
Tinnitus (ringing in ears)			
Panic attacks			
Cough			
Day sweats			
NIGHT SWEATS			
Frequent yawning or sighing			
VIVID OR VIOLENT NIGHTMARES			
Very dark (maple colored) urine			
Skin extra sensitive, burning pain			
SEVERE HEADACHES ALL OVER			
Eyes sensitive to light			
NAUSEA			

Babesia (bold items above are most predictive of a Babesia infection)

* * *

LYME DISEASE (BORRELIA BURGDORFERI)

- Multiple red rashes
- Fever
- Chills
- Malaise
- Fatigue
- Headache
- Myalgia
- Arthralgia
- Lymphadenopathy
- Joint swelling and/or pain

Untreated or unnoticed early Lyme disease will progress to disseminated disease for about 60% of patients, with diverse clinical manifestations:

- Neurological manifestations
- Cranial neuritis, most commonly Bell's palsy (facial paralysis, can be bilateral)
- Gastrointestinal symptoms
- Lymphocytic meningitis
- Painful peripheral motor and sensory neuropathy (mononeuritis multiplex)
- Intracranial hypertension
- Cardiac manifestations
- Lyme carditis
- Cognitive dysfunction
- Rheumatologic manifestations
- Lightheadedness, fainting
- Oligoarticular arthritis: transient, migratory arthritis and effusion in one or multiple joints, often large joints; may cause Baker's cyst
- Migratory pain in tendons, bursae, muscles, and bones
- Neuropathic symptoms: nerve pain, numbness, hot/cold sensations, tingling
- Sensitivity to light
- Meningitis
- Memory impairment
- Inflammation of the brain and spinal cord
- Psychiatric symptoms: including depression, anxiety, and mood changes
- Severe headaches and neck stiffness
- Numbness and tingling in hands and feet
- Palpitations or chest pain, shortness of breath
- Unprovoked pain which may interfere with sleep
- Encephalitis
- Seizures

- Death

TICK-BORNE RELAPSING FEVER

- High fever (e.g., 103° F) with relapses
- Headache
- Muscle and joint aches
- Symptoms can reoccur, producing a telltale pattern of fever lasting roughly three days, followed by seven days without fever, followed by another three days of fever
- Myalgia/arthralgia
- Meningoencephalitis
- Cranial neuritis
- Ocular manifestations
- Acute respiratory distress syndrome (ARDS)
- Dry cough
- Sweats
- Dizziness
- Nausea/vomiting
- Facial palsy

ALPHA-GAL SYNDROME (AGS)

- AGS reactions can be different from person to person. They can range from mild to severe or even life-threatening. Anaphylaxis (a potentially life-threatening reaction involving multiple organ systems) may need urgent medical care.
- People may not have an allergic reaction after every alpha-gal exposure.
- Hives or itchy rash
- Nausea or vomiting
- Heartburn or indigestion
- Diarrhea
- Cough, shortness of breath, or difficulty breathing

- Drop in blood pressure
- Swelling of the lips, throat, tongue, or eyelids
- Dizziness or faintness
- Severe stomach pain

EHRLICHIOSIS

- Fever
- Chills
- Headache
- Malaise
- Muscle pain
- Gastrointestinal symptoms (nausea, vomiting, diarrhea, anorexia)
- Altered mental status
- Rash (more commonly reported among children)
- Toxic or septic shock-like syndrome
- Hepatic (liver) failure
- Coagulopathies
- Renal (kidney) failure
- ARDS (acute respiratory distress syndrome)
- Delay in treatment may result in severe illness and death

BABESIOSIS

- Fever
- Chills
- Sweats
- Malaise
- Fatigue
- Myalgia
- Arthralgia
- Headache
- Air hunger

- Gastrointestinal symptoms, such as anorexia and nausea (less common: abdominal pain, vomiting)
- Dark urine
- Dry cough
- Sore throat
- Photophobia (light sensitivity)
- Mild splenomegaly (enlarged spleen)
- Mild hepatomegaly (enlarged liver)
- Jaundice

Severe Cases of Babesiosis:

- Thrombocytopenia
- Disseminated intravascular coagulation
- Hemodynamic instability
- Acute respiratory distress
- Renal failure
- Hepatic compromise
- Altered mental status
- Death

BARTONELLA

- Neurological symptoms
- Myalgia
- Joint pain
- Muscle twitching
- Bone pain
- Progressive arthropathy
- Fever
- Brain fog
- Skin resembling stretch marks
- Pains in the soles of feet

- Irritability/rage
- Numbness/pins and needles
- Swollen lymph node
- Infection of eye
- Infection of liver
- Infection of spleen
- Infection of bone
- Infection of heart valve
- Skin rash or lesions
- Endocarditis

ANAPLASMOSIS

- Fevers & chills
- Myalgias
- Severe headaches
- Nausea, vomiting, diarrhea, loss of appetite
- Respiratory failure
- Bleeding problems
- Organ failure
- Death

*This is not a complete list of all of the symptoms. Nor are these all of the co-infections/complications that you can get from a tick. There are several more: Rocky Mountain spotted fever, Powassan virus, tularemia, mycoplasmas, and others. The ones listed above are the specific infections my mother and I are suffering with. You can learn more about the different symptoms and co-infections through ILADS.org or CDC.gov. (**I used those websites to compile this information for you.**)*

* * *

My Lyme center recommends ILADS.org for finding a doctor and researching treatment for each disease.

35

What Is It Like to Be Chronically Ill, and What Can You Do to Help?

What is it like to be chronically ill?
It kind of feels like you are drowning.
It feels like waves rushing in, crashing into you.
Like a current you will never escape.

Do you have a loved one with chronic illness and
want to know what you can do to help?

I want you to think about the time that you were the sickest you have ever been. Now, think about feeling that way every single day, with no relief from the pain. Next, imagine watching everyone else around you live normally while you are stuck on the sidelines. Then, add on medical professionals neglecting you, and everyone around you abandoning you or not believing you. Sounds lonely, doesn't it? That is chronic illness. Empathy goes a long way. Be patient, kind, and offer a listening ear or a warm embrace.

- If your loved one who is struggling with chronic illness is being short-tempered with you, don't take it personally. Pain significantly reduces tolerance and patience. Perhaps ask them if they need a heat pack or something that can help take the edge off.

- Most likely, people with chronic illness are not showing themselves compassion. Sometimes acts of love and reminders that they are doing enough can be helpful.

- It can be really hard to empathize if you haven't gone through the issues yourself. Taking time to educate yourself on the conditions they have can be helpful. We don't expect you to understand all of the conditions, but it is nice when we don't have to explain ourselves multiple times. Explaining the situation repeatedly can spike a stress response from talking about the trauma.

- Invite your chronically ill friends to places, even if they have said no before, and be understanding if they have to cancel. They cannot predict their symptoms, and just because you see them doing certain things one day, that does not mean the next day will be the same.

- Try to be understanding if certain tasks get forgotten or go undone. Having a chronic illness can cause severe forgetfulness, especially when the mind is under stress or overwhelmed with the burden. Small upsets can really be hard on a person who is experiencing extreme symptoms daily. Let it go.

- Help them grieve over the loss of their previous self, and let them know it's okay to feel sad. Embrace them. Many times, nothing at all needs to be said and they just need to feel safe.

- Encourage them in their grounding and healing exercises, and maybe even involve yourself in some of them if they don't want to do it alone. It is very isolating to try and heal and have a positive mind frame during extreme suffering.

- Cry together sometimes.

- If your partner wants to research a possible underlying cause, perhaps do it together. It's so hard to carry that burden internally and worry about your partner being upset that there may be a different avenue to investigate.

- Take time to look at old photo albums or memories together. Talk about the happy times and the things that you want to do together on good days or when the disease is in remission.

- Watch happy movies together.
- Embrace.
- Gentle touch can sometimes be helpful in pulling your partner out of a bad cycle of thoughts on a hard day. A foot massage, back massage, or gently pulling your fingers through your partner's hair can be helpful.
- Pray together.
- If you see your loved one really struggling, it's okay to stop them and say, *"I know you are struggling right now, and I am here. You are not alone."* Hug them if they can tolerate touch in that moment.
- Give them space if they can't tolerate any more touch because of the overstimulation or pain they already feel.
- Help them as much as you can with meal prep, and find out what they can eat. Food can feel extremely overwhelming and impossible. If your loved one gets a food list they have to follow, take it and research meals yourself that you can make to freeze for them for later. Meal prepping is huge when someone is going through treatment for certain chronic illnesses.
- Saying things like, *"You are doing the best you can and that's enough. No matter how bad you are feeling, you are not alone,"* can be helpful. Tell them, *"I am proud of you for making it through every dark day so far,"* or *"Whatever you are feeling right now is very real and valid. You are not a burden, your illness is."* We need to hear words of affirmation.
- If you notice your partner in a depression, please draw close to them, even if no words are spoken. Sometimes human touch is enough to bring them back.
- Don't scream and be overstimulating around them. They are already feeling overstimulated.
- If you are the spouse of a person with chronic illness, accept help offered from others. Chronic illness already makes your loved one feel like they are a burden, especially financially.
- If you see laundry in piles or toilets that have been dirty for too long, it's probably a good idea to take care of the tasks.

- Remind your partner that they are not a burden, the chronic illness is a burden on them.
- If you have children, please take them to the zoo or do other activities that are now difficult or impossible for your loved one to do. The one going through the illness already feels very guilty that your children are missing out on what they used to do together. If your partner is feeling guilty about missing out on that day because of the chronic illness, say it is okay and reassure them that you can go together on an easier day.
- Sometimes your partner will not want to be alone because of the symptoms they are experiencing. If you can't be there, try to find someone else that can.
- If your partner is struggling with the symptoms and has an emotional breakdown—*"I can't do this anymore!"*—the best thing you can do is just embrace them and let the tears come out. Cry together if you want to. Your partner is not expecting you to be able to solve all of the problems at that moment, but is just feeling defeated. A lot is held in emotionally with chronic illness. Sometimes a good cry and embrace can make them feel safe in that vulnerability.
- Finally, help them by *helping yourself.* The health condition is a burden for the person suffering, but also for the one witnessing it. The person experiencing the symptoms know this. They often feel like they are a burden. If you do not find an outlet for this trauma, the anger will expand, making everything feel unbearable. The one suffering physically does not mean to cause stress, but they will confide in you a lot about how they are feeling. They do not do this to constantly be negative or complain, but they are often experiencing symptoms that they are unsure are safe. If they have someone to confide in, they may feel more at ease if something *does* happen. Most things are held in, but it can become unbearable to hold it all in, and if you are their safe person they feel a need to tell you. This can cause great stress on the person witnessing the suffering. Find time for yourself, or confide in others concerning what you are going through. Go to therapy, do a

Bible study, or do something in nature to destress. Easing the burden by asking for help can allow you to get a break. If you don't do this for yourself, life can start to feel very hopeless, you'll feel trapped, and you may begin to experience deep distress yourself.

Chronic illness is not just a few days off of work. It is broken friendships, forgotten passions, lost friends, lost hobbies, all while feeling as if you have no value or purpose in life anymore. Please consider this before casting judgment on those suffering with chronic illness. People are walking around every day hanging on by a single thread. Choose kindness and empathy.

What does it feel like to have POTS/dysautonomia and Lyme disease?

- *They have compared the quality of life that a POTS patients has to those suffering with congestive heart failure, COPD, and to patients on dialysis for kidney failure.*
- Imagine waking up every day and feeling hung over. You have a headache, are nauseous, and your head is pounding, but you still have to work or take care of screaming children. Every day.
- Imagine if you went and donated blood and they took too much and now you feel really dizzy and lightheaded, but you just have to go on with your normal tasks.
- Imagine if you got out of bed but you are sprinting as soon as you stand up. Your heart is racing. But you are not really sprinting, you are just standing there.
- Imagine standing up to give a huge presentation all of the time. Do you feel breathless or have air hunger from the anxiety? That's all day with POTS.
- Imagine feeling like you are having a panic attack every time you go up a step on a staircase.
- Imagine that every day when you eat you feel like you are going to have a heart attack because of heart palpitations.
- Imagine being hooked up to an electrical current and your whole body

is vibrating. Stand on your cell phone while it's vibrating. That's what the buzzing feels like.

- Imagine the feeling you get right before developing a cold, that's how you feel every day now.
- Imagine you are fighting an infection and have a terrible fever every day.
- Spin around in circles for thirty seconds and lie on your back. This what a vestibular POTS episode feels like.
- Imagine being stabbed over and over again in your abdomen and back, and blood is pooling into your lungs, making it hard to breathe. This is what the GI issues feel like.
- Have you ever lost a lot of blood and needed an emergency blood transfusion? This is what an acute flare feels like.
- Imagine having food poisoning every day, but you actually don't and that's just your life.
- Imagine you just missed a step. How do you feel? That happens a lot with POTS. But there was no missed step.
- Imagine being put on a merry-go-round after running a marathon.
- Imagine someone shining a flashlight in your eyes all day, but then you remember you are just looking outside or you've walked into a room lit with florescent lights.
- Imagine you drank too much coffee and your body is shaking . . . oh wait, you didn't . . . you have POTS.
- Lie on your back and have someone push on your chest. Now try to breathe. That is what an air hunger flare feels like.
- Imagine the feeling you get right before vomiting: you are cold and clammy, your heart is racing, and you feel weak and nauseated. This is how it feels when you get up in the morning, after a shower, after getting overheated, or when you try to exercise. Every time.
- *Now* imagine POTS was from a chronic infection that could have been treated, but you were left to live that way. Now . . . wouldn't you be angry?

36

What Can You Do in a Flare?

What you can do in a flare to improve your mental health:

I t can be incredibly hard on your mental health when you experience a regression in your physical health from an acute illness or other factors. Some feel these regressions after starting certain treatments that cause herxheimer reactions. You may start to go deeper and deeper into darkness and wonder if this is going to be your "new normal." You may feel hopeless and like a failure. These feelings of despair and worry can make you feel worse physically and emotionally. These are the things that I have found most helpful when experiencing another flare.

***

TECHNIQUES TO TRY

- Listen to meditations. There are many free meditations on YouTube. I used the *Insight Timer* app quite often. There are a lot of faith-based meditations, too, if that helps you most.
- PowerThoughts Meditation Club on YouTube is very helpful.
- Pray. Cry. Or scream out to God. *Maybe you feel he does not hear you.*
- Listen to uplifting music.

- Write a gratitude list.
- Cry . . . maybe you need to let it out. It's okay.
- Take a bath. Adding some lavender essential oil may help too.
- Ask your partner to gently rub your skin. It can be enough to pull your mind out of dark thoughts.
- It helps me to ask God to be with me. I say it over and over. *Please be with me.*
- Go outside and just sit in the sun. Breathe the fresh air, even if it's winter. If you are too weak to put winter clothes on, throw a blanket on and just sit for a while.
- Hug yourself.
- Hug a loved one.
- Look at happy memories of pictures and videos.
- Listen to a funny podcast.
- Watch one of your favorite movies.
- Sleep. Your body needs more rest.
- Ask for help when your body is really needing it. If you don't have good support at home, perhaps reach out to a friend or find others online that can relate and build you up.
- Do some light stretching, even if you have to do it lying down. You hold yourself a certain way while experiencing extreme suffering, and that can make you have more pain.
- Practice the 4-7-8 breathing exercises multiple times a day for as long as you can tolerate it.
- Practice tapping exercises. That can help stimulate your nervous system to calm down.
- If you have enough energy, do something you enjoy that you can do while resting. Draw, write, play a video game.
- If it helps you, imagine in detail a happy memory or things that you would do again if your body allowed it.
- Stand in front of your mirror. Tell yourself all of the powerful things you have overcome. Tell yourself you are strong. Remind yourself who you are.

No one will ever be able to fully understand the internal battles you had to endure just to be diagnosed, just to heal, just to make it where you are at today. Be proud of the way you fought to save your life. Be proud of the way you survived while everyone else was living. Give yourself grace.

* * *

SONG LIST
Songs that helped me during dark times.

Hallelujah (Pentatonix)

Healing (Riley Clemmons)

Sound Mind (Melissa Helser)

Gratitude (Brandon Lake)

Breath of Heaven (Leanna Crawford)

Battle Belongs (Bethel Music)

Honest (Kyndal Inskeep)

Spirit Lead Me (Hillsong United)

In Jesus Name (Katy Nichole)

You'd Never Know (Blü Eyes)

Healing Hurts (Blü Eyes)

Landslide (Fleetwood Mac)

Fighting For Me (Riley Clemmons)

Heal (Tom Odell)

Lord (Shaya Zamora)

One Name (Jesus) (Naomi Raine)

The Story I'll Tell (Naomi Raine)

Faithfully (TobyMac)

Highs & Lows (Hillsong Young and Free)

Hold On To Me (Lauren Daigle)

Graves Into Gardens (Brandon Lake)

I Will Carry You (Ellie Holcomb)

Counting My Blessings (Seph Schlueter)

Don't Stop Believin' (Journey)
My Story (Big Daddy Weave)
Head Above Water (Avril Lavigne)

* * *

POSITIVE AFFIRMATIONS FOR HEALING

I can heal. I will heal. I will surround myself with loving people. Miracles happen every day. I will nourish myself. I will seek outlets for creativity. I will be my own health advocate. I will put music on and dance. I will speak healing words to myself. I will focus on what brings me joy. I will keep moving forward. I will *trust* my instincts when choosing treatments. I can do this. There's a divine force guiding this journey. I will laugh, any chance I get. I am worthy of healing.

Now tell yourself these things while looking in the mirror.

* * *

WHAT GETTING SICK HAS TAUGHT ME
(from a fellow Lyme Warrior in remission)

- Treat everyone you meet with kindness. You never know what they are going through. Pain is invisible.
- Not everyone is your friend for a lifetime, and that is okay.
- You will change so many times in your lifetime, and that should be embraced. It is beautiful.
- Everything we go through is meant to teach us something.
- You are stronger than you think you are.
- We all have the amazing ability to self-heal. Our time frames are all different.
- Never compare your journey to anyone else's.

- Healing is not linear. A setback is not failure.
- Gratitude for what we already have is a magnet for more positive changes.
- Things *do* happen for a reason. It is up to us to take the lesson and turn it into something beautiful.
- You can do hard things.
- You are resilient.
- You are strong.
- Healing is possible.

* * *

VAGUS NERVE STIMULATION
How to help a heart rate flare.

You wake up suddenly, your heart rate is through the roof, you feel delirious with severe air hunger . . . what can you do?

- Hum. Humming stimulates the vagus nerve. *I always start here.*
- Rub alongside the back of your ears, down to your neck. Use ice cubes if not working.
- Put your arms, up to your elbows, in ice water.
- Gargle water.
- Flush your face with ice water.
- Bear down as if having a bowl movement.
- Breathing exercises. Breathe in for 4, hold for 7, exhale for 8. Do this twenty times in a row.

* * *

SIMPLE DETOX METHODS

Your body detoxes naturally, but sometimes it needs help. Certain factors can affect how well your body is detoxing, such as how much toxic buildup you have, genetic factors, and if your immune system is overloaded. Just remember this . . . just because you have a genetic factor does not *mean you cannot detox. It just means you need* help.

- Dry brushing.
- Detox baths. You can find *Epsoak* Epsom salt on *Amazon*.
- Infrared sauna. If you have heat intolerance, bring ice cubes into the sauna with you and run them up and down your chest, on your vagus nerve, and along the sides of your neck. This can slow your heart rate, making the heat more tolerable. If you experience more head pressure from the heat, rub the ice along your face and temples. *I have found that the more times I have used the sauna, the less trouble I have with the heat. I no longer need ice cubes when I go in.*
- Red light.
- Liver support: Find a certified health provider who can offer you infusion therapy if suggested by your doctor. *I go to a local medical infusion clinic that offers IV therapy to help support the liver, and they can* ensure *that the quality is safe.*

* * *

LET GO

I lived with *anger* for a long time, and one day it revealed itself to me as *grief*. I still feel *grief* over what has happened to me. Parts of me died when I experienced the things that I did, and I am still trying to gain my whole self back. I believe that *someday* I can rebuild those parts that were destroyed within me. I believe that *someday* I may actually love the person I have become from this experience. But healing is not linear. I am trying. Being angry forever at doctors really doesn't get me anywhere, though, so I have chosen to *let go*.

You may wonder if I feel any anger at my functional medicine doctors. My answer is *no*. They are only human, and I truly believe they did the best they could with our circumstances. *They truly cared about me.* They were on the right path. They found many parts that caused *the perfect storm*.

The problem is not what may have been *missed*. The problem has been the disconnect between doctors. I truly believe that if all of the different specialists I had got together and shared the things they have learned, we could reform our health care system. That is *the true problem*. Our health care system. Throughout my journey, I was disappointed to find that the real medical system is *nothing* like they depict on-screen, nothing like the TV series *House*. No one is coming to save you. *You have to do it yourself.* The doctors that want to help simply don't have the time to work together on one case. Rates of chronic illness are rising at a scary pace every day, and these doctors are overloaded and overwhelmed.

Because of the reality that I wasn't going to be evaluated like they do on *House*, I spent hours researching by reading books or medical journals and by talking with others who had experienced similar conditions. A lot of times, you have to become your *own doctor* and your *own advocate* in this situation.

It is *not their fault*. I know there are doctors and nurses who truly care. My biggest wish is that all would come together. My entries show the real and raw emotions of what a person goes through with chronic illness. *Letting go* of anger is one step in the healing journey.

Know that you are not alone.

These suggestions are not medical advice. I share these suggestions because they are what work for me. I strongly caution my readers to not rely on my suggestions alone for their own unique medical problems. The reader should find care and advice from qualified medical professionals.

37

Bible Verses That Helped Me

All verses (except for two from the NKJV) taken from the New
International Version [NIV] using the website biblegateway.com. (Italics
added for emphasis by author.)

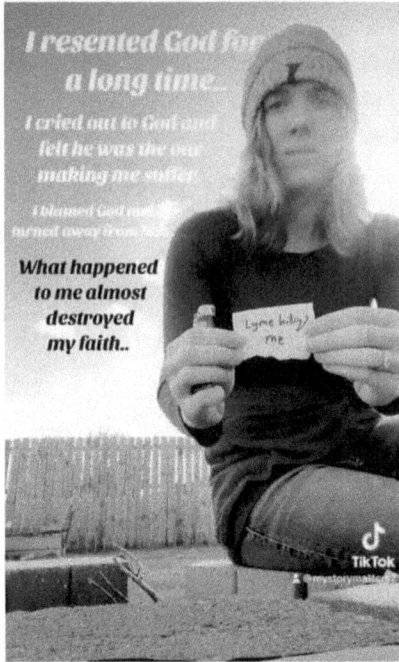

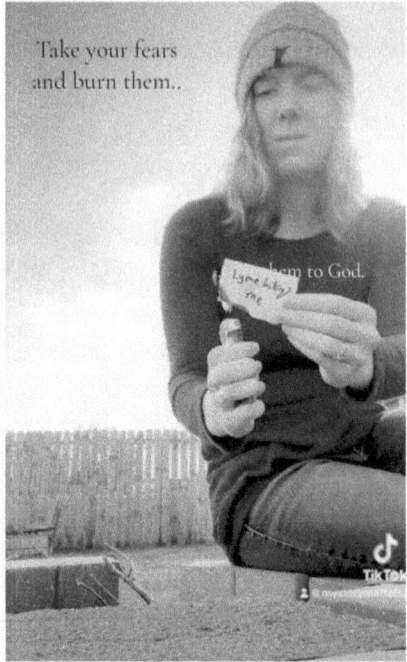

Philippians 4:13 (NKJV) - I can do all things through Christ who strengthens me.

PSALM 143
A psalm of David.
[1] Lord, hear my prayer,
listen to my cry for mercy;
in your faithfulness and righteousness
come to my relief.
[2] Do not bring your servant into judgment,
for no one living is righteous before you.
[3] The enemy pursues me,
he crushes me to the ground;
he makes me dwell in the darkness
like those long dead.
[4] So my spirit grows faint within me;

my heart within me is dismayed.

⁵ I remember the days of long ago;

I meditate on all your works

and consider what your hands have done.

⁶ I spread out my hands to you;

I thirst for you like a parched land.

⁷ Answer me quickly, Lord;

my spirit fails.

Do not hide your face from me

or I will be like those who go down to the pit.

⁸ Let the morning bring me word of your unfailing love,

for I have put my *trust* in you.

Show me the way I should go,

for to you I entrust my life.

⁹ Rescue me from my enemies, Lord,

for I hide myself in you.

¹⁰ Teach me to do your will,

for you are my God;

may your good Spirit

lead me on level ground.

¹¹ For your name's sake, Lord, preserve my life;

in your righteousness, bring me out of trouble.

¹² In your unfailing love, silence my enemies;

destroy all my foes,

for I am your servant.

ISAIAH 41:10

So do not *fear*, for I am with you;

do not be dismayed, for I am your God.

I will strengthen you and help you;

I will uphold you with my righteous right hand.

REVELATION 21:4

"'He will wipe every tear from their eyes. There will be no more death' or mourning or crying or pain, for the old order of things has passed away."

JEREMIAH 29:11–13

"For I know the plans I have for you," declares the Lord, "plans to prosper you and not to harm you, plans to give you *hope* and a future. Then you will call on me and come and pray to me, and I will listen to you. You will seek me and find me when you seek me with all your heart."

2 CORINTHIANS 1:4

[The Lord] comforts us in all our troubles, so that we can comfort those in any trouble with the comfort we ourselves receive from God.

1 John 1:5

This is the message we have heard from him and declare to you: God is light; in him there is no darkness at all.

PSALM 56:3

When I am afraid, I put my *trust* in you.

JOHN 16:22

So with you: Now is your time of grief, but I will see you again and you will rejoice, and no one will take away your joy.

MATTHEW 11:28–29

"Come to me, all you who are weary and burdened, and I will give you rest. Take my yoke upon you and learn from me, for I am gentle and humble in heart, and you will find rest for your souls."

2 TIMOTHY 1:7 (NKJV)

For God has not given us a spirit of *fear*, but of power and of love and of a sound mind.

PSALM 23

A psalm of David.

[1] The Lord is my shepherd, I lack nothing.
[2] He makes me lie down in green pastures,
he leads me beside quiet waters,
[3] he refreshes my soul.
He guides me along the right paths
for his name's sake.
[4] Even though I walk
through the darkest valley,
I will *fear* no evil,
for you are with me;
your rod and your staff,
they comfort me.
[5] You prepare a table before me
in the presence of my enemies.
You anoint my head with oil;
my cup overflows.
[6] Surely your goodness and love will follow me
all the days of my life,
and I will dwell in the house of the Lord
forever.

PHILIPPIANS 4:13 (NKJV)

I can do all things through Christ who strengthens me.

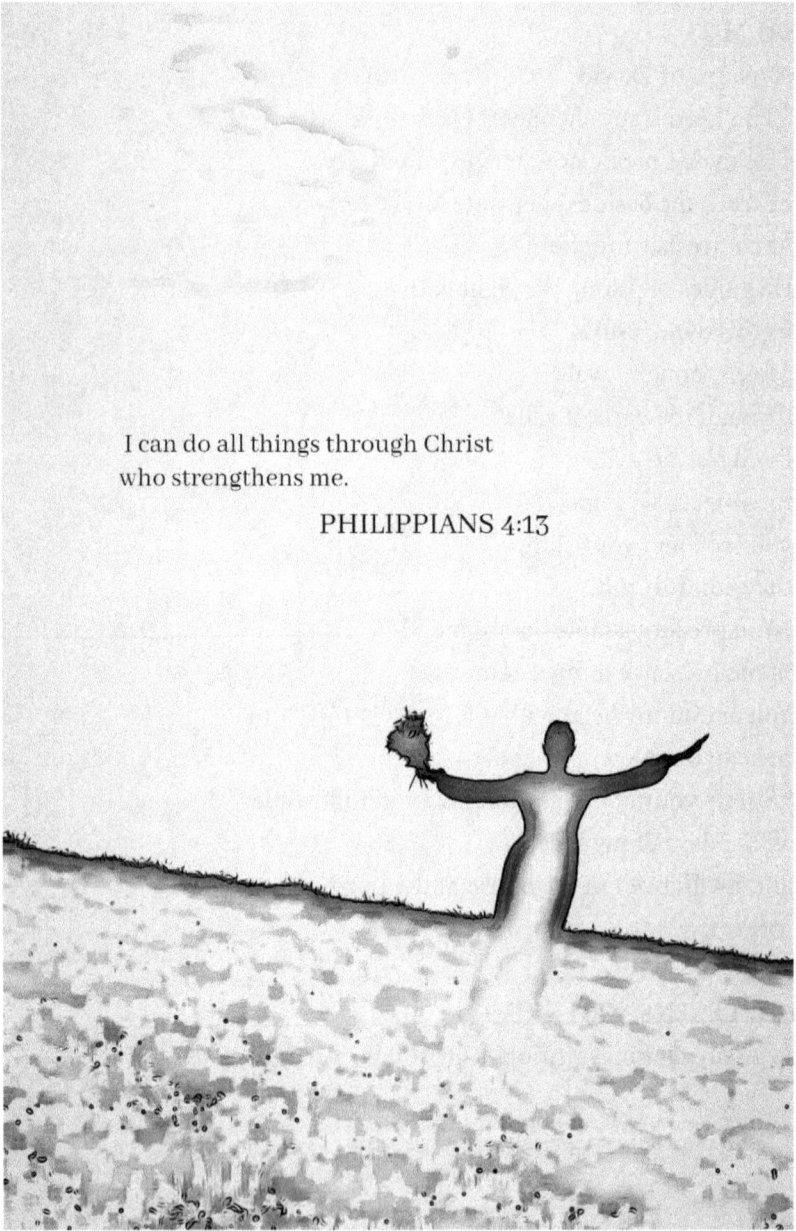

I can do all things through Christ
who strengthens me.

PHILIPPIANS 4:13

"Loving God, I pray that you will comfort me in my suffering, lend skill to the hands of my healers, and bless the means used for my care. Give me such confidence in the power of your grace, that even when I am afraid, I may put my whole trust in you; through our Savior Jesus Christ. Amen."

Conclusion

I have debated for a long time whether I should write my book now or wait until I have healed my body. I even debated for countless months on the title. *Chronic* Lyme disease? Some would roll their eyes and think *Isn't that pseudoscience?* The medical establishment would approve of the term *untreated late-stage Lyme disease* or *post-treatment Lyme disease syndrome.* In a recent CDC update, they are acknowledging long-term issues after a Lyme *infection,* but are *denying* the possibility that it can be from a *persistent* infection.

I *understand* the concern with being on long-term antibiotics, *but* there is also great concern if there is a *persistent* Lyme bacteria invading the body. There is also the concern that I struggle with: perhaps the condition keeping one sick with Lyme is mold, candida overgrowth, or other factors. If those factors were keeping someone sick, and it was *not* from persistent Lyme bacteria, then antibiotics may not be beneficial. This is why you need a Lyme-literate doctor who considers all factors.

The medical establishment does *not* look at environmental factors in Lyme disease patients. There is such a disconnect between providers and what should be done. It makes me go back to the time when my endocrinologist called my hormone specialist a *quack* . . .

I feel that if doctors could come *together,* instead of battling each other over who is right and who is wrong, we could achieve better medical care for these conditions.

Chronic illness from Lyme and chronic persistent bacteria does exist. It's important to find the factors as to what is keeping you sick. Is it a *persistent* infection? Is it *mold*? Is it *heavy metals*? Is it candida? Are your *cells hurting*? Or is your *nervous system dysregulated*? I don't want to be hurt by long-term antibiotics, either, if one of the other factors is what is keeping me in this condition. *But* if the condition is a *persistent infection* I want it *gone*. And, as a person suffering with chronic Lyme, we have to navigate these outcomes very carefully.

Yes, there are risks to long-term antibiotics, but there are also risks involved with cancer treatment. Cancer is looked at very differently. There is risk with chemo and radiation, but we do not hear doctors saying, "We cannot give you any treatment because the chemo or radiation may kill you. Sorry, you are out of luck." No. They do *everything* in their power to provide a positive outcome, despite the risks involved. Why isn't Lyme disease given the same thought process?

After my recent diagnosis, I have chosen to share my story now because *my story matters* too. Many Lyme patients have encouraged me to write it while I am healing. I have been told that it may help progress my healing. I already feel like it has . . . I have been able to put so many things into perspective while digging deep into my past, *the past I wanted to bury*. So many are suffering, and so many are going through chronic illness with no answers. *I didn't want to write this book until I was healed . . .* but I think it is important to talk about the ups and downs of having Lyme disease go undiagnosed for so long. I think it is important to share while I am *still healing.*

I want to be real.
I want people to know that perseverance *can* lead to answers and the *peace in knowing.*
This is why I have chosen to write this book, and I *hope* it helps someone like *you.*

* * *

You may have noticed that I often said I just wanted to *"give up."*

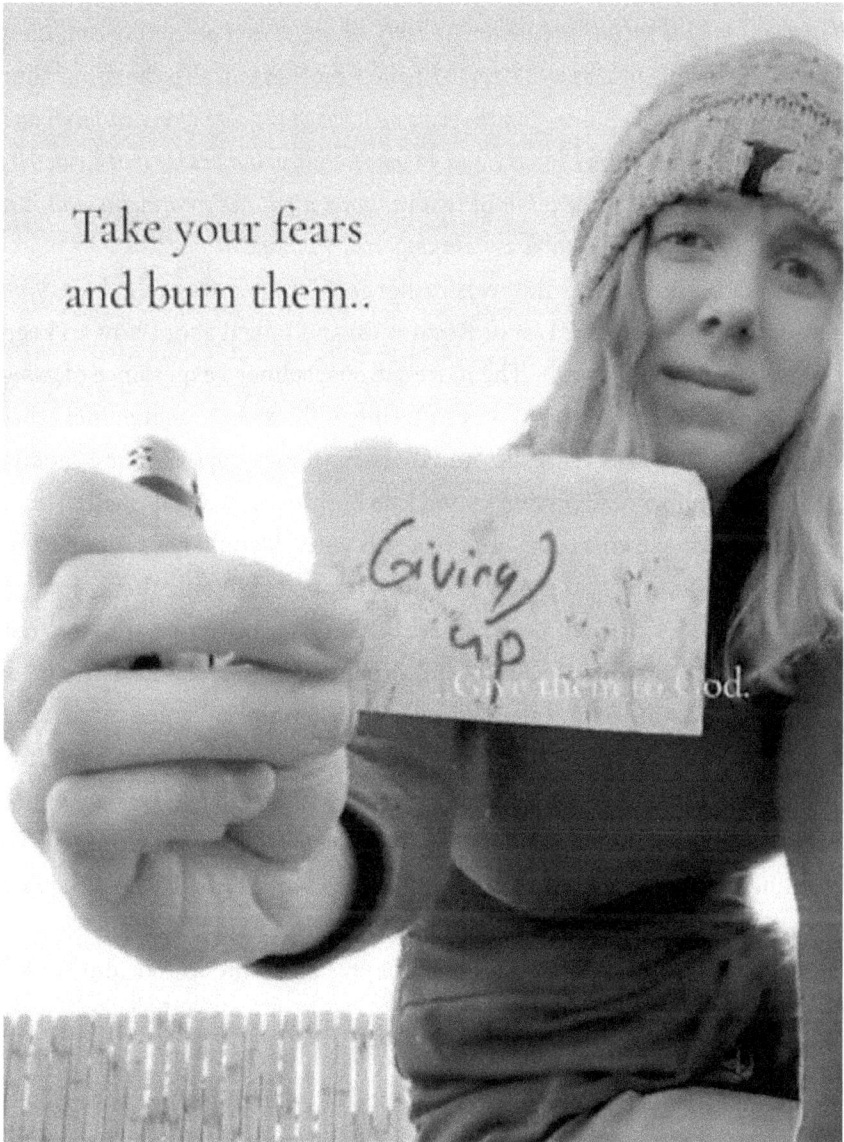

Take your fears
and burn them..

Give them to God.

Giving up

What did it mean for me . . . ?

Giving up meant a lot of different things in my world, not what you may think. Medical burnout is *real*. Healing burnout is *real*. *Giving up* could have meant a lot of things to me, depending on what I was going through. *I just want to give up on these protocols. I just want to give up on the testing. I just want to give up on finding the underlying cause and accept my condition.* Having a chronic illness while trying to be a mother can also cause burnout. *"Maybe I just need to tell my family I can no longer take care of my children and ask for help. Maybe I need to try and go on disability and accept that Lyme has destroyed my body. Maybe I need to give up on all of the treatments and just focus on my PTSD and limbic system impairment alone."*

I read a book recently that was rather inspiring. It was called *"Staying Away from the Edge"* (see List of Resources) and talked about how to keep yourself from going over it. The more serious feelings I experience of *going over the edge* occurred when I was suffering with extreme acute illness that caused a regression in my chronic disease. Those days of being mostly bedbound again would send my mind into hopelessness and despair. Those were the most extreme times, and that was when I would have thoughts of ending my life. But nothing ever serious happened during those times. I don't have any stories of how I drove off and attempted anything. What kept me from that was always my children. I could not abandon them.

My battle was different. I would battle with an internal voice that would tell me to *end it.* And I would feel like I was in a *frozen* state of being for some time. I would go on like this over and over again and be *stuck* there. *Frozen* in time. And when I finally gained *enough strength,* I would break free and cry out to *God to save me.* And then I would finally cry. I *couldn't* cry for months because the pain was so overwhelming. *Please God be with me,* I would cry out. And then all the thoughts of my life would come at me in *waves.* I would see my children. I would remember all of the happy times we have had together. I would be *pulled back* into the happiest memories with my husband and my mother. My family and friends. And it was like a slideshow of my life that I would *lose in the darkness* and finally be able to *see again when I was pulled out.* And it was *enough* to help me fight again.

During the darkest times, I didn't think I could get back to the light. *But I have.* Many times, and it was God that put me there again and again. That doesn't mean I don't still battle it. I still do. Because I am still fighting this disease. But now I always say, *Please be with me.* And I know that I am *not alone.* I know that God can pull me out *again.* And I remember, *again,* the poem, *"Footprints in the Sand,"* and how *profound* of an *influence* that has had in *my life*. Time and time again, God has had to *carry me,* and I never even realized it. *We are not meant to carry these burdens on our own.* It will tear us up inside. And God did not do this to me. I *do not* blame God for the state of my condition. I blame a world full of greed and a broken medical system . . . *but . . .* I cannot harbor anger and hate in my heart either. I cannot *heal* in that state of mind. So I practice *forgiveness* and tell *my story* to others who have lost all *hope*. I want to encourage all of you, that even if you have lost all *hope, new hope can* be found again.

Epilogue

We go through life in such a rush to get things. A new house, a new baby, a new car. We often compare our life accomplishments and status with those around us. We fail to live in the moment and enjoy life in its simplest of forms. I have learned through chronic illness that the most important thing in life is your health and those around you . . .

The things you want should not be rushed after. Enjoy the time in between. You cannot enjoy any of those things, anyway, if you don't have your health. Sit down in the sunshine and hold your loves one's hand while you enjoy an ice cream together. Life can drastically change overnight. You cannot predict life struggles, so why not enjoy the simplicity, even if it's not exactly where you want to be. And when you choose your people, do so wisely because if you do have a health struggle, the person you chose will either make or break you. My perspective in life has changed drastically, from wanting more to being *grateful* in simplicity.

My husband and I often ask each other, *"Do you sometimes miss when life was more simple . . . like when we were in the trailer?"*

We both answer yes, and because of our experience we will go on being happier in the now and *grateful* for answers and healing. True happiness lies in the people you spend your time with, in the sunrises and sunsets, in the cool breeze against your cheek, in the ability to get out of bed, and sitting together with your loved ones without your body internally screaming at you. Happiness is all about perspective. And always listen to your internal voice because that may actually be God's.

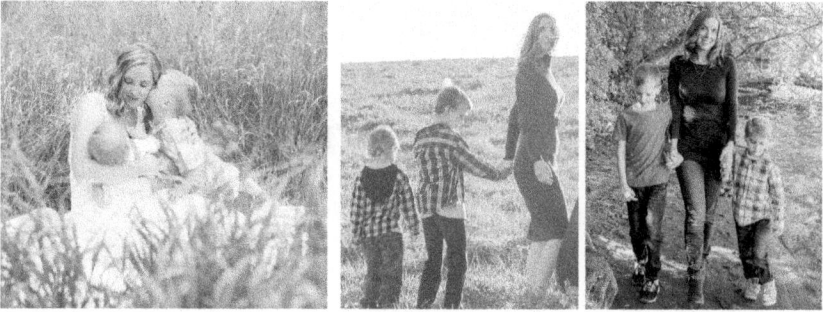

Hope

I *hope* that my children will mostly remember the happy moments and not the moments when Mom was overwhelmed. I *hope* that someday they get the healed version of me. That is what I keep fighting for. I *hope* we can end the cycle of suffering.

I think when something bad happens to us we have to search for a purpose for our pain and suffering. We obsess over the thought that there has to be a reason we are going through this. Or we think *"Why me?"* I have found that sometimes really bad things just happen to good people. Depending on what type of person you are, your attitude will show how you respond to the situation and will determine what you are going to do with it.

I do *hope* that my story can help others, but I grieve deeply when I imagine anyone going through this like I did. You do not deserve this. Any of it. But, unfortunately, others *will* go through this if nothing changes, and I don't want them to be as lost as I was. What I really *hope* is that someday our medical system concerning chronic illness and Lyme disease changes, and then we won't have to continue this endless cycle of suffering.

Lyme Warriors

The suffering I hear on my social media accounts.

Some of these may be hard for fellow Lyme Warriors to read, but our words matter.

- "I will heal even if it brings me to death."
- "My ghost is myself."
- "Sleep is the only escape from this kind of suffering."
- "I had no idea life would be this way."
- "Please God be with me."
- "Please let me die."
- "Please heal me."
- "I do not feel human."
- "The torture is endless."
- "If I stay, let it be to help others."
- "I want my mind back."
- "I don't know who I am any longer."
- "I lost everything."
- "God has abandoned me."
- "I cannot be a father. I cannot support my family."
- "I want to get out of this isolation, but my body keeps me trapped."
- "How am I still alive?"
- "I am sad and alone . . . isolated."
- "I just want my life back."
- "How many more suicides will occur before there is help?"
- "Death would be merciful."
- "The able-bodied people in my life don't want me to die . . . but they

watch me slowly rot in my room as I plead that I cannot heal this way."
- "The ringing in my ears . . . I could end it all so easily . . . jump in front of a bus."
- "The hardest part is feeling that there's no one to turn to for love and support that touches my soul."
- "When I look in the mirror I no longer see myself, just a shadow of who I once was."
- "I feel that I have lost my soul."
- "I am in darkness and I cannot escape it."
- "Lyme is attacking my brain."
- "Get me out of this body!"
- "It is so hard to live this way."
- "The isolation in this depth of suffering is breaking me."
- "I beg for death almost every waking moment that I live enduring this pain."
- "My brain is burning and my soul goes with it."
- "It feels like I am floating in an eternal abyss of darkness."
- "Every day on this earth I am just surviving."
- "No one can help me."
- "The way we are treated is inhumane."
- "I thought I could do it alone, but the darkness won."
- "I don't want to do this anymore."
- "I am a fraction of the person I once was."
- "Lyme has destroyed my dreams."
- "I am a shadow of the mother I wanted to be."
- "Neurological Lyme is torture."
- "This severe chronic illness has caused me extreme isolation. Loneliness is all that I feel."
- "*Loneliness* is all that I know."
- "I called the assisted suicide line . . . I cannot do this anymore."
- "I gave up *hope* for healing a long time ago."
- "Every day I spend in torture. Neurological Lyme is destroying every part of me."

- "The layers of torture from Lyme are many. The only time we feel heard is by others who are suffering."
- "He abandoned me."
- "You are lucky your husband stayed . . . mine left me."
- "The ringing in my ears is so loud I can hardly hear myself scream anymore."
- "Death is inviting."
- "Please don't leave me."
- "My family doesn't understand."
- "My friends think I am faking this."
- "I am trapped in a torture chamber, and that chamber is my own own body and mind."
- "Everyone expects me to be normal again after one treatment . . . I feel like a failure."
- "Everyone needs me, but I can barely take care of myself."
- "Everyone has abandoned me and I have no one to turn to."
- "I no longer recognize who I am."
- "My number one job right now is staying alive."
- "I miss life, but I'll miss it even more if I don't take this time to heal."
- "Every minute I feel a new pain and my brain loudly whispers, 'Is this it?'"
- "Our loved ones say they care about us, but no one outside of our fellow Lyme community fights for us. We are on our own."
- "When Lyme is known and accepted for what it is, the world will be in outrage."
- "I wish they could live in my body for one day . . . then they would *know* that *chronic Lyme is real.*"

MEDICAL PTSD

- "When I was in my 20s, suffering symptoms, the doctor said to me, 'You're young and look like you're in good shape, so you probably just have anxiety.'"

- "Before I had my diagnosis, I went to the hospital because I had passed out in the shower. My dad took me to the ER and my husband stayed home with our young daughter. The doctor closed the door and said, 'What's wrong at home, why are you always here?' 'What?' I said, confused. 'What is the real reason you are here?' he retorted. I said, 'Because I just passed out in the shower.' He wasn't having any of that and didn't believe me."

- "After explaining all of my symptoms to my primary care doctor, he said, 'It's not that I don't believe you, I just think you'd benefit from talking to someone.' . . . He then sent me to a psychiatrist."

- "When I got my Lyme disease diagnosis, I went into the hospital because my heart rate on the monitor was 172bpm. The doctor came in and looked at me and looked at my file and began to question why I was on antibiotics '*because you know you only need two weeks of doxycycline and you are fine.*' She began to lecture me about Lyme disease and said all of this stuff was unnecessary. By this point, I knew what I was talking about. I looked at my husband and I looked at her and said, 'Excuse me, I am not here for a diagnosis or treatment for Lyme disease. I am here because if you look at the heart monitor my heart rate is 172bpm, that is why I am here. I am not looking for treatments or antibiotics. I am not looking for a diagnosis. I want you to make sure there is nothing wrong with my heart.' This doctor turned and looked at her resident, nodded and left and she never came back in. Anytime anything needed to be said or done, it was through her resident."

- "I was told I am too pretty to be sick and must be an anxious girl."

- "After I got diagnosed with Lyme disease from an ER doctor and proceeded to not get better, I waited three months to see a 'top infectious disease doctor.' I was then told that there was *no* such thing as chronic Lyme and there was nothing he could do for me and I must have other issues going on."

- "I don't know where I would be without my doctor who believed my Lyme disease diagnosis. That doctor had good intentions by referring me to my very first neurologist. I had lost some weight, because

373

when you are sick you don't eat as much and you lose weight. I was also following a specific diet in an attempt to reduce gut issues and inflammation through a naturopathic doctor. In the notes the neurologist wrote, 'Even though the patient denies being anorexic, the weight she has lost has led us to believe it's either a case of bulimia or anorexia. She just wants to be one of these Lyme people who want an IV of antibiotics in them.' That's what this doctor took out of the situation while I was sitting there crying, thinking that I wasn't going to live to see my children."

- "This is what we deal with while fighting a terrible disease in this medical system. Because of my experiences, I don't go to the hospital unless I absolutely have to. There are many that don't have a voice and get labeled as Lyme loonies or drug seekers."

- "I have declined pain meds, even when I broke my hand and foot, because I know if I take that pain med it is written in my chart and if I go back in for a different acute reason, as a Lyme sufferer, I don't want to be labeled as a drug seeker. That is PTSD. I am worried about what will happen if I go to the hospital, how I will handle it, and what they will say to me."

- "Once a doctor told me it was normal to have heart rates in the 180s while making my bed because it was from anxiety."

- "I will probably die at home before I go to the hospital again."

- "I was diagnosed with anxiety before I could even get one word out concerning my condition."

- "The system has failed us time and time again. We have to fight for everything we want or need. It is not even a want, we don't want this. This happened from a tick that bit us, we didn't do anything wrong to deserve this."

- "If you come across a Lyme patient who is quiet and they don't talk much about their disease or they are just not okay . . . it's not always because of you, we deal with a lot of negativity in our community and outside our community. The doubts, the naysayers, the doctors, the specialists. They always have us pegged as these crazy people who want IV antibiotics. I will never in my life understand why we are treated so poorly."

* * *

These are only *some* of the words I have heard from fellow people suffering with Lyme disease and tick-borne illnesses.

Something needs to be done
to help us all.

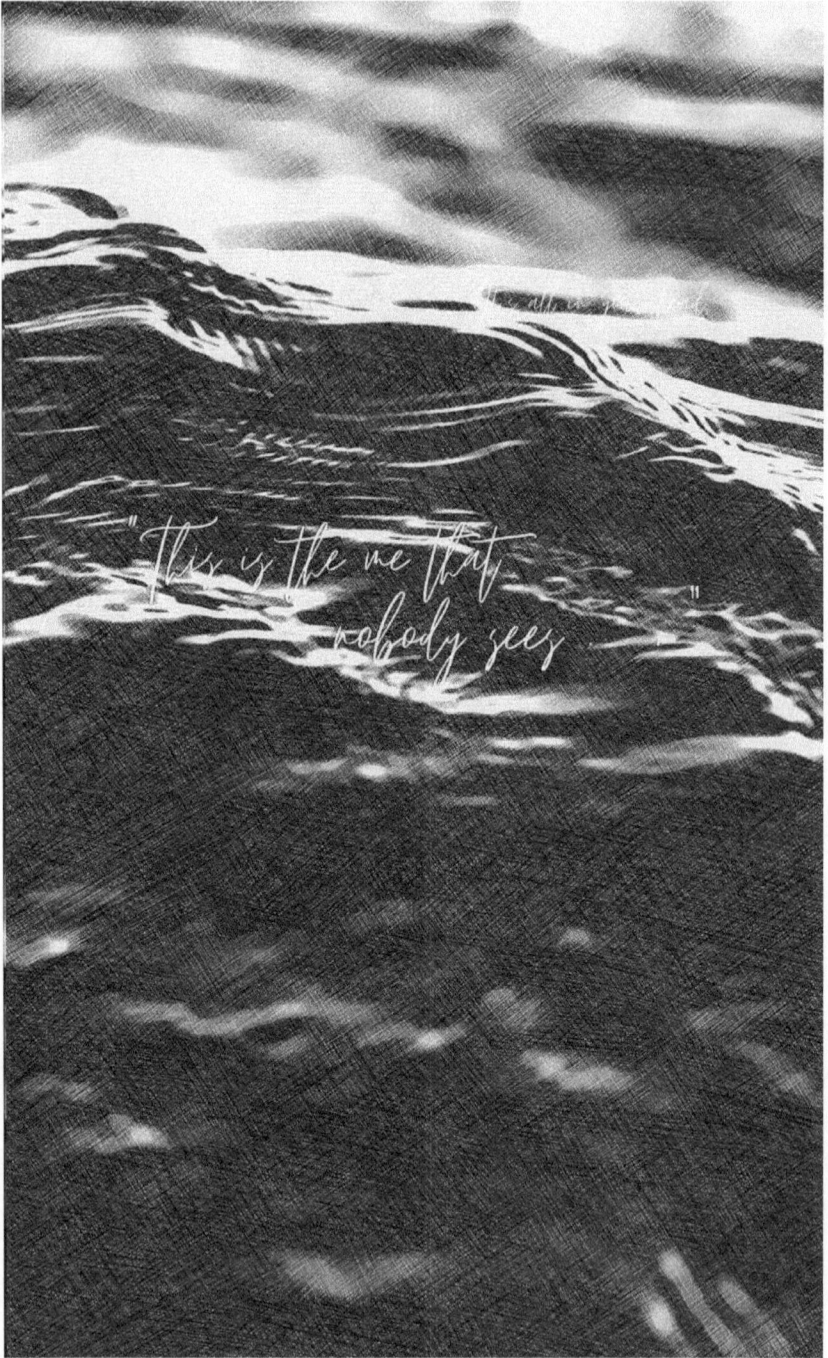

"This is the me that nobody sees"

"May light enter into all who suffer and wash our grief into *waves* of love."

List of Resources

You may be thinking,
"None of this makes sense to me. Where do I start?"
Here are some resources that may help.

DOCUMENTARIES

- *The Quiet Epidemic*. Co-directed by Lindsay Keys & Winslow Crane-Murdoch. New York: First Run Features, 2022.
- *Under Our Skin*. Directed by Andrew Abrahams. San Rafael: Open Eye Pictures, 2008.
- *The Monster Inside Me*. Directed by Tony C. Silva. Phoenix: Kreate Productions, 2022.
- *I'm Not Crazy, I'm Sick*. Directed by Elle Brooks-Tao. New York: Fieldhouse Productions, 2023.
- *Behind the Visible*. Directed by Ashley Rippentrop. Petoskey: Petoskey Productions, 2021.

BOOKS
Lyme disease & chronic illness

- *Rewire Your Anxious Brain: How to Use the Neuroscience of Fear to End Anxiety, Panic, and Worry* by Catherine M. Pittman, PhD & Elizabeth M. Karl, MLIS (New Harbinger Publications 2015)
- *Wired for Healing: Remapping the Brain to Recover from Chronic and Mysterious Illnesses* by Annie Hopper (Friesens 2014)
- *The Ultimate Guide to Methylene Blue: Remarkable Hope for Depression,*

COVID, AIDS & other Viruses, Alzheimer's, Autism, Cancer, Heart Disease, Cognitive Enhancement, Pain & The Great Transition to Metabolic Medicine by Mark Sloan (Endalldisease Publishing 2021)

- *Rebuild Yourself: Whole Body Practices to Heal Your Brain and Nervous System* by Jen Donovan (Whole Body Healing Media 2023)
- *Victory: A Lyme Story* by Aimee Goodwin (AuthorHouse 2014)
- *Unlocking Lyme: Myths, Truths, & Practical Solutions for Chronic Lyme Disease* by William Rawls, MD (Vital Plan, Inc. 2017)
- *Mast Cells United: A Holistic Approach to Mast Cell Activation Syndrome* by Amber Walker (Amber Walker 2019)
- *Cure Unknown: Inside the Lyme Epidemic* by Pamela Weintraub (St. Martin's Griffin; Second Edition, Revised 2013)
- *My Promise to Alex* by Jody Hudson and Penelope Childers (Independently published 2022)
- *Healing Lyme: Natural Healing and Prevention of Lyme Borreliosis and Its Co-infections* by Stephen Harrod Buhner (Raven Press 2005)
- *Defeating Dysautonomia* by Tara Smith Johnson (Redemption Press 2021)
- *The Trifecta Passport: Tools for Mast Cell Activation Syndrome, Postural Orthostatic Tachycardia Syndrome and Ehlers-Danlos Syndrome* by Amber Walker (Amber Walker 2021)
- *Little Bite, Big Trouble: A Bird's Eye View of Lyme Disease* by Sarah Schlichte Sanchez (Vigor For Life 2017)
- *My Crazy Life: A Humorous Guide to Understanding Mast Cell Disorders* by Daniel & Pamela Hodge (Lulu.com 2015)
- *Love, Hope, Lyme: What Family Members, Partners, and Friends Who Love A Chronic Lyme Survivor Need to Know* by Fred Diamond (Fred Diamond 2022)
- *The Essential Guide to Alpha-Gal Syndrome: Tips & Advice for Coping* by Lauren Iseley (Independently published 2021)
- *The Cellular Wellness Solution: Tap Into Your Full Health Potential with the Science-Backed Power of Herbs* by Bill Rawls, MD (Vital Plan, Inc. 2022)

- *The Gratitude Curve: Using the Lessons of Chronic Illness to Reach Personal Empowerment* by Gregg Kirk (CreateSpace Independent Publishing Platform 2018)
- *Toxic: Heal Your Body from Mold Toxicity, Lyme Disease, Multiple Chemical Sensitivities, and Chronic Environmental Illness* by Neil Nathan, MD (Victory Belt Publishing 2018)
- *Why Can't I Get Better?: Solving the Mystery of Lyme and Chronic Disease* by Richard I. Horowitz, MD (St. Martin's Press 2013)
- *Out of the Woods: Healing from Lyme Disease for Body, Mind, and Spirit* by Katina Makris (Helios Press 2015)
- *The Brain That Changes Itself: Stories of Personal Triumph from the Frontiers of Brain Science* by Norman Doidge, MD (Penguin Life 2007)
- *The Sensitive Patient's Healing Guide: Top Experts Offer New Insights and Treatments for Environmental Toxins, Lyme Disease, and EMFs* by Neil Nathan, MD (Cypress House 2024)
- *Finding Resilience: A Teen's Journey Through Lyme Disease* by Rachel Leland and Dorothy Kupcha Leland (River Grove Books 2023)
- *Brain on Fire: My Month of Madness* by Susannah Cahalan (Simon & Schuster 2020)

ADDITIONAL BOOKS

- *Jesus Calling: Morning & Evening* by Sarah Young (Thomas Nelson 2015)
- *Staying Away from the Edge: Help and Hope for Living after a Mental Health Diagnosis* by Robyn Mulder (Start Living Press 2024)
- *It's Not Supposed to Be This Way: Finding Unexpected Strength When Disappointments Leave You Shattered* by Lysa TerKeurst (Thomas Nelson 2018)
- ESV Illuminated Bible (Crossway 2017)

About the Author

Who am I?

I am not Lyme.

Whitney Helen Goetsch grew up in small-town South Dakota. She spent most of her childhood with her dad and family outside of Hill City. She saw the many struggles that her aunt went through with rheumatoid arthritis, and the determination that she showed while raising her children inspired Whitney. She grew up with a love for animals and nature and spent most of her time reading.

There was an abundance of artistic qualities on Whitney's mother's side of the family. Her mother and aunts inspired her to start drawing, and later Whitney became the illustrator and author of the children's book series: *Boomer* (*Boomer's Little Library* can be found on *Facebook*). Whitney also practices the art of photography and believes that so much beauty can be found in the world by simply capturing one photo. She would say that her biggest accomplishment, though, has been raising her children.

Her health decline began in December of 2018, which forced her into a pattern of finding a diagnosis to save her life and end her suffering. Later, she was thrown into the world of chronic Lyme disease upon its diagnosis in May of 2023.

She lives in South Dakota with her husband while she homeschools their two children. She is happiest in the presence of family and friends, and she is not only a proud mother but also a proud aunt. Whitney continues to battle chronic Lyme disease and has *new hope* that the future will bring more knowledge to the condition and help for those suffering. She still relies on God to carry her through the hardest days.

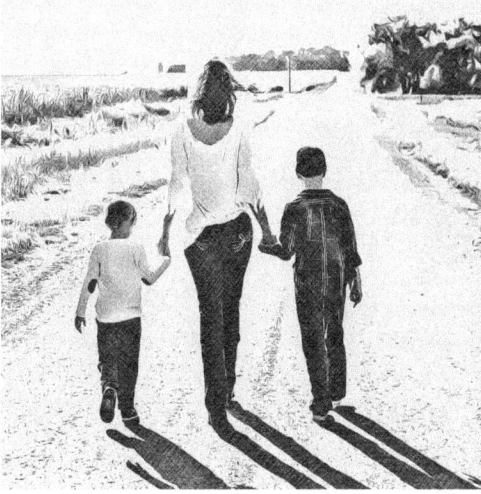

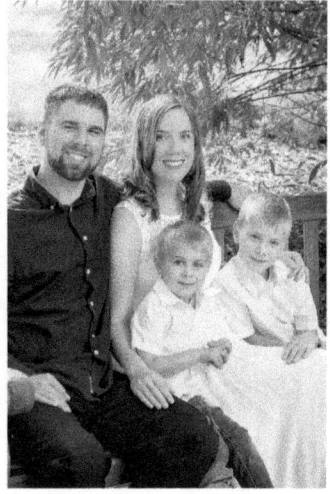

My greatest accomplishments . . .

@MYSTORYMATTERS2

You can follow Whitney's story on Instagram

WAVES

mystorymatters

Let others follow you by scanning your QR code

♪ TikTok

Or TikTok

https://mystorymatters.my.canva.site/

Afterword

. . . "What is your name!?!"
You will scream in desperation.
"Bartonella, Babesia, and I am *LYME*."
You pray that you have found me in just the right time.

* * *

. . . but Behold, I am *Alpha* and *Omega*
The *Beginning* and the *End*.
I will part the *waves* . . .
and you will *never* suffer alone again.

. . . *I* will give you answers
and guide your path.
I will wipe *every* tear
and Lyme will feel *my* wrath.

You *will* tell your story . . .
and *many* will relate.
Your prayers *will* be answered . . .
and you will finally understand *why* you had to wait.
-God

Whitney Helen Goetsch

Waves

a Memoir of Perseverance

in Battling

Chronic Lyme Disease

by Whitney Goetsch

Perseverance . . .

www.ingramcontent.com/pod-product-compliance
Lightning Source LLC
Chambersburg PA
CBHW031544260326
41914CB00002B/266